ABORIGINAL HEALTH IN CANADA:
HISTORICAL, CULTURAL, AND EPIDEMIOLOGICAL
PERSPECTIVES

Second Edition

Numerous studies, inquiries, and statistical analyses undertaken over the years have demonstrated the poor health status of Aboriginal peoples relative to the Canadian population in general. This situation has led to charges of neglect, indifference, and even genocide against the federal government by Aboriginal groups and their supporters. While several books have addressed specific aspects of this issue, *Aboriginal Health in Canada*, originally published in 1995, set the standard for studies in Aboriginal health. Now available in a fully up-to-date second edition, this book provides a comprehensive historical review that is national in scope, and combines the methodologies and perspectives of a number of fields, including epidemiology, history, and anthropology.

Aboriginal Health in Canada discusses the complex web of physiological, psychological, spiritual, historical, sociological, cultural, economic, and environmental factors that contribute to health and disease patterns among the Aboriginal peoples of Canada. The authors explore the evidence for changes in patterns of health and disease from prior to European contact to the present. They discuss medical systems and the place of medicine within various Aboriginal cultures and trace the relationship between politics and the organization of health services for Aboriginal peoples. They also examine popular explanations for Aboriginal health patterns today, and emphasize the need to understand both the historical-cultural context and the diverse circumstances that give rise to variations in health problems and healing strategies among Aboriginal populations. Finally, the book addresses the role of Aboriginal healing traditions in a contemporary context, and the place of health care in Aboriginal peoples' struggle for self-determination.

JAMES B. WALDRAM is a professor in the Department of Psychology at the University of Saskatchewan.

D. ANN HERRING is a professor in the Department of Anthropology at McMaster University.

T. KUE YOUNG is a professor in the Department of Public Health Sciences in the Faculty of Medicine at the University of Toronto.

JAMES B. WALDRAM, D. ANN HERRING, AND
T. KUE YOUNG

Aboriginal Health in Canada: Historical, Cultural, and Epidemiological Perspectives

Second Edition

UNIVERSITY OF TORONTO PRESS
Toronto Buffalo London

© University of Toronto Press Incorporated 2006
Toronto Buffalo London
Printed in Canada

Reprinted 2007, 2011, 2012

ISBN-13: 978-0-8020-8792-8 (cloth)
ISBN-10: 0-8020-8792-2 (cloth)

ISBN-13: 978-0-8020-8579-5 (paper)
ISBN-10: 0-8020-8579-2 (paper)

Printed on acid-free paper

Library and Archives Canada Cataloguing in Publication

Waldram, James B. (James Burgess)
  Aboriginal health in Canada : historical, cultural, and epidemiological
  perspectives / James B. Waldram, D. Ann Herring and T. Kue Young. –
  2nd ed.

  Includes bibliographical references and index.
  ISBN-13: 978-0-8020-8792-8 (bound)
  ISBN-10: 0-8020-8792-8 (bound)
  ISBN-13: 978-0-8020-8579-8 (pbk.)
  ISBN-10: 0-8020-8579-2 (pbk.)

  1. Native peoples – Health and hugiene – Canada.   2. Native peoples –
  Medical care – Canada.   I. Herring, Ann, 1951–   II. Young, T. Kue
  III. Title.

  RA449.W35 2006   362.1′ 089′ 97071   C2006-900539-7

University of Toronto Press acknowledges the financial assistance to its
publishing program of the Canada Council for the Arts and the Ontario Arts
Council.

University of Toronto Press acknowledges the financial support for its
publishing activities of the Government of Canada through the Book
Publishing Industry Development Program (BPIDP).

Contents

Figures

Preface to the Second Edition

The state of health and health care for Canada's Aboriginal peoples has often been the subject of controversy. Numerous studies, inquiries, and statistics accumulated over the years have demonstrated the poor health status of Aboriginal people relative to the Canadian population in general. This state of affairs has led to charges of neglect, indifference, and even genocide against the federal government and the larger Canadian society by Aboriginal groups and their supporters. In defence, government agencies responsible for health care often point to the extensive network of health facilities in the remotest corners of the country and the high level of health expenditures allocated to Aboriginal communities. The discrepancy in perception has at times led to confrontation between the users and the providers of health services, incidents that have attracted considerable media and public attention.

Much of the debate on Aboriginal health services to date has focused on their current availability, adequacy, accessibility, effectiveness, comprehensiveness, quality, and sensitivity to community needs and aspirations. The current system, however, did not come about spontaneously, but has been shaped over the years by specific policies reflecting the social and political realities of the time and influenced by the changing demographic and epidemiological picture of the population.

In the first edition of this book, published in 1995, we lamented the fact that much of the literature on Aboriginal health and health care in Canada was scattered in the biomedical and social science literatures, as well as in relatively inaccessible 'grey literature' or unpublished documents. What a difference a few years have made! Since 1995, there has been a notable expansion in research and publication on Aboriginal health issues and, equally noteworthy, a proliferation of health-oriented websites on the Internet that have made the research and its policy implications much more widely available. In addition to the National Aboriginal Health Organization and the Institute for Aboriginal People's Health, an institute within the Canadian Institutes of Health Research, there are now dozens of Aboriginal health research centres and/or training programs across the country. There has been an explosion in the attention provided to Aboriginal health research, making this attempt to revise our book all the more daunting.

We believe that there remains a place for a generalist historical and contemporary review that is national in scope and combines the methodologies and perspectives of epidemiology, history, and anthropology. We realize that we cannot come close to providing adequate attention to all the health research that has been done recently, but we do hope at least to flag some of the most important work in selected areas and, perhaps just as importantly, draw out some of the critical issues that seem to be emerging. We have attempted to address some of the flaws that characterized the first edition and that were so kindly pointed out in the many published reviews. However, in an effort to keep the book roughly the same length, and therefore as widely accessible as possible, we have had to make some difficult decisions.

This second edition, then, remains an entry point into the field of Aboriginal health in Canada, an introduction for the uninitiated, or the researcher who seeks a broader perspective on the topic he or she is investigating. We still hope to satisfy the need for materials suitable for both graduate and undergraduate students in medical anthropology, Native studies, and the health sciences. This volume should also appeal to health practitioners, planners, and administrators in agencies (federal, regional, and Aboriginal) involved in health care delivery to Aboriginal people.

This book brings a broad, interdisciplinary perspective to the topic of Aboriginal health, reflective of the diverse backgrounds of the authors and of the need to present as comprehensive a picture as possible. To this end it is important for the reader to understand the academic backgrounds of the authors and their specific involvement in the book. Dr James Waldram is a medical anthropologist who has undertaken research among both northern and urban Aboriginal people, and with Aboriginal offenders. As a cultural anthropologist, he lends a broad understanding of Aboriginal health matters from a cultural perspective. He is responsible primarily for chapters 5, 6, 7, 9, and 10. Dr Ann Herring is also a medical anthropologist, but she approaches her research from the perspective of biological anthropology and the anthropology of infectious diseases. Her work in historical epidemiology, as evident in chapters 2 and 3, is informed by her expertise in assessing the effects of past disease processes from archaeological remains and historical sources. Dr Kue Young, a public health physician who also has a doctorate in biological anthropology, lends the 'medical' perspective, and that of contemporary epidemiology, to the book in chapters 4 and 8. He has worked extensively as a practitioner, administrator, and researcher in various Aboriginal communities in northern Canada, as well as internationally in the circumpolar zone.

This book in no way pretends to offer an 'Aboriginal' perspective on issues of health and health care. Actually, we do not think such a singular perspective exists, given the diversity of background and experience of Aboriginal people across the country. The authors are committed to sociocultural and biomedical scholarship and have extensive research in the areas covered in this book. It is from these perspectives that the book is offered. While individual authors have prepared specific chapters, as indicated above, we have reviewed and critiqued each other's work extensively to ensure the smooth flow of ideas, consistency in prose style, and avoidance of duplication.

We have not taken a strictly chronological approach in this book; however, we try to cover the major issues and events from the time of early contact with Europeans to the beginning of the twenty-first century. We strive for national coverage whenever possible, recognizing the cultural diversity of Aboriginal people in Canada and the limitations of our expertise. We also consciously include data and materials, where available, from status and non-status Indians, Métis, and Inuit, and from both urban and rural/remote areas.

A NOTE ON TERMINOLOGY

In keeping with the terminology used by the Royal Commission on Aboriginal Peoples, we use a variety of terms to refer to the indigenous inhabitants of Canada. We use the term 'Aboriginal people' or 'Aboriginal' to refer in a collective sense to Inuit, First Nations, and Métis people. This is consistent with the Constitution of Canada, which recognizes Aboriginal people as the descendants of the original people of North America. More specific labels are used where appropriate; however, we do not alter historical usages, such as the term 'Indian,' to be compatible with contemporary trends.

xii Preface to the Second Edition

We also use the general terms 'non-Aboriginal' or 'Euro-Canadian' to refer to those who settled in what would become Canada, while acknowledging that these labels also overgeneralize. Nevertheless, European colonization remains the most significant historical fact in our analysis, and the institutions that govern the country (and, indeed, the people who govern it) remain of European heritage.

ACKNOWLEDGMENTS

Many individuals assisted us in the preparation of the second edition of this book. We are indebted to Virgil Duff of the University of Toronto Press, for giving us the opportunity to revise our work. Margaret Allen and Anne Laughlin provided expert guidance in the copy-editing and publication process. Katherine Minich at the University of Toronto helped organize the bibliography and index. Countless readers – colleagues and students – have offered their opinions, not always complimentary but always helpful, and thus contributed to the revision and, we hope, improvement of this book.

ABORIGINAL HEALTH IN CANADA:
HISTORICAL, CULTURAL, AND EPIDEMIOLOGICAL
PERSPECTIVES

1

An overview of the Aboriginal peoples of Canada

This book is about health, the fundamental human condition. It takes as axiomatic that the health of any human population is a product of a complex web of physiological, psychological, spiritual, historical, sociological, cultural, economic, and environmental factors. In Canada, one of the most telling examples of how these factors interact can be found in the health of the country's Aboriginal people. Long considered to be the most disadvantaged group in an otherwise affluent society, Aboriginal people today paradoxically experience the kinds of health problems most closely associated with poverty, problems linked to their historical position within the Canadian social system. This book seeks to explain the current health problems being experienced by Aboriginal people, to provide an overview of health and health care from a historical perspective, and to look to the future as fundamental changes to the health care system attempt to grapple with the most pressing problems.

According to the 2001 census, slightly more than 1.3 million people in Canada considered themselves to have some Aboriginal ancestry, almost 4.5 per cent of the total Canadian population.[1] Among Aboriginal people, the First Nations population is the largest (958,000), followed by the Métis (266,000), and the Inuit (51,000). The growth in the Aboriginal population in Canada since the beginning of the century is shown in figure 1, and it is clear that the period between 1951 and 2001 is characterized by a marked sevenfold increase in population size. This stands in stark contrast to the near doubling of the Canadian population as a whole over the same period (Statistics Canada 2003). The complexities of Aboriginal Canada seem to grow by leaps and bounds, as events rapidly alter existing perspectives and understandings. It is essential for readers to be aware of these complexities in order to understand prop-

Figure1. Increase in Aboriginal population in Canada according to the census, 1901–2001

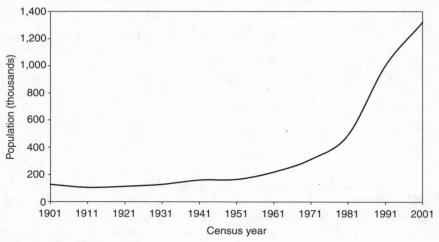

Source: Statistics Canada 2003

erly the many issues dealt with in this book. The aim of this first chapter, therefore, is to provide background information that helps to explain current conditions.

WHO ARE THE ABORIGINAL PEOPLES?

There are three broad dimensions fundamental to understanding the Aboriginal people of Canada, with particular reference to health and health care. These are the biological, cultural, and legal dimensions.

The biological dimension

One of the central questions within anthropological research relates to the origins of living populations worldwide. This is part of a larger area of inquiry that seeks to understand the history of humanity and to do so from the perspective of the remains, both biological and cultural, that have survived to be analysed by scholars in the present. There is, therefore, a long tradition of investigation into the bio-archaeological past of the people of the Americas as part of this project to understand the long trajectory of human history on a global scale. Over the years, archaeologists, linguists, and physical anthropologists have developed a large body of information that indicates that the earliest ancestors of contemporary Aboriginal peoples came to the Americas from Asia, as did the people of the Pacific (Kirk and Szathmary 1985). Several lines of evidence point to the Asian origins of Aboriginal Americans, among them phenotypic characteristics such as dental morphology (Turner 1985) and skeletal features (Szathmary and Ossenberg 1978), as well as a host of genetic characteristics (see Szathmary 1985, 1993, for excellent reviews).

In addition, an influential synthesis of linguistic, archaeological, and molecular genetic evidence (Greenberg, Turner, and Zegura 1986) put forward the proposition that, beginning some 12,000 years ago, three separate waves of people migrated from Asia, with each wave giving rise to one of three major linguistic groups in the Americas (Amerind, Eskimo-Aleut, and Na-Dene).[2] According to this analysis, people moved westward into the Americas via a now submerged landmass in the Bering Strait, known as Beringia or the Bering Land Bridge (Greenberg, Turner, and Zegura 1986). Geological evidence shows that the Bering Land Bridge was exposed during periods of glaciation when the sea level dropped by about fifty metres, uniting the two continents. This wide expanse of open grassland and tundra periodically allowed the easy movement of plants, animals, and people between northeast Siberia and Alaska from about 60,000 to 11,000 years ago (Hoffecker, Powers, and Goebel 1993). Movement southward was postulated to have been on foot, via an inland route through an ice-free corridor east of the Rocky Mountain Front. Scholarly disagreement with this proposition centred on whether the expansion of populations over this prairie-like region occurred very early or whether it was a relatively recent phenomenon, on the order of 12,000 to 14,000 years ago (see Zegura 1985).

Over the past two decades, however, the picture of the origins of the indigenous people of the Americas has become far more complicated as increasing evidence from living and past populations has accumulated and as new techniques of analysis have been developed. In particular, the recognized potential for molecular genetic studies to clarify many of the details of this process has led to a proliferation of research in this area. Further support for the Asian origins of indigenous people has come from studies of mitochondrial DNA (mtDNA)[3] and the Y chromosome of Siberian and Native American populations (Eshleman, Malhi, and Smith 2003).

Much of the new research focuses on the analysis of mtDNA genetic sequences in the Americas, their distribution in living and past populations, and how these distributions compare with those found elsewhere in the world. From these studies, it is now generally accepted that there were five founding lineages of mtDNA in the Americas. They are shared with Asian populations and were present in the pre-Columbian Americas.[4]

Although the genetic evidence continues to confirm that the ancestors of contemporary Aboriginal people entered North America from Asia, there is still considerable discussion about how many migrations there were, where the migrants came from, the routes through which the Americas were colonized, and the timing of the process (for a very readable review, see Eshleman, Malhi, and Smith 2003). Some generalizations nevertheless can be made about the current state of opinion, bearing in mind that this is a hotly debated and rapidly changing area of inquiry. Following Schurr and Sherry (2004), an emerging view contends that the earliest movement of ancestral Asians into the Americas likely occurred between 20,000 and 15,000 years ago. Early Amerindian people emanated out of south-central Siberia, and their population expanded and covered the 10,000-kilometre distance to South America by about 14,500 years ago.[5] This initial movement was probably *not* characterized by big-game hunters slowly following animal movements along an inland passage east of the Rockies; rather, the route of passage was likely maritime, with people moving southward, and relatively quickly, along the western seacoast. Why maritime? Because Beringia and the ice-free corridor were closed at this period of time, and a biologically productive and accessible sea route was open (Mandryk, Josenhans, Fedje, and Mathewes 2001). A subsequent expansion of Asian people via the ice-free corridor may have occurred around 12,500 years ago, followed by the later arrival of circumarctic peoples (Eskimo-Aleuts and Na-Dene) after the last glacial maximum. Throughout this process, Aboriginal populations increasingly differentiated in biological and social dimensions, giving rise to unique societies and civilizations, but maintained contact between regions through trade and other forms of social interaction.

Some Aboriginal peoples have different understandings of how they came to be, and these often involve a 'creation' in areas more or less identical to where they live today. Some have even speculated about a reverse migration, from North America to Siberia via the Bering Land Bridge. Their rich oral traditions link the existence of peoples with specific territories and define both secular and spiritual places. Oral histories of people such as the Haida include descriptions of treeless land, lower sea levels than exist today, exposed land where there is none now, and narrow strips of shoreline (Harris 1997, cited in Mandryk et al. 2001:307). Yet others speak of migrations, some of epic proportions, from earlier North American homelands to new ones. Nevertheless, a sense of place and of relationships to the land is invariably rooted in these traditions. Well-being, as broadly understood, is a product of this connectedness in the eyes of many Aboriginal people.

The pre-contact cultural dimension

Prior to the arrival of Europeans on this continent, there were thousands of autonomous Aboriginal bands, tribes, or First Nations, as many are referred to today, living in what would become Canada. Linguists have identified within this diversity eleven different language families – that is, groupings of related, though separate, languages. There were as many as fifty or sixty different languages in Canada at the time of European contact in the fifteenth century; today, many of these languages are con-sidered threatened or in danger of disappearing. The Cree, Inuktitut, and Ojibwa languages, which have the largest number of speakers and are spoken across much of Canada, may well be the only ones that are truly safe, for the time being. Many Aboriginal groups are working diligently to save their languages, however, and the process of language loss may ultimately be reversed. In 2001, about 20 per cent of individuals who identified themselves as Aboriginal reported having an Aboriginal mother tongue, while 24 per cent claimed to have enough knowledge of an Aboriginal language to carry on a conversation (Statistics Canada 2003).

It is important to realize just how different Aboriginal languages are, both from European languages such as English or French and from each other. This point is often misunderstood by Anglophones and Francoph-ones. The structural differences between, say, Cree and Mohawk (both found in Quebec) are much greater than those between French and English! There are also regional and local dialect differences that are detectable by speakers of the particular language, such as the Cree dia-lects spoken on the east and west sides of James Bay

Out of a concern for the development of typologies, anthropologists initially grouped Aboriginal peoples into 'culture areas.' The concept of cultural area was defined by Harold Driver as 'a geographical area occu-pied by a number of peoples whose cultures show a significant degree of similarity with each other and at the same time a significant dissimilarity with the cultures of the peoples of other such areas' (Driver 1969:17). The following culture areas have been identified for Canada: Arctic, Western subarctic, Eastern subarctic, Northeastern Woodlands, Plains, Plateau, and Northwest Coast. These culture areas corresponded to a great extent to the boundaries of the language families, most of which correspond well to natural geographic features, such as vegetation patterns. It has become common to speak of historical patterns of adaptation and inter-action, rather than culture areas, an approach that emphasizes the manner in which human groups exploited and managed available resources and the ways in which they interacted with each other. Hence, for instance, the pre-contact Cree, Ojibwa, and Inuit of the Subarctic and Arctic culture areas can be thought of as hunter-gatherer and forager societies (although this still does not imply that the cultures were identical). The ecological base of Aboriginal cultures is easily established, and the role of language as a cultural marker is self-evident.

Given the variability of the environmental zones found in Canada, from the tundra in the north to the wetlands in the east and the mountains in the west, it is not surprising that Aboriginal cultures developed in a diverse manner. But it is also true that the sharing of certain ecological zones, combined with cultural diffusion (or the exchange of ideas and materials as well as the movement of people), resulted in similarities among neighbouring groups.

What did the cultures of these peoples look like at the time of contact? Through anthropological and ethnohistorical inquiry, we have been able to develop some profiles for this period. However, the reader is cautioned that the evidence for pre-contact cultural formations is fragmented, and that there was extensive cultural diversity even within the ecological zones.[6]

For much of Canada, including the Arctic and Subarctic areas, Aboriginal peoples lived primarily by hunting small and large game, fishing, and gathering plant foods, berries, lichens, nuts, and other seasonally available land foods. Peoples such as the Cree, the Ojibwa, the Chipewyan, and the Inuit covered large territorial ranges on foot and by dog team, hunting and fishing on a seasonal basis at known locales. The primary social unit, the band, was relatively small, often consisting of only 50 to 100 people. When resources were plentiful, a number of these bands might temporarily join together into a larger entity, the regional band; however, during times of hardship, the band might break up into its constituent parts – nuclear and extended families. Hence, each family existed within a delicate balance, containing all of the essential skills to exist, at least for short periods.

These northern hunters can be contrasted with the peoples of other areas, whose environments allowed for greater aggregates of people and different forms of social organization. The peoples of the Northeastern Woodlands, for instance, were horticulturalists, producing a variety of crops (including maize or corn, beans, and squash) as the staple of their diet. Greater certainty in food supply allowed peoples such as the Huron and the Five Nations of the Iroquois (Mohawk, Seneca, Cayuga, Oneida, and Onondaga) to establish permanent villages, and areas of southern Ontario and Quebec are dotted with the ancestral remains of many of these. In the Plains region, Aboriginal peoples such as the Plains Cree, Saulteaux, Assiniboine, and the nations of the Blackfoot Confederacy (Blackfoot, Blood, and Peigan) developed a reliance on the bison as the staple, a reliance that became even more significant as horses, introduced by the Spanish in the sixteenth century in the southern part of the continent, began to make their way onto the northern Plains by the mid-eighteenth century. Iroquoian villages often numbered in the high hundreds, and even thousands, while Plains groups often spent the summer bison-hunting season in equally large encampments. Unlike the Iroquoians, however, the Plains Indians tended to split into smaller units – bands – for the harsher winter months.

The Northwest Coast Aboriginal peoples, such as the Haida and Kwakiutl, often lived in permanent villages along the coastal areas, or inland along the many rivers, and survived primarily by hunting sea mammals and by fishing. Their societies were perhaps the most diverse and complex among all the northern Aboriginal peoples, and their impressive artistic traditions are perhaps the best recognized throughout the world.

In contrast to these Aboriginal groups, the Métis emerged as a 'new people' as a result of intermarriage with Europeans, primarily fur traders (Brown 1980). With their roots in both northern Aboriginal peoples, such as the Cree, Ojibwa, and Dene, and European peoples, especially the English, Scottish, and French, the Métis blended languages and cultures to create a unique identity and role in the developing northwest throughout the eighteenth and nineteenth centuries.

It is crucial to reinforce at this stage that the culture area formulation was designed solely to allow scholars to generalize between cultural formations and environmental niches primarily in the pre-contact and early post-contact eras. In our view, culture areas, and the brief cultural generalizations presented here, are of limited utility in understanding contemporary Aboriginal health issues.

Contemporary cultural orientations and experience

There have been a great many changes to Aboriginal cultures since the time of first contact with Europeans. Legislated attempts to destroy these cultures, combined with more subtle pressures that result from culture contact, have resulted in a situation where Aboriginal people today display a range of cultural orientations of a different sort. There are still many individuals, especially on reserves and in settlements in rural and remote areas, who are fluent in their Aboriginal language but may speak little or no English or French and may have had little formal education. Their contact with the larger, Euro-Canadian society will have been minimal. In contrast, there are also many Aboriginal people who have little or no knowledge of their heritage cultures. These individuals may have been adopted into Euro-Canadian families at a young age (an all-too-common phenomenon in Canada until recently), or they may have spent large portions of their formative years in Euro-Canadian foster homes or residential schools. Even where they may have had sustained contact with their Aboriginal parents, they may not have been exposed to their Aboriginal language or culture to any great extent, as a result of conscious efforts by their parents to prepare them for the 'White' world. Yet others are effectively bilingual, able to speak both their Aboriginal language and English or French, and bicultural or multicultural, with extensive experience in both Aboriginal and non-Aboriginal worlds. Some Aboriginal communities today can be found on the borders of large cities, and new 'urban' reserves are beoming more common, especially in western Canada (Barron and Garcea 1999).

   Much social and medical scientific research has combined Aboriginal peoples together into an 'Aboriginal' variable, to be contrasted with the Canadian population according to a variety of dimensions. The preceding, and necessarily brief, discussion of the cultural and legal complexity of Aboriginal Canada brings the legitimacy of this practice into question. How Aboriginality, broadly conceived, affects health in a contemporary sense, remains poorly understood. The reader should keep this in mind throughout this book. While a work of this nature must necessarily generalize, we are mindful of the problems inherent in so doing.

The legal dimension

The cultural context of contemporary Aboriginal Canada is complicated by Canadian government legislation and other policies. There are two broad legal categories of Aboriginal peoples: those with Indian 'status,' and those without. 'Status' or 'registered' Indians are those individuals legally recognized by the federal government to be 'Indians' for purposes of the Indian Act. First passed in 1876, the Indian Act was designed to facilitate the administration of programs to Indians, as well as to facilitate their assimilation into mainstream Canadian society. It included definitions of who constituted an 'Indian,' and how such status could be gained or lost. Many Aboriginal people of Indian ancestry who lost their 'Indian' status for a variety of reasons (or who never had it in the first place) are often referred to as 'non-status Indians.' Every registered Indian in Canada has a unique registration number; this actually facilitates the gathering of social, economic, and health data for this population, and for this reason many of the contemporary data referred to in this book pertain to them.

Many Aboriginal groups in Canada signed 'treaties' with the British and Canadian governments, although only some were preserved in writing. These individuals are often referred to as 'treaty Indians.' From the perspective of the government, the intent of the treaties, which cover much of western Canada including northern Ontario but excluding most of British Columbia, was to remove the Indians' title to the lands, and to remove Aboriginal people themselves, to allow for settlement and exploitation of the natural resources by European immigrants. There are many controversial issues regarding the signing of the treaties, and many treaty Indians argue that the promises made have not been fulfilled. Some First Nations accept that their ancestors never intended to surrender the land, but rather agreed to share it. Chapter 7 of this book examines the treaty promises in the area of health care.

The federal government is responsible for both the registered and the treaty Indians under the Indian Act, including areas related to their health. However, much of the federal responsibility has centred on registered Indians on reserves. Reserves are parcels of land held by Canada on behalf of the First Nations. In practice, in many areas the federal government does not take responsibility for Aboriginal people who move off the reserves to live elsewhere but leaves them to seek services under provincial or municipal jurisdiction.

The Inuit are separate from the registered Indians, and there is no legislation comparable to the Indian Act defining them. The federal government has nevertheless assumed primary responsibility for these people and provides or delegates many services to them as if they were registered Indians. The Métis and non-status Indians have a legal status that is, in many ways no different from that of other Canadians, the Constitution notwithstanding. The provinces or territories wherein they live deliver programs to these people as part of their obligations to all their citizens, although some special programs may also be developed in recognition of their special needs or circumstances.

Currently, the Indian, Inuit, and Métis peoples are recognized as 'Aboriginal peoples' under Section 35 of the Constitution, and their 'existing Aboriginal and treaty rights [are] recognized and affirmed.' While the courts and politicians continue to wrangle about the legal implications of this section, clearly the Constitution establishes the Aboriginal peoples as unique, with special status within Canada.

ABORIGINAL-EUROPEAN POST-CONTACT HISTORY

When Aboriginal and European peoples first encountered each other in what would become North America, the 'first peoples' of the continent exhibited a wide variety of political entities, which at the time were construed by Europeans to be 'nations.' These nations of Aboriginal people had been here for a very long time.

Although the earliest contacts between Aboriginal people and Europeans occurred along the eastern coasts and were related to the fishery, for most of Canada the history of contact is linked to the fur trade and to missionary activities. In these endeavours, the British and French gained ascendancy over the other European powers, such as the Dutch, Portuguese, and Spanish, who were also carving out stakes in their 'New World.'

When in 1604 the beaver felt hat became a popular fashion item in Europe, the vast and apparently unused fur resources of the Canadian wilderness beckoned. In 1670, the 'Company of Adventurers Trading into Hudson Bay,' or Hudson's Bay Company (HBC), was formed. Under a charter granted to the company by King Charles II of England, the HBC was granted a monopoly to trade in all of the territory drained by all of the rivers that emptied into Hudson Bay, an enormous expanse of land the boundaries of which were not even known in 1670. Initially, the HBC showed little inclination to explore and preferred to establish posts or 'factories' along the coasts of Hudson Bay and James Bay. The Indians brought their furs to the posts via a vast network of trade involving coastal and interior groups. However, it was not long before other European and eastern Canadian interests saw the lucrative profits to be made in the fur trade, and many defied the charter to establish rival operations in the interior. Indeed, it was many of the traders of these other companies, most notably the North West Company (NWC), who charted much of the interior of Canada in search of new sources of furs.

Aboriginal peoples became involved in the fur trade because it was to their benefit. They were able to exchange a common commodity – beaver pelts – for items of European manufacture – such as knives, pots, and guns – that greatly improved their livelihoods. In the early years of the trade, little disruption of their lifestyles ensued, since it was their skills in the bush as hunters that also made them successful in the fur trade. But over successive generations, they became increasingly and irreversibly dependent on European technologies. This posed little real problem as long as there were various companies and 'free' traders competing for their furs, a strong European market, and plenty of animals. However, when in 1821 the HBC and the NWC amalgamated to form a new, leaner HBC, the position of the Indians engaged in the fur trade deteriorated dramatically.

When Canada was formed in 1867, a legislative basis for dealing with the Indian peoples as 'nations' already existed. The Royal Proclamation of 1763, a piece of British legislation, had referred to the 'Nations or Tribes of Indians,' and implied fairly clearly that they had some form of land title recognizable by British law. The Royal Proclamation established the basis by which the Crown could secure that title, to allow for settlement, by purchase or cessation. The British North America Act in 1867 granted to Canada jurisdiction over Indians and the lands reserved for Indians, which bound Canada to the Royal Proclamation notion of Indian title and the need to obtain proper surrender of Indian lands. Hence was born the treaty process.

'Treaties' are normally thought of as international agreements, signed between 'nations.' Between 1871 and 1930, treaties and 'adhesions' were signed between Canada and the Indian peoples over much of the country. There is still argument today about whether or not Canada was explicitly recognizing Indian bands and tribal groupings as 'nations' in this international sense (and hence as having all the rights, privileges, and powers of 'nations'). The government's intent in so doing was clear: to secure title to the land and resources. While the Indians made efforts to negotiate good deals, the evidence suggests that the odds were clearly stacked against them. For instance, by the time the so-called numbered treaties commenced in the west in 1871, Aboriginal people were becoming destitute and ever mindful of encroaching settlement that appeared to be accelerating even without the treaties. In the west they were often presented with a pre-written treaty, by a treaty commissioner, with instructions not to alter the provisions in any way. Treaty commissioners frequently threatened to move on without signing the treaty if the Indian bands continued to dissent. In fact, one of the few treaties where it is clear that the Indians were able to have new clauses inserted was Treaty Six, signed in 1876 in central Saskatchewan and Alberta. In this instance, the clause referred to a 'medicine chest' and government assistance in the event of 'famine or pestilence,' two references related to health care that are discussed in chapter 7.

During the period of the fur trade, some Indians found work around the trading posts, hunting or doing other chores for the traders. Eventually, greater numbers of them began to establish more or less permanent residences around the posts. These people became known as the 'Homeguard,' and their dependence on the European traders for both technology and wages dramatically increased. The legacy of the Homeguard is still with us today. Many northern Aboriginal communities can be found at the sites of old fur trade posts, as is evidenced by such names as Nelson House, Moose Factory, and Cumberland House. Perhaps more significant is that these permanent settlements allowed for extensive intermarriage with the inherently single French, English, and Scottish traders. Out of these unions came mixed-blood children and eventually an entirely new population, the Métis.

The Métis developed essentially as a labouring class in the fur trade. Able to speak both Indian and European languages (typically a combination of Cree, Ojibwa, French, and English – eventually a synthesis language, called 'Michif,' developed), they were equally able to function in the bush and at the posts. Some began to work their way into southern areas, particularly into what would become Manitoba, and by the early 1800s there was a sizeable population there involved in wage labour, farming, fishing, and bison hunting.

The missionaries also had a profound influence on Aboriginal people in the New World. The desire of European powers to save their 'souls' through conversion to Christianity was a dominant theme in the post-contact historical period. Indeed, much of the seizing of Indian lands and resources, as well as the attempts at forced assimilation, were often couched in humanitarian, Christian terms. Simply put, the missionary perspective was one in which Indians lacked knowledge of the Christian 'God,' Jesus, the Holy Sacraments, and so on, and therefore by definition were considered 'savages'; they required careful, paternalistic care until they could become 'civilized'. Of course, this meant being assimilated into Euro-Canadian cultural patterns and belief systems.

While the early efforts of the missionaries reaped mixed success (due, in part, to Indian views that their own religious systems were better), inroads were made throughout Canada as Indian people began to sink into the poverty and despair that accompanied the collapse of the fur trade after 1821. With their populations seriously eroded by European-introduced diseases, and their economies collapsing (both the beaver and the bison were severely depleted in many areas by the third quarter of the nineteenth century), Aboriginal people were less able to resist the efforts of the missionaries. But the greatest effects of missionization came after the formation of Canada, in 1867, when the churches were given control of Indian education.

The treaties in western Canada included promises that education would be provided; indeed, Indian leaders at the time recognized that their children required new skills within the changing political and economic context of the west. Hence the 1880s saw the development of residential schools in the west. As Miller (1989:196; 1996) notes, the assimilationist underpinnings of the new schooling system required that the children be separated from their families and, therefore, their cultures; the Catholic, Anglican, Methodist, and Presbyterian churches took the lead in this regard. Although only a minority of children ever experienced these schools (Miller 1989:198), and although resistance to their operation was extensive, many children in effect became 'deculturized,' losing both their ability to be culturally 'Indian,' and the ability to provide good parental role models to their own children as they reached adulthood. Some students also experienced severe emotional, physical, and sexual abuse, a fact that the Canadian government and many churches have now recognized. Litigation, mediation and compensation processes to provide restitution to Aboriginal survivors of the residential schools are now in place.

The church-run residential schools clearly did serious damage to the lives and cultures of Aboriginal people. The fact remains that the residential schools played a significant role in engendering irreversible changes within Aboriginal society, and many of these changes are now seen to have a direct impact on the mental and physical health and well-being of Aboriginal people today. Indeed, the notion of a 'residential school syndrome' pervades contemporary Aboriginal health discourse, regardless of both historical fact and individual experience, as we shall see later in this book.

The missionaries were active in other ways as well. In 1884, the Northwest Coast feasting ceremonial system known as the 'potlatch' was banned, largely at the insistence of the missionaries. In 1886, the Plains

Indian 'Sun Dance' was effectively banned as well. Both these ceremonies included practices considered by missionaries and government administrators to be essentially heathen and repugnant, and therefore roadblocks to civilization (Miller 1989; Pettipas 1994; Dickason 2002). The ultimate effect of such laws was to drive these and other religious (and related healing) practices underground. They have survived, in altered forms, until today, but one legacy of these oppressive acts has been to make Aboriginal people very secretive about what were once public activities. There are many Aboriginal people today, for instance, who feel that Euro-Canadians should not be taught about their traditional medicine. But there are also many Aboriginal people, devout Christians, who are sincerely opposed to the revitalization of these traditions.

The history of the Inuit people reflects that of the Indians to the south, although extensive contact with Europeans occurred later, as did federal government administration programs. However, social change, when it did begin to accelerate in the 1950s and 1960s, came rapidly and caused many social problems. This unfortunate fact allowed medical scientists to develop a more detailed understanding of the health implications of European contact.

The Inuit were active in the fur trade, and some were also involved in commercial whaling for many years. But by the 1950s, neither industry was actively supporting the Inuit. Some groups were still hunting extensively, especially in the interior, and although many had been missionized, at least marginally, there were still many bands living more or less as they had in the past (Fossett 2001; Dickason 2002).

In 1939, the Supreme Court of Canada ruled that the Inuit were included in the more generic term 'Indian' for purposes of federal government jurisdiction, although they were not to be classified as 'Indians' under the Indian Act. In an effort to provide administrative services (including health care) to them, in 1941, the government began attempts to register the Inuit in a manner similar to that for registered Indians; in this instance, however, special 'disks' were issued to some people, with unique numbers stamped thereon, that the individuals were to wear at all times. Given that most Euro-Canadians could not pronounce Inuit names (and made no effort to learn), the 'disk list' system provided a convenient, bureaucratic method to identify individuals. However, the system was not widely accepted by the Inuit and soon fell into disuse (D.G. Smith 1993). Nevertheless, the federal government has continued to develop policies for the Inuit that mirror those for the registered Indians.

The post-Confederation years were a period of great change for the Indians, Inuit, and Métis of Canada. There were occasional flourishes of concerted resistance by some, most notably in the Red River settlement in 1869–70 and in Saskatchewan in 1885, events that galvanized Canadian opinion about the French-speaking Métis in particular. As the Indians were settled on reserves, the Métis were pushed farther and farther from their 'homeland' in Manitoba, through Saskatchewan and Alberta, with some even making new homes for themselves in the Territories. The Inuit stayed mostly out of the public eye until the 1950s, when government turned its attention northward in the wake of the Cold War. Government attempts to assimilate Aboriginal people continued unabated, and met with some success. Nevertheless, a strategy of passive resistance by Aboriginal people throughout this era ensured that some elements of language and culture would remain intact.

While periodic wage labour activities were available (the Plains Indians were noted agricultural workers, and the Indians of British Columbia were actively involved in the commercial fishery in the early years of the settlement of the west; see Elias 2002 and Knight 1996), these Aboriginal groups slowly became more economically and socially marginalized. For northern Indians and Inuit, hunting, fishing, and trapping activities continued. The Iroquoian peoples in southern Ontario and Quebec started to become more involved in the industrial economies of surrounding Euro-Canadian communities. Indians and Métis on the western plains continued to participate to some degree in the agricultural economy, although their own operations were often marginal because of problems with government agricultural policies (N. Dyck 1986; Carter 1990). And out on the Northwest Coast, salmon and other river and ocean resources remained the staples of the local economies. But times were changing, and widespread poverty became the norm. By 1945, it seemed as though Aboriginal people in Canada had all but disappeared from the national conscience.

It was in the 1960s that Aboriginal people in Canada began once again to be heard. The seminal event that launched what is known today as the Aboriginal rights movement was the federal government's White Paper on Indian policy (Weaver 1981).[7] This 1969 policy statement proposed, among other things, to make Indians 'equal' to other Canadians by eliminating the Indian Act, and therefore their separate legal distinction, as well as eliminating reserves and turning over administrative jurisdiction of Indian programs to the provincial governments. What was at issue was not the question of the oppressive nature of federal administration of Indians (the Indians agreed with this), but rather Indian fears that this form of 'termination' without recognition of their special rights and unique status would lead to even greater assimilation and oppression by the provinces.

The federal government never formally adopted the White Paper on Indian policy, but the legacy of that failed effort was to shape First Nations-federal relationships for decades to come. Many Aboriginal people grew increasingly suspicious of Canada's motives whenever any new programs were announced. Fears that inherently assimilationist policies would be developed, perhaps under the rhetoric of 'equality,' remained constant. Such remains the case today, as the federal government continues its attempts to introduce new legislation on First Nations governance.

An opportunity to entrench the rights of Aboriginal peoples within the Canadian federation came when Canada attempted to patriate the constitution. Prior to the early 1980s, Canada's constitution was actually a piece of British legislation, the British North America Act. When it became evident that then-Prime Minister Pierre Trudeau was going to be successful in developing a new, 'made in Canada' constitution, the Aboriginal peoples realized that the opportunity was at hand to have their 'Aboriginal' rights recognized as well. After a great deal of political activity, they were actually able to secure these ill-defined rights in the 1982 Constitution Act. Section 35 (1) states that 'The existing Aboriginal and treaty rights of the Aboriginal peoples of Canada are hereby recognized and affirmed.' What exactly these rights are remains contentious to this day.

Since the mid-1970s, the federal government has embarked on a program to affirm its view of self-government, predicated on the notion of delegated powers and the creation of municipal-style Indian governments. In 1975, the James Bay and Northern Quebec Agreement was signed between the Cree and Inuit of northern Quebec and the federal and Quebec governments. The subsequent Cree-Naskapi (of Quebec) Act of 1984 gave these northern Aboriginal peoples the authority to govern a wide variety of areas, such as education and health, although only as a result of delegated powers. Some hailed the agreement as a model; others condemned it as simply Aboriginal management of federal and provincial programs.

By 1986, the Sechelt Band in British Columbia had devised their own model of self-government and had obtained approval of the federal government via Bill C-93. The bill allowed the band to take over many of the powers that the federal government had under the Indian Act, including obtaining fee simple ownership of reserve lands and the ability to control education, health and social services, taxation, public order and safety, natural resource utilization, and infrastructure developments. Again, this model was criticized in some quarters as being insufficient, since the federal government still, in effect, maintained legislative control over the band.

The 1980s saw the federal government develop many joint ventures with First Nations, and many took delegated control of areas such as social services, education, and health under 'transfer' programs. In some instances, these programs involved the cooperation of provincial governments. Today, most First Nations have acquired at least some control over their own affairs.

In contrast to First Nations, the Inuit have gained a form of public self-government with the creation of the new territory in the eastern Arctic known as Nunavut. By virtue of their demographic majority, the Inuit are now able to exercise political will over their traditional lands. For their part, the Métis continue to struggle to develop appropriate forms of self-government, hampered in part by the fact that they lack a land base and are scattered throughout the various provinces.

In 1991, a royal commission was established to investigate a variety of Aboriginal issues in Canada, and one of its priorities was to learn the truth about residential schools. The Royal Commission on Aboriginal Peoples (RCAP) had a sweeping mandate, essentially to investigate the evolution of the relationship among Aboriginal peoples (Indian, Inuit, and Métis), the Canadian government, and Canadian society as a whole, and concluded that nothing short of a complete restructuring of Aboriginal/non-Aboriginal relations in Canada was required. While health issues, including those related to the residential schools, were included in the commission's work (e.g., RCAP 1993), the extent to which its findings have had a real impact remains questionable. One of its legacies is worthy of mention in this book, however, and that is the Aboriginal Healing Foundation (AHF). Endowed in 1998 with $350 million, the AHF's mandate is to 'encourage and support Aboriginal people in building and supporting sustainable healing processes that address the legacy of physical and sexual abuse in the residential school system, including intergenerational impacts' (AHF 1999:1; see chapter 10).

Finally, it would be fitting to conclude this overview of Aboriginal legal history by noting that the development of the Canadian Institutes of Health Research, and especially its Institute for Aboriginal People's Health (IAPH), in 2000, represents the beginning of a new era in Aborig-

Figure 2. Selected socio-economic indicators, 2001 census

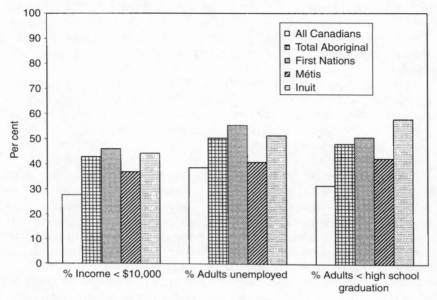

Source: Statistics Canada census tables. See endnote 1.

inal health research. The product, in part, of intense and effective lobbying by activists and health researchers, the IAPH has sparked renewed attention to the importance of Aboriginal health research and the training of Aboriginal health researchers.

CURRENT SOCIO-ECONOMIC CONDITIONS

Despite its limitations, the census remains the best and most comprehensive database from which to examine Aboriginal social and economic conditions on a national level. Figure 2 summarizes several key socio-economic indicators based on the 2001 census, comparing different categories of Aboriginal people with the Canadian national population.

Demographically, the Aboriginal population is quite young. According to the 2001 census, the median age of Aboriginal individuals was about twenty-five years, compared to thirty-eight years in the non-Aboriginal population. Perhaps more striking is that about one-third of the Aboriginal population is under the age of fifteen, compared with only 20 per cent nationally. The overall Aboriginal birth rate by 2001 was 1.5 times higher than the non-Aboriginal rate (Statistics Canada 2003). The average number of children for the on-reserve registered Indian population was almost double that for the national population, at 2.1 children per family. The prevalence of female lone-parent families is also roughly twice that for Canada (23 per cent, compared to 12 per cent) (DIAND 2000). Although the data suggest clearly that the Aboriginal population is relatively young, the number of Aboriginal seniors has increased dramatically in recent years, some 40 per cent between 1996 and 2001, the largest increase in all age categories (Statistics Canada 2003). This, of course, represents a new challenge for Aboriginal health practitioners and policy makers.

Significant strides have been made in recent years with respect to improvements in access to education for Aboriginal people, although some important gaps still remain between them and the national population. Only 4 per cent of the Aboriginal population had achieved a university degree in 2001 compared with 15 per cent nationally. Furthermore, while only 31 per cent of the national population had not completed high school, such was the case for 48 per cent of the Aboriginal population. The data also demonstrate that on-reserve registered Indians lagged behind other Aboriginal populations in terms of educational attainment (Statistics Canada 2003).

The trend towards increasing urbanization for Canadian Aboriginal people remains significant. In 2001, roughly half of the Aboriginal population lived in urban areas, and the proportion of Aboriginal people, primarily registered Indians, living on reserves and settlements was barely 30 per cent. One-quarter of the Aboriginal population now lives in ten major cities, with Saskatoon, Winnipeg, and Edmonton having the highest proportion (Statistics Canada 2003). The Aboriginal cultural and experiential complexity that continues to emerge within our cities presents unique challenges to those concerned about health issues, and especially the provision of services deemed to be 'culturally appropriate.' This will be discussed in greater detail later in the book.

The Aboriginal population continues to be bedevilled by relatively high unemployment rates. According to the 2001 census, 62 per cent of Canadians were employed, compared to just under 50 per cent for Aboriginal people. The proportion of adults employed full time for a full year was similarly much lower among Aboriginal people (26 per cent) than Canadians nationally (37 per cent). The registered Indian population continues to have the highest unemployment rates in comparison to the Inuit and the Métis, and unemployment on reserves is especially high. The Aboriginal population also experiences significantly lower incomes than non-Aboriginal Canadians. While 43 per cent of the Aboriginal respondents reported an annual income in 2000 of less than $10,000, only 28 per cent of Canadians as a whole belonged to this category (which also includes individuals who reported earning no income). And while 24 per cent of Canadians reported an income in excess of $40,000, only 12 per cent of Aboriginal people did as well. As is the case for most socio-economic variables, there are significant discrepancies when we examine specific Aboriginal categories. In general, on-reserve Indians and Inuit tend to be the least well off economically, while the Métis reported incomes closest to the Canadian national average. Government transfer payments constitute a higher proportion of the income of Aboriginal people (21 per cent) than of other Canadians (12 per cent).

Housing conditions also remain a problem, especially for on-reserve residents, and are implicated in many of the health problems people experience. In general, the housing and living conditions of Aboriginal people have consistently been poor and remain below national standards. However, many initiatives by both federal and provincial governments to provide electricity, proper sewage disposal, potable water, and better quality housing have resulted in improvements in recent years. For instance, while 21 per cent of on-reserve houses in 1991 had more than one person per room, by 1996 this had declined slightly to 19 per cent. Of course, this still dwarfs the national figure of just 1.7 per cent of houses with more than one person per room. Similarly, the 1996 figure of 0.7 persons per room, down slightly from 0.8 per cent in 1991, is still double the national average of 0.4 per cent. On a more positive note, by 1996 almost 92 per cent of homes on reserves had adequate sewage disposal facilities, and 96 per cent had water supply services (DIAND 2000).

It should be noted that the socio-economic data presented in this chapter mask the considerable regional and intercommunity differences within the Aboriginal population. Aboriginal communities are not homogeneous, and they are not all uniformly affected by poverty, unemployment, and economic underdevelopment. McHardy and O'Sullivan (2004) developed a First Nations Community Well-Being Index, based on the 2001 census, that combines education, labour force, income, and housing indicators. In general, communities in the Lower Mainland of British Columbia and in southern Ontario are the best off, while those located in the prairie provinces and the Canadian Shield tend to have the lowest levels of community well-being.

CONCLUSION

This introductory overview of Aboriginal people in Canada has been necessarily brief. It has not been possible to examine individual cultural groups, communities, or local or even major historical processes to any great extent. Such an understanding is nevertheless important for those who wish to appreciate current health issues affecting Aboriginal people. In an era of increasing globalization, we must nevertheless keep sight of the fact that people live their lives at the local level of families and communities, and it is at this level that many health determinants have the greatest impact. While we would direct the reader's attention to the literature referred to in this chapter and elsewhere for more comprehensive treatment of issues of culture and history, we also encourage you to do so with a critical eye, with the realization that any broad, generalizing statements may not be directly appropriate at *any* local level.

What we have tried to establish here is that the Aboriginal people of Canada today are exceptionally diverse, culturally, linguistically, socially, economically, historically, and in other ways. The recognition and acceptance of such diversity is essential to an appreciation of developments in the health care field and to an appreciation of the myriad processes that have affected the health status of Aboriginal people in both the pre-contact and post-contact periods. The remainder of this book examines these aspects in greater detail.

2

Health and disease prior to European contact

It is no easy task to construct a coherent picture of health and disease in the past. The project is acknowledged to be largely inferential, based on limited information and analytic methods (Johansson 1982:134–5). The recovery of prehistoric disease patterns depends on the careful weighing and patching together of several lines of evidence by various researchers working independently on diverse questions, rather than on a single grand synthesis by a lone researcher. To appreciate the pitfalls in the endeavour and to develop a healthy respect for its limitations, it is necessary to be fully aware of the problems facing investigators of ancient disease patterns.

Chief among these is the daunting time span over which health and disease must be appraised, over the huge geographical expanse of present-day Canada.[1] If a new generation is produced every twenty to thirty years, a truly comprehensive survey of health and disease must be based on archaeological evidence for some 600 to 1,000 generations of people who lived at different times and places, in a variety of social and environmental circumstances. After all, there is no reason to suppose that pre-contact American societies were any less complex, dynamic, diverse, or subject to social change than societies elsewhere in the world, even if they have often been represented as static and unchanging until European contact (Dobyns 1983:25).

But it is unrealistic to expect this fine degree of texture and historical detail, so broad generalizations about disease over time and space are made out of necessity. This makes small-scale studies of local sites more meaningful by connecting them to larger-scale regional and chronological patterns of health and disease. An ambitious interdisciplinary project, for instance, evaluated the history of health and nutrition in the

Americas over several millennia, drawing on a database of more than 12,500 skeletal remains from sixty-five sites (Steckel and Rose 2002d). Their overall analysis based on a health index developed specifically for the project showed health inequalities in which hunter-gatherer populations were the healthiest and large communities sustained by agriculture were the least healthy. They also identified a long-term decline in health during the pre-Columbian period as 'societies evolved from simple to complex and hierarchical' (Steckel and Rose 2002a:587). Yet generalizations drawn from such large-scale assessments should not be assumed to have been replicated at the community level. Although long-term change in health and disease was heavily conditioned by subsistence activities and population size, Steckel and Rose (2002a) note that other aspects of the environment, such as topography and proximity to the coast, also influenced health profiles.

In Canada, bio-archaeological work is spread unevenly across the country. Some regions have longer and more extensive records than others, either because of preservation conditions, length of time of occupation, a history of archaeological interest in the area, the pace of urban development, or just plain luck. Deep concerns of Aboriginal groups about the removal, study, and reburial of ancient human remains has effectively limited pre-contact skeletal research in some regions.

But the body of available evidence on pre-contact health and disease in Canada continues to expand through ongoing bio-archaeological research that aims to assess the quality and length of life of the members of past societies. Special attention is paid to the quality of life of children, who are the most vulnerable members of any society, and to the degenerative processes associated with aging and labour seen among adults. We turn now to the nature of the evidence for ancient health and disease and the inferences that can be made from even scanty bio-archaeological remains.

EVIDENCE FOR HEALTH AND DISEASE IN THE PAST

The clearest available signs of pre-contact health and disease come from autopsies of intentionally or accidentally mummified human remains. Just such an examination led to the identification of acid-fast bacilli of *Mycobacterium tuberculosis*, the micro-organism associated with tuberculosis, in the lungs of a young Peruvian boy whose death is estimated to have occurred in the eighth century, some 800 years before European contact (Allison, Mendoza, and Pezzia 1973). Many other infectious and non-infectious diseases, antigens, and evidence of medical treatment have been identified from autopsies of pre-contact mummies (cf: Allison 1976; Bernardo, Salo, et al. 1995; Konomi et al. 2002).

Preserved human feces, known as coprolites, provide information on pre-contact parasitic infestations and nutrition. Roundworms have been found in archaeological sites in the Colorado Plateau dating from 1100 BC to AD 200 (Fry 1974), and pinworms come from many other sites as well (Rheinhard, Ambler, and McGuffie 1985). Hookworms may have debilitated people from the American Southeast prior to 200 BC (Rheinhard 1992). Parasite burdens, however, tend to decrease with increasing latitude and thus were probably less of a threat north of forty degrees latitude. On the other hand, animal food consumption tends to increase with latitude, heightening the risks of meat-borne parasitic infections (Cohen 1989:98). In just such a way, roundworms, trematodes, and tapeworms of domestic dogs and wolves were transmitted to pre-contact Alaskans (Fortuine 1989:60) and, presumably, to other arctic dwellers. Human roundworm (*Ascaris lumbricoides*) and fish tapeworm (*Diphyllobothrium* spp) dating as far back as 5,500 years ago have been identified in shell midden sediments from the Pacific coast of Canada (Bathurst 2004).

Lest worm infestations be taken lightly, Riley (1993) points out that roundworm larvae can infect the lungs, producing pneumonia or symptoms of asthma; they can also lodge in and cause damage to the central nervous system. Adult roundworms inhabit the lumen of the alimentary tract, inducing nausea, vomiting, and sleeplessness; they produce abdominal distension in children and inhibit normal growth. Hookworm and roundworm infections provoke iron deficiency anaemia in both adults and children and can compromise the immune system's ability to cope with other infections. In other words, these were seriously debilitating parasites that afflicted past Aboriginal populations, a fact that is borne out by evidence that some Aboriginal healing traditions contained information on how to eliminate them with, among other things, *Chemopodium* (goosefoot or lamb's-quarters) (Riley 1993).

Mummified human remains and coprolites are quite rare in the Canadian context. An exception is the discovery by three hunters in 1999 of a preserved body in the vicinity of a glacier in Tatshenshini-alsek Park in British Columbia, within the traditional territory of the Champagne and Aishihik First Nations (Beattie et al. 2000). Dated to about 550 years ago via the radiocarbon method, the remains are those of a young man in his late teens to early twenties, referred to as Kwäday Dän Ts'inchí in the Southern Tutchone language. Apart from the rarity of ancient mummified remains in Canada, the discovery is noteworthy because of the ongoing research collaboration established between the Champagne and Aishihik First Nations and academic researchers. Such collaborations are becoming increasingly common (cf: Williamson and Pfeiffer 2003), enriching scholarship through the shared perspectives of complementary knowledge traditions.

More often than not, skeletal and dental remains provide the only clues to past diseases. Much of the skeletal evidence is non-specific in nature, showing up as general inflammations of bone such as osteomyelitis and periostitis. Aspects of dental form and structure, tooth wear, dental caries, periodontal disease, and developmental defects help skeletal biologists recover past lifestyles (Mayhall 1992). In fact, dental pathology is considered to be a reliable general marker of disease loads and nutritional stress. Evidence of shifts in the frequency of dental disease over time and space allows valuable inferences to be made about episodic or altered disease stress and malnutrition, but it is difficult nonetheless to take such observations to a more precise level of disease specificity. It may be necessary to turn to epidemiological studies of dental disease in living people to sort out the impact of cultural differences and change on pre-contact peoples (Skinner and Goodman 1992).

Because of the scarcity and non-specific nature of most of the skeletal and dental evidence, only the barest epidemiological outlines can be sketched for the pre-contact period – what Ortner (1992:5) calls 'probabilities, possibilities, and impossibilities.' It is virtually impossible to outline a clearly defined suite of specific diseases for particular times and places, let alone to determine what the leading causes of illness and death were or the magnitude of disease. Acute infectious diseases rarely leave signs on bone, so their effects must be deduced from other indirect clues, such as unusual age profiles in skeletal samples (Jackes 1983; Larocque 1991), or from bone tissue responses to the presence of infection (Stuart-Macadam 1992).

The diagnostic process is made even more complex because different micro-organisms produce similar effects on bone. The similarities between osseous lesions resulting from tuberculosis and those produced by pathogenic fungi, for instance, led Shadomy to dub their associated micro-organisms as 'the great mimics' (Shadomy 1981:25). *Blastomyces dermatitidis*, the fungal agent of blastomycosis,[2] today is found in cool, moist areas such as southern Manitoba, southwestern Ontario, and the St Lawrence River region of Quebec. Although rare, this fungus produces bone lesions similar to those of tuberculosis, and investigators in these parts of Canada must eliminate it as a possibility before provisionally diagnosing tuberculosis (see Pfeiffer 1984:188). Knowledge of the contemporary geographic distribution of micro-organisms and their ecological affinities also assists with the detective process. Coccidioidomycosis is yet another fungal disease whose effects on bone can be confused with those of tuberculosis; however, since it is endemic to the arid and semi-arid regions of the Americas (Long and Merbs 1981), it can be dropped from consideration when suspicious lesions are found in archaeological sites in Canada.

There is also a very marked bias in the kinds of infectious conditions that are expressed and detectable in bone. Most skeletal lesions result from chronic bacterial infections that have followed a protracted course from which, ironically, the individual survived owing to adequate immunological resistance. In other words, there is a paradoxical tendency for the palaeopathological evidence to come from the remains of *healthier* individuals (Wood et al. 1992). There is some optimism that antibodies to viral diseases may eventually be extractable from archaeological bone and thus expand the array of identifiable diseases in the past, but the results so far are mixed. Measles, smallpox, scarlet fever, and influenza, to name a few, are important infectious diseases that cannot be detected in bone.[3]

Because the symptoms and soft tissue evidence needed for provisional diagnoses are not visible in bone, investigators essentially must evaluate distinctive *patterning* of bone lesions throughout the skeleton to narrow down the range of possible underlying conditions. This is particularly important, for instance, for distinguishing leprosy from the treponemal infections of yaws and syphilis (Steinbock 1976). Following such a protocol, and in partnership and consultation with Aboriginal communities, Merrett and colleagues (2003) assessed the health of eleven archaeologically recovered adults and children from the Whaley Cairn site in southeastern Manitoba. By carefully analysing the type, frequency, and distribution of skeletal lesions, the team concluded that treponemal infection, probably yaws, affected boreal forest people some 2,000 years ago (Merrett et al. 2003).

Their study highlights the issues of completeness, preservation, and sample sizes in the analysis of skeletal populations. Depending on the conditions of deposition, a skeleton, or more frequently *parts* of a skeleton, may survive taphonomic and diagenetic processes. The latter refer collectively to the effects of climate, moisture, soil conditions, plant roots, farmers' ploughs, rodent gnawing, animal scavenging, or any other post-mortem environmental factor that may alter skeletal remains to such an extent that meaningful analysis cannot be undertaken. The surface and internal composition of the bones may be well preserved, permitting a detailed examination of morphological features, or they may be so worn or pitted that much of their exterior and microstructure have been obliterated. Sometimes post-mortem disturbances by plants and animals create the illusion of pathogenic processes. Henderson (1987) describes a misdiagnosis of syphilis made on the basis of cranial lesions that were produced by post-mortem chewing by beetles!

The small size of many skeletal samples lowers the statistical probabilities of detecting the presence of a disease in bone. Tuberculosis is a case in point. If tuberculosis is manifest in bones and joints in from 1 per cent (T.M. Daniel 1981) to 7 per cent of cases (Steinbock 1976), then the chances of finding it in a skeletal sample are low, even if the disease was common when the population was living. Indeed, while large skeletal samples increase the odds of finding examples of pathological lesions, there is still the difficulty of translating their presence into meaningful statements about a community's experience of the disease. In her study of the pre-contact Uxbridge ossuary (AD 1490 +/– 80 years) from southern Ontario, for instance, Pfeiffer (1984) identified a minimum of eight children and eighteen adults with tubercular lesions out of a possible 457 individuals. These people represent a population that was extant over many years. However, because the age structure of mortality from tuberculosis changes over time (Frost 1939) as the population experiences the epidemic wave (Grigg 1958; J. Bates 1982), we can only speculate what these results might mean in terms of the Uxbridge people's history of exposure to and death from tuberculosis.

Sampling problems also influence our understanding of non-infectious conditions in the past. Because no large skeletal samples have been excavated in the Cree-Ojibwa territory, we cannot ascertain whether congenital dislocation of the hip was as common in the pre-contact period as the unusually high prevalence of 6 per cent suggests for the region in the twentieth century (Pfeiffer 1991:14). The identification of developmental anomalies of the axial skeleton in several individuals from Manitoba, over perhaps 2,000 years or more, may be evidence for a genetic condition among related people in the region (Meiklejohn 2002; Meiklejohn and Merrett 2002, 2004). But the individuals expressing the condition are single cases dispersed through time, making it difficult to establish a genetic relationship among them. Clearly, the calculation of basic epidemiological measures such as prevalence and incidence is difficult, if not impossible, for the pre-contact and much of the post-contact period, as is the charting of epidemic waves.

Although the issues of sample size and representativeness are troubling, advances in the analysis of bone tissue at the microscopic and molecular levels are helping circumvent some of the problems associated with morphological assessments of skeletal pathology. The use of polarizing optics, various sophisticated forms of microscopy, and digital imaging make it possible to distinguish the cellular structure of normal bone from that disrupted by underlying disease states (Rothschild 1992; Von Hunnius 2004). Other sophisticated methods for going beyond surface marks on bone to cellular, chemical, and genetic levels have further expanded the amount of information that can be gleaned from human remains.

Microscopic analysis of thin sections of bone, for instance, makes it possible to compare adult bone mass and cortical bone density between populations and, hence, the risks of fracture (Pfeiffer 1991; Southern 1990). Evaluation of the chemical constituents and trace elements in bone and teeth offers a means of assessing diet and nutritional stress. The introduction of maize into the Great Lakes region of southern Ontario, for instance, has been well documented through the analysis of stable carbon isotopes (Schwarcz et al. 1985), and attempts have been made to link this dietary change to specific disease indicators (Katzenberg 1992). At the molecular level, analysis of ancient bacterial DNA is beginning to clarify and supplement skeletal studies of human disease expressed in bone, providing information on acute and chronic diseases such as tuberculosis, leprosy, treponemal infection, malaria, Chagas disease, plague, syphilis, diphtheria, and gastro-intestinal infection (Cohen and Crane-Kramer 2003; Zink et al. 2005:32). Current research, in fact, stresses the use of multiple methods and sources of information, rather than relying on a single source of evidence or analytic method.

New ideas about the origins and spread of infectious diseases in the Americas have arisen from just such a cosmopolitan approach. Consider the transformation in the debate about the origins, transmission, and spread of tuberculosis. In the early twentieth century, high rates of tuberculosis morbidity and mortality among Aboriginal people led scholars to conclude that tuberculosis was recently introduced from Europe to the Americas (Hrdlicka 1908; D.A. Stewart 1936). Subsequently, the identification of tuberculosis in mummified tissue (Allison et al. 1973) and bone lesions consistent with a differential diagnosis of tuberculosis forced scholars to conclude that tubercular disease was endemic in the Americas prior to European contact (Buikstra 1999; Ramenofsky 1987). Now there are more than 133 pre-contact cases of tubercular-like lesions dated to a period of at least two millennia (Prat and de Souza 2003). Some diagnoses in human and animal bone have been buttressed by the identification of *IS6110*, the diagnostic fragment of DNA from the *Mycobacterium tuberculosis* complex (Arriaza et al. 1995; Braun et al. 1998; Konomi et al. 2002; Rothschild et al. 2001; Salo et al. 1994). There is good potential for an ancient DNA approach to studying the history of tuberculosis because characteristics of *Mycobacteria* make them more likely to have been preserved than other bacteria (Zink et al. 2003).

A fascinating new array of questions about the origins and evolution of tubercular disease, on a worldwide scale, has arisen from this multi-method approach (cf: Pálfi et al. 1999). Considering a map of the distribution of cases in the Americas, for instance, Jane Buikstra asks why there are no cases from Mesoamerica when they are abundant in North and South America (Buikstra 1999:482). Did low-grade tubercular infections accompany the earliest inhabitants of the Americas and only become acute when people began settling in large groups? Did animal herds in the Americas, such as bison, acquire tubercular infections from humans, or were they transmitted in the other direction (see Stead 1997)? Ramenofsky wonders whether the high post-contact morbidity and mortality from tuberculosis observed among Native Americans results from the introduction of new, more virulent strains from Europe compared to those already endemic in the Americas (Ramenofsky et al. 2003:250). In other words, the debate about tuberculosis in the Americas is no longer simply about whether it was present prior to European contact but about what strains of the *Mycobacteria tuberculosis* complex were present in the Americas, how the strains may have been transmitted and have interacted with each other, and how they may have interacted with strains brought by Europeans (Braun et al. 1998). Clearly, more research needs to be focused on the evolution of host-pathogen interactions, on the evolution of the pathogens themselves, and on environmental circumstances that affect the spread of infection and the expression of disease (Ewald 2003; Ramenofsky et al. 2003).

Reframing the debate about tuberculosis also highlights the significance of human-animal relationships, acknowledging that they have far-reaching implications for human disease ecology and for the kinds of infections that may be present in a society (Armelagos, Barnes, and Lin 1996). It is a central premise of contemporary epidemiological theory that zoonoses – animal diseases – are a key element in the appearance of new diseases among humans. Many of the emerging infectious diseases[4] that afflict human populations today have their origins in animal diseases, or the 'zoonotic pool' (Morse 1993:15). For example, strains of influenza that infect pigs and fowl can give rise to virulent new strains that, in turn, infect humans. This process precipitated the devastating pandemic of Influenza A in 1918 (Scholtissek 1994).

It is therefore imperative to incorporate zoo-archaeological evidence – the remains of non-human animal species at archaeological sites – into studies of ancient human disease. Fortunately, archaeological sites often yield abundant faunal remains (animals), even when human remains are absent. Additionally, the study of animal bone is not subject to the same sensitivities and ethical considerations that appropriately constrain the study of human bone (Cannon, Schwarcz, and Knyf 1999:405). Much can be discovered about human nutrition and disease, for instance, from the study of domesticated animals, such as dogs. Dogs scavenge the remains of human meals, forage in middens, steal or are intentionally fed human food. Because of this, dogs have similar chemical signatures to the humans with whom they live. Canine remains at archaeological sites are therefore a rich source of information on broad classes of food in the human diet wherever they are found (see Katzenberg 2000). Analysis of a sample of fifteen dog bones from the site of Namu, located in the traditional territory of the Heiltsuk nation on the central coast of British Columbia, confirmed an early reliance of humans on maritime foods (Cannon, Schwarcz, and Knyf 1999). Close contact with domesticated animals also creates the opportunity for their diseases to spread to humans, and vice versa. As the first domesticated animal, dogs may have been transferring diseases to humans for some 15,000 years (Mitchell 2003:173, table 2). Skeletal lesions and molecular evidence for *IS6110* (the diagnostic fragment of DNA from the *Mycobacterium tuberculosis* complex) in dog remains from a sixteenth-century Neutral site in Ontario suggest that tubercular disease was transmitted back and forth between dogs and humans, as occurs today (Bathurst and Barta 2004). The study of human-animal relationships, concentrating on the potential for cross-species transmission of pathogens, represents perhaps the most significant new direction for approaching the problem of ancient disease in the Americas and elsewhere.

Another important direction involves integrating local evidence for health and disease into the larger framework of epidemiological transition theory. In its classic formulation, epidemiological transition theory refers to the shift away from a disease profile that features the predominance of acute infectious diseases towards one that emphasises chronic, degenerative diseases. This transformation was understood to have accompanied the process of industrialization in Europe and elsewhere and has been described within the context of several hundred years (Omran 1971). An expansion of the concept considers the health history of humanity in the thousands of years that elapsed from the Palaeolithic (Old Stone Age) to contemporary society, noting that three major shifts in subsistence practices were accompanied by concomitant changes in disease profiles (Armelagos et al. 1996). In this scheme, the first transition marks the shift of hunting and foraging economies to those based on food production (sometimes referred to as the Neolithic revolution, dating to 10,000 years ago). This process was associated with a cascade of other changes, including increasingly sedentary settlement patterns, population growth, permanent common water sources, accumulation of human and other forms of waste, exposure to the pathogens of domesticated animals, accelerating social inequalities accompanied by growing health inequalities, and so on. Together, they are believed to have increased parasite loads, and hence disease loads, in settled agricultural communities.

The point to be taken from this is not that hunters and foragers were disease-free (they weren't, as we shall see shortly), but that there has been a long-term relationship between human behaviour and pathogens 'which demonstrates the profound importance of human social and ecological change on disease organisms' (Cohen and Crane-Kramer 2003:79). Paying attention to the full environmental context within which ancient populations lived is crucial for developing local and regional chronologies of diseases and how these changed through time.

It should be evident nevertheless that a true 'palaeoepidemiology' of the Americas has yet to be developed and that it may never be possible to discuss fully the dynamics, determinants, and distribution of ancient diseases.

We can never know what specific physiological, immunologic, or genetic characteristics prevailed in earlier human populations which may have influenced the invasiveness, virulence, or pathogenicity of infectious agents. Similarly, we do not know what specific physiological or genetic characteristics prevailed in prehistoric bacteria, viruses, or fungi which may have conditioned their effect on human hosts. Simply put, the specific nature and course of host-parasite relationships, as revealed and understood in modern clinical and epidemiological studies, may not be exactly the same as in the past. (Widmer and Perzigian 1981:100)

Despite these important caveats and limitations, a great deal is known about many facets of pre-contact disease in what has become present-day Canada. This is illustrated with examples drawn from three areas: southern Ontario Iroquoia, the Arctic, and the Northwest Coast.

PRE-CONTACT DISEASES IN CANADA

Southern Ontario Iroquoia

Archaeological excavations in southern Ontario have produced some of the most extensively studied collections of Aboriginal skeletal remains in Canada. While many of the sites have yielded relatively small and poorly preserved samples, others are ossuaries consisting of thousands of individual bones, representing the remains of hundreds of individuals. Most of these sites were excavated more than twenty years ago, owing to a voluntary research moratorium in this region on all but salvage sites (Pfeiffer and Fairgrieve 1994). This extraordinary abundance of information has stimulated intense interest and analysis by a large cadre of skeletal biologists over several decades.[5]

Equally important to the enterprise is a strong and well-defined archaeological record that includes whole village plans, controlled dating of sites based on artifact and radiocarbon analyses, and detailed regional sequences. Without reasonably good appraisals of the socio-ecological context of the living population, it is difficult to evaluate its skeletal remains and develop hypotheses about prevailing diseases and causes of death. Fortunately, the archaeological sequence for southern Ontario is quite solid and offers insight into changes over time in subsistence activities, trade routes, population size and density, patterns of migration and other forms of interpersonal contact, village sanitation and relocation practices, seasonal resource availability, and the presence of reservoirs and possible vectors for the spread of infection (Starna et al. 1984; Fecteau et al. 1991; Williamson and Pfeiffer 2003). The accumulated evidence makes it clear that there were significant social and health changes in the region well before European contact.

Of course, the question of what actually constitutes 'contact' needs to be addressed at this point. Even though AD 1492 has become a powerful metaphor for the cascade of processes set in motion as a result of the first contact between people from the western Mediterranean and the Americas, direct and regular contact between ethnically diverse groups of Europeans and North Americans began at different times, in different places. For southern Ontario, the onset of the beaver fur trade around AD 1580 essentially represents the point at which intense and habitual direct contact occurred between Europeans and Aboriginal groups. The pre-contact period for this region therefore ends in the last decades of the sixteenth century, although European influences reached the area before this time.

Much of the research on skeletal remains from pre-contact sites falls into three categories: identification of nutritionally mediated disease stress associated with the introduction of maize from the sixth to the fourteenth centuries; evaluation of time trends in the incidence of non-specific disease indicators, such as caries and bone density; and detection and assessment of the impact of specific infectious diseases.

Considerable attention has been paid to the relationship between a nutritional shift towards increased incorporation into the diet of carbohydrates in the form of maize and concomitant changes in disease over time (Katzenberg and Schwarcz 1986; Schwarcz et al. 1985; Katzenberg, Saunders, and Fitzgerald 1993). It is not known exactly when maize entered the diet or became a widely cultivated food source, but the combined results of carbon isotope[6] and archaeological analysis indicate that maize consumption increased significantly between AD 500 and 1200. Maize became a major food source between AD 900 to 1300 (Schwarcz et al. 1985) and among some groups may have accounted for as much as 70 per cent of the energy value of the diet (van der Merwe et al. 2003). Certainly, heavy reliance on maize is linked to a high frequency of caries, abscesses, and tooth loss (Crinnion et al. 2003). Over roughly the same period, the consumption of animal protein remained quite stable, and the subsistence base of pre-contact Iroquoian villages involved mixed swidden horticulture, hunting, fishing, and collecting, from the fifth century to the contact period.

The impact of the temporal trend towards an increasingly large maize component in the diet on the health of pre-contact Iroquoian peoples is difficult to assess. There is a large anthropological literature, discussed earlier in this chapter, that equates horticultural and agricultural societies with higher pathogen loads, largely because settled village life is associated with the accumulation of wastes, increased contact with domesticated animals, and higher population densities, all of which enhance the opportunities for infectious disease transmission. Heavy reliance on cultigens, moreover, makes a population vulnerable to starvation from periodic crop failures and from nutritional deficiencies, depending on the extent to which monoculture is practised and essential amino acids (tryptophan and lysine) and metals, such as zinc, are missing from the diet (Armelagos et al. 1996; Cohen 1989). This sets up the well-known synergistic cycle of malnutrition–infectious disease–malnutrition so common in less developed countries today.

In this regard, the regular relocation of Iroquoian villages at twelve- to twenty-year intervals has been attributed to soil and other local resource depletion as well as to crop infestations; but deteriorating village conditions, dreams, and misfortune may also have contributed to the relocation cycle (Starna, Hammell, and Butts 1984; Fecteau et al. 1991). Yet it cannot be denied that pre-contact Iroquoian villages exploited a wide range of nutritional sources and never relied completely on cultivated crops. Katzenberg's (1992) stable isotope analysis suggests nonetheless that bone lesions from infections were highest when maize consumption was highest, although this may have been influenced by concomitant increases in population density that would have enhanced the chances of disease transmission. The Moatfield people who lived just north of present-day Toronto between AD 1280 and 1320,[7] for instance, frequently had tuberculosis. On the other hand, they showed no growth stunting (Dupras 2003) and little in the way of anaemia (Pfeiffer 2003), probably because the high nutritive content of the fish in their diet countered the deficiencies of maize (van der Merwe et al. 2003).

Support for a link between maize horticulture and infectious disease comes from the skeletal remains of twenty-nine individuals from the MacPherson Site, a pre-contact Ontario Neutral Iroquoian village site dated to AD 1530–80.[8] Two young children aged three to four years of age present the only known cases of circular caries detected so far among the southern Ontario skeletal remains (Katzenberg et al. 1993). Circular caries is a defect in the enamel that develops during deciduous tooth formation; later, caries form in the portions of the tooth where the enamel is thin. Such lesions are particularly prevalent today in children from less developed countries and are often a consequence of malnutrition following chronic diarrhoea. This led Katzenberg and co-workers to hypothesize that the circular caries in the MacPherson children were the scars of nutritionally mediated infection during early childhood. The nitrogen isotope ratios indicate that the diet onto which these children were weaned was high in maize. Since high-carbohydrate weaning diets may contribute to child mortality, the combination of nutritionally mediated infection and a high-carbohydrate weaning diet may have created insurmountable stress for these two children. However, like most of the data that bear on the question of pre-contact disease, this evidence, though persuasive, is still non-specific and indirect. There is no way to determine which infectious diseases might have afflicted the children, for how long, or how often.

Other indirect evidence for nutritionally related conditions in pre-contact southern Ontario Iroquoia is summarized by Pfeiffer (1991) and Pfeiffer and Fairgrieve (1994). One of the more intriguing conditions found at a number of pre- and post-contact adult Iroquoian sites is relatively thin childhood and adult cortical bone (an exception is the Moatfield ossuary; see Stock and Willmore 2003). This is significant because growth in cortical bone thickness can be retarded during nutritional and disease stress. In fact, adult Iroquoian bone density appears to have decreased over time and reached subnormal values by the late fifteenth century (Southern 1990). Although thin cortical bone has been interpreted as possible evidence for disease stress (Saunders et al. 1992), it is difficult to disentangle the relative contributions that diet, disease, nutrition-disease interaction, or other factors may have made to the phenomenon (Pfeiffer and Fairgrieve 1994).

The presence of porotic hyperostosis in skeletal remains from a number of pre-contact sites is additional evidence for the action of infectious disease. Porotic hyperostosis is a condition of the skull vault visible to the unaided eye as small holes of varying size on the surface of the bone. There is general agreement among skeletal biologists that it is often a manifestation of acquired iron-deficiency anaemia. The condition was once considered to be a nutritional stress indicator, but it is now recognized that the withholding of iron (hypoferrin), which porotic hyperostosis expresses, is more properly viewed as successful adaptation to pathogen stress (Stuart-Macadam 1992). Regardless of the source of stress, there is solid evidence of porotic hyperostosis from a number of pre-contact sites, with the Fairty ossuary sample showing an especially high prevalence of 38 per cent among juveniles (Pfeiffer and Fairgrieve 1994). Chronic sinusitis was present at the fourteenth century Moatfield site. Over half of the people, especially adults, suffered from the condition. While acute and chronic exposure to respiratory pathogens can lead to sinusitis, in this case it is more likely a result of chronic exposure to wood smoke (Merrett 2003).

Although the discussion so far has emphasized non-specific indicators of disease, there is also clear evidence for the pre-contact presence of specific infectious diseases in southern Ontario. Several cases of treponemal disease have been described (Molto and Melbye 1984; Saunders 1988) and bacteria such as *Staphyloccus*, *Streptococcus*, *Moraxella*, and *Actinomyces* species were ubiquitous and endemic (Pfeiffer and Williamson 2003). A great deal of attention has been paid to tuberculosis, which leaves scars on bone and affects life expectancy, and which has been identified at sites in the region that date from AD 100 to 1650 (Hartney 1981). At the fourteenth-century Moatfield site, for instance, at least four adults were diagnosed with chronic tuberculosis, although the prevalence of the disease may have been lower than that seen at later sites, such as Uxbridge (Pfeiffer and Williamson 2003). Nevertheless, tuberculosis epidemics may have occurred in the region prior to European contact (Pfeiffer 1984).

Southern Ontario Iroquoia, especially just prior to direct European contact, appears to have been a particularly fertile ground for infectious disease. From the eight to the seventeenth centuries there are clear trends to increasing population density, larger and more numerous villages, and increased population density within villages. Crowding within villages was quite high, and longhouses were rarely separated by more than three metres. Refuse dumps, consisting mostly of organic waste, dotted the villages, usually no more than eight metres from the longhouses (Warwick 1984). By the second half of the fifteenth century and certainly by the time that trade goods appear in Ontario Iroquoian sites, these sociodemographic changes had increased the opportunity for infectious disease outbreaks (Saunders et al. 1992). These conditions probably enhanced the spread of the series of devastating, historically documented epidemics that swept through Huronia between AD 1634 and 1650.

The Arctic

In contrast to the relative wealth of skeletal information on pre-contact health and disease in southern Ontario Iroquoian populations, very little is known about Arctic populations. Vanast claims, in fact, that 'scholars have almost completely avoided the medical aspects of arctic history' (Vanast 1991b:76). What evidence there is comes from studies of Aleutian mummies and from skeletal remains from sites throughout the Arctic, but especially from Alaska and the Aleutian Islands. Speculation based on climatic and demographic patterns and references to health and disease in early contact narratives figure prominently in current reconstructions of pre-contact epidemiologic patterns in the Arctic.

The arctic regions occupy a particularly important intellectual space in the thinking about pre-contact disease in the Americas. The idea of a disease-free America, in fact, is predicated upon the idea that a 'cold screen' filtered out Old World diseases during the peopling of the Americas via the Bering Land Bridge.[9] Popularized by T. Dale Stewart in his influential book *The People of America*, Beringia and the northern regions leading to and from it came to be conceptualized 'as a germ filter that served to hold back the diseases of the people who passed through it' (Stewart 1973:19). This ensured that 'the men who passed through this cold zone in effect passed through a germ filter, leaving behind whatever disease germs there were in the old world' and that 'only the fittest survived the harsh northern climate that existed over the whole distance' (Stewart 1973:20). In Stewart's vision, ice and glaciers acted as significant barriers to pathogens and prevented contact with Eurasian populations. The cold climate, moreover, was 'unfavourable to the spread and perpetuation of disease germs' (Stewart 1973:19). This depiction of the northern regions as inimical to infectious disease has some merit. Parasite burdens tend to decrease with increasing latitude, and the relatively simple arctic ecosystem supports lower species diversity than in tropical regions (Dunn 1968:226–7). Fewer viruses are found in temperate than in tropical zones (van Rooyen 1968:548). Diseases caused by parasites that spend part of their life cycle outside of the host, such as hookworms, are substantially less common in the north (Cohen 1989:98). Cold climates are inhospitable for many insect vectors and hence preclude infection with the pathogenic micro-organisms they harbour (Newman 1976:668).

But Stewart's idealization of the health of Arctic peoples is not supported by current evidence, and it is clear that they were anything but disease-free prior to European contact. Robert Fortuine (1989, 2005), in particular, refutes many of the traditional contentions about a natural or genetic tendency to good health in the pre-contact Arctic. He draws attention to the presence of environmental hazards, such as toxic substances in water hemlock and the presence of other poisonous plants; the potential for paralytic shellfish poisoning; and the danger of ingesting environmental type E *Clostridium botulinum* in soil, associated with marine mammal butchering (Fortuine 1989:53–6).

As for the purported lack of insect vectors, it is worth remembering that the necessary conditions for the reproduction of biting insects are created whenever surface water accumulates in tundra and taiga climates. Mosquitoes (*Culicidae*), black flies (*Simulidae*), snipe flies (*Leptidae*), punkies (*Heleidae cubicoides*), and house flies (*Tabanidae*) multiply profusely in the Arctic (van Rooyen 1968:548):

No one who has passed a summer in Alaska has failed to notice – sometimes in unprintable language – the myriads of biting insects that swarm around any warm-blooded creature, including humans ... Mosquitoes, although present throughout Alaska, were a particular curse in the coastal areas ... Continuous scratching of bites usually led to skin infections such as impetigo, which could then be spread to other parts of the body or to other persons. (Fortuine 1989:57)

Lice and their eggs are commonly found in pre-contact Aleut mummies, and early contact narratives confirm that Arctic peoples sustained heavy infestations of head and body lice. The combination of crowded living and sleeping conditions, heavy fur clothing, and a shortage of water created 'almost perfect living conditions' for them (Fortuine 1989:64).

Exposure to pathogenic micro-organisms also occurred simply because northern populations were in frequent and close contact with mammals (domestic and feral), birds, fish, and insects, as well as with their waste products (Cohen 1989). Bacterial diseases such as brucellosis (caribou reservoir), tularemia (probable muskrat reservoir), and salmonellosis (birds) found in arctic wildlife today may have infected pre-contact communities. Although rabies has long been endemic in arctic foxes and wolves, it is not yet possible to determine whether these animals acted as its reservoirs prior to European contact (Fortuine 1989:62–3).

The heavy emphasis on animal foods in the diet of Arctic peoples also resulted in enhanced exposure to food-borne parasites, especially in uncooked meat. Trichinosis, roundworms, trematodes, and the tapeworms of domestic dogs and wolves can be acquired through eating ungulates such as moose and caribou (Fortuine 1989:59). Not surprisingly, Eskimos in Alaska have been observed to suffer from trichinosis and tapeworms (Cohen 1989:98). Careful autopsies of Aleutian mummies have confirmed the presence of a variety of infections, including trichinosis and fish trematode infestations, prior to European contact. Respiratory diseases, such as pneumonia and anthracosis,[10] and a possible case of the fungal infection associated with histoplasmosis, have also been identified. There are clear cases of chronic otitis media and mastoiditis as well (Zimmerman, Yeatman, Sprinz, and Titterington 1971; Zimmerman and Smith 1975; Zimmerman, Trinkaus, LeMay, et al. 1981; Zimmerman and Aufderheide 1984).

Early contact narratives from the Arctic also provide a glimpse of some of the health problems prevalent at the time. They contain many references to skin ulcers, sores, boils, carbuncles, and throat infections (Fortuine 1989:65–7). In contrast, diarrhoeal diseases receive scant mention, but 'the record of a brief or casual encounter with Alaska Natives

would not be expected to include observations on the frequency or character of their stools' (Fortuine 1989:70). Of course, the brevity of such
contacts and the heavy clothing of Arctic peoples would have hidden all
but the most obvious signs of illness, so only particularly noticeable
symptoms would have been mentioned. The very sick would have
stayed behind in the village, further skewing the impressions of health
and disease formed by early explorers (Fortuine 1971).

In any event, virtually none of the infections, infestations, or intoxica-
tions mentioned so far can be diagnosed in bone. This explains to a great
extent why much of the skeletal research on pre-contact Arctic populations has emphasized more readily observable dental pathology, trauma,
cribra orbitalia/porotic hyperostosis, spondylolytic and osteoarthritic
lesions, and evidence for non-specific infections, treponemal disease, and
tuberculosis (T.D. Stewart 1932, 1979; Merbs, Wilson, and Laughlin 1961;
Merbs and Wilson 1960; Merbs 1963; Way 1978; Salter 1984). It fails to
explain why there have been so few systematic skeletal analyses of temporal changes in the health of Arctic populations (Keenleyside 1993; an
exception is Laughlin, Harper, and Thompson 1979). Schindler (1985) has
taken the provocative stance that skeletal biologists working on arctic
material have been preoccupied with the antiquated and long-aban-
doned anthropological enterprise of race classification, instead of exploring the dynamic interaction between culture and biology. It should be
noted however that most arctic skeletal remains date to the post-contact
or late pre-contact periods, prior to which sample sizes are exceedingly
small (Cybulski, personal communication).

In her analysis of osteological collections held at the Smithsonian
Institution in Washington, Anne Keenleyside (1993, 1994) documents a
number of health problems diagnosable in the skeletal remains of 193
Alaskan Aleuts and northern coastal Eskimos from five pre-contact
sites. As one would expect, most of the infectious lesions were of non-
specific origin, although active periostitis on the pleural surfaces of the
ribs of one young adult male indicates some form of pre-contact respiratory infection. The presence of cribra orbitalia and porotic hyperostosis
in the cranial remains was also noted, evidence of bone tissue response
to pathogen load. Fractures of the crania, ribs, clavicles, hands, and feet
were the most common type of trauma observed.

As other researchers have noted, and in contrast to southern Ontario
Iroquoia, there is no conclusive evidence for treponematoses in the pre-
contact Arctic. In fact, there is general agreement that they were likely to
have been acquired by Arctic people recently, probably through contact

with nineteenth-century European whalers (Keenleyside 1990:7–8; Holcomb 1940). On the other hand, tuberculosis may have been endemic for thousands of years before European contact (Fortuine 2005:2–3). The rarity of dental caries, enamel hypoplasia, dental abscesses, and periodontal disease also stands in stark contrast to the situation found in pre-contact southern Ontario (Keenleyside 1993:4). This difference is likely explained by dietary differences between the two regions, with the higher-carbohydrate diet associated with maize horticulture in southern Ontario resulting in greater nutritionally mediated dental disease.

Perhaps the most interesting feature of this work is the documentation and discussion of significant differences in health between the pre-contact Aleut and Eskimo samples. The Aleut skeletal remains showed significantly more trauma and infection than those of the Eskimos. The higher frequency of trauma among adult Aleut males may reflect the greater involvement in warfare that is suggested by the archaeological record for Aleuts during this period. Although there is probably a complex of factors that underlie the phenomenon, Keenleyside suggests that housing differences between Aleuts and Eskimos may have contributed to it. Since Aleuts lived in large, semi-subterranean dwellings estimated to have accommodated anywhere from 30 to 300 people, the opportunity for the spread of infection was substantially higher than it was for the Eskimos, who occupied much smaller houses containing 8 to 12 individuals (Keenleyside 1993:5–6). In other words, it appears that differences in the pre-contact social contexts of the two groups produced divergences in their health profiles, just as one would expect.

In a comparison of health and disease among pre-contact and post-contact Aleuts, Keenleyside (2003) notes that Aleut health declined in concert with contact with Russian fur traders, shown in a significant increase in the prevalence of infection. Introduced diseases, such as smallpox, influenza, and measles, surely contributed to this observation. But she notes that their effects were nevertheless exacerbated by dietary changes that increased nutritional stress and by brutal policies practised by Russian traders, including forced labour, resettlements that compelled Aleuts to travel increasingly great distances to hunt waning sea otter populations, and hostilities among Aleuts and Russian traders.

The Northwest Coast

The early contact period for the Northwest Coast peoples generally spans the late eighteenth to mid-nineteenth centuries. While it has been argued that introduced diseases diffused over large geographical expanses and infected Aboriginal groups that had no direct contact with Europeans (Dobyns 1983, 1992), archaeological, historical, and oral tradition sources indicate that this was not the case for the Northwest Coast. Old World diseases appear to have been introduced to this region quite late, after 1774 (Boyd 1992, 1999). The pre-contact period for this area, therefore, is not located in the distant past but hovers several generations beyond living memory.

The best known Northwest Coast archaeological and osteological sequences come from coastal British Columbia (Cybulski 1994) from the results of systematic, controlled excavations carried out in the 1960s and 1970s (Cybulski 1990:55). The earliest human remains date to about 5,500 years ago and coincide with the onset of shell midden build-up that typifies most prehistoric sites in coastal British Columbia. There are thirty pre-contact sites where preservation and completeness are sufficient to allow analysis of the skeletal remains of 759 individuals. The skeletal remains, however, do not represent all areas or times, and about three-quarters of them are dated between 3,500 and 1,500 years ago (Middle Developmental Stage), and come from sites at Prince Rupert Harbour and the Strait of Georgia (Cybulski 1994). Complete skeletons are not always available, narrowing the accuracy of differential diagnosis in such cases because assessment of lesion patterns is critical for discerning the likelihood that infectious diseases such as tuberculosis or the treponemal diseases were present (Cybulski 1990).

Much of the writing about prehistoric coastal British Columbia emphasizes cultural continuity in the various regional sequences and depicts gradual social change over the 5,000 or so years that precede European contact. Other interpretations emphasize the dynamic relationship between the various groups of people and their socio-ecological environment (Cannon 2001). Evidence from dental abrasion facets caused by the use of labrets and from diversity over time and space in head-shape modification practices suggests greater degrees of social change in the pre-contact period than previously suspected. There is, however, broad agreement that human populations used a variety of maritime species, and there is ancient DNA evidence for a well-established multi-species salmon fishery at the site of Namu by 7,000 years ago (Yang et al. 2004).

The social system encountered in the southern coastal area at contact, for instance, may have been 5,000 years old, while that known for the north appears to have been as recent as 1,300 years old. Changes in burial rituals may signify or be part of larger sociocultural transformations that might have occurred at that time. Below-ground burial of single individuals in shallow pits in shell middens, for example, was commonly practised until about AD 1000, in contrast to the above-ground burial practices typical of the historic period. The latter form of mortuary treatment may have begun 500 years before contact (Cybulski 1994).

Differences in the sex ratio of mortuary remains signal other forms of cultural diversity in the pre-contact period. The Prince Rupert Harbour remains, for example, contain almost twice as many males as females. Cybulski (1990) hypothesizes that since females periodically made up a large proportion of the slave population in consequence of intertribal warfare, their remains and those of other low-status individuals would have been interred elsewhere. He further speculates that the Prince Rupert Harbour people had a very different sociocultural context from the Strait of Georgia people, where there was little evidence for selective burial practices or warfare.

This speculation is supported by differences in fracture frequencies at the two locales. At Prince Rupert Harbour almost 40 per cent of the individuals had limb and/or spinal fractures; the Strait of Georgia region shows a much lower frequency, around 11 per cent. Interpersonal violence associated with tribal warfare at Prince Rupert Harbour likely accounts for most of the trauma. This is because almost 60 per cent of the traumatic injuries at the site consisted of depressed skull fractures from club blows, parry fractures, various defensive and disarming fractures of the hands and forearms, and cases of decapitation (Cybulski 1990).

The pre-contact maritime subsistence economy of the Northwest Coast is typically depicted as rich and plentiful. Intensive harvesting of almost the full range of marine resources, but with particular emphasis on salmon, provided the economic foundation for social organizational complexity; dense, sedentary village populations; and diverse forms of artistic expression (Suttles 1968). Cannon (1995) makes a case, however, for fluctuations in village prosperity in conjunction with periods of local marine resource failure, signalled by increased proportions of starvation foods (deer and ratfish) in archaeological assemblages. This interpretation is consistent with Suttles's (1968) observation that serious food shortages frequently occurred for the Northwest Coast area in the wake of episodic resource failures.

Attained adult stature is considered to be a good indirect measure of health and nutrition during childhood. Studies of growth and development in developing countries support the contention that stunting and wasting in children, brought about through severe and prolonged nutritional and/or disease stress, can produce permanent reductions in achieved adult height (King and Ulijaszek 1999). In this regard, the apparent stability in stature among coastal peoples over a 3,000- to 4,000-year period is striking. Average heights of 162.4 cm estimated for skeletal remains for the Early Stage (3500–1500 BC) compare favourably to Boas's average measure of 164.2 cm for living people in the area in the late nineteenth century (Cybulski 1990, 1994). The consistency of the stature estimates suggests that, periods of scarcity notwithstanding, the Northwest Coast people who survived to adulthood probably did not experience prolonged bouts of malnutrition or chronic and debilitating infectious disease during childhood growth. On the other hand, regional differences in the frequency of porotic hyperostosis have been detected, despite its coast-wide prevalence of 13 to 14 per cent (Cybulski 1977, 1990). This suggests that there was local variation in pathogen loads, the sources of which remain unexplained and which undoubtedly embrace a complex of sociodemographic factors (Stuart-Macadam 1992). It is evident, nonetheless, that coastal peoples were challenged by micro-organisms to varying degrees but not sufficiently to produce irreversible growth stunting.

The discovery of intestinal parasites in coastal shell middens from several sites of the Northwest Coast peoples indicates that people suffered from fish tapeworm (*Diphyllobothrium* spp) and human roundworm (*Ascaris lumbricoides*) as early as 5,500 years ago (Bathurst 2004). These intestinal parasites may explain, at least in part, the unusually high frequency of skeletal indicators of anaemia found in Northwest Coast skeletal remains (Bathurst 2005). Such parasite infections are usually chronic, persisting within the infected individual for years, leading to anaemia that can be severe and that lowers resistance to other infectious agents. Interestingly, large numbers of *Diphyllobthrium* eggs were recovered from the small intestine, descending colon, and rectum of Kwäday Dän Ts'ìnchí, the young man whose preserved body (dated to about 550 years ago) was found in Tatshenshini-alsek Park in British Columbia. Such tapeworms are common in fish-eating societies (as well as birds and mammals) and often infect humans through the eating of uncooked, infected fish (Dickson et al. 2004).

Dental health in the pre-contact period also seems to have been quite good, with dental caries affecting less than 1 per cent of all teeth (Cybulski 1990:57).[11] In contrast to southern Ontario Iroquoia, caries are notably absent in Northwest Coast populations until the twentieth century, when the diet of fish, plant foods, and sea and land mammal meats began to be supplemented with foods rich in carbohydrates (W.A. Price 1934). Abscessed jaw sockets, which must have been quite painful, were common in the pre-contact period and affected upward of 50 per cent of all adults. This marked tendency towards abscesses probably resulted from a combination of dietary and cultural practices. Traditional food preparation techniques introduced grit into the food, and this contributed to tooth wear. Trauma and wear to the front teeth sustained through use of the lower jaw by women as a tool, and associated with a high frequency of head and facial fractures among males, probably contributed to the prevalence of abscessed anterior teeth in the upper jaws of both sexes (Cybulski 1990:58).

Skeletal studies to date have failed to turn up any evidence for pre-contact tuberculosis or malignant bone tumours, even though both of these diseases are present in historic Northwest Coast skeletal remains (Cybulski 1990). While it is conceivable that they were unknown to pre-contact coastal people, their absence may equally reasonably be an artifact of poor bone preservation and age-related sampling (Cybulski 1994).

There is clear evidence, nonetheless, for treponemal infection well before AD 1492 from two Middle Development Stage sites (1500 BC to AD 500). Four out of ten skeletons from the Duke Point site near Nanaimo (1490 BC +/− 125 years) show classic symptoms of treponemal infection, and as many as six individuals, including a fetus, may have been affected. The widespread nature of the infection suggests endemic non-venereal syphilis, at least in this sample. One female at the Boardwalk Site at Prince Rupert Harbour (325 BC +/− 90 years) shows clear signs of *caries sicca* (Cybulski 1990), the classic 'worm-eaten' cranial lesions considered to be 'the only reliable and pathognomonic lesion of syphilis' (C. Hackett 1983:113).

CONCLUSIONS

The study of human remains from various regions in Canada provides substantial evidence for disease and nutritional compromise, of varying degrees and kinds, prior to European contact. Fungal, bacterial, and parasitic infections afflicted pre-contact peoples to varying degrees, depending on local socio-ecological conditions. Health patterns changed over time well before contact, as illustrated by the prehistory of southern Ontario Iroquoia, and there was much diversity within and between regions, typified by the Arctic and Northwest Coast sequences. The concurrent infectious disease load supported by pre-contact Aboriginal groups, moreover, likely influenced the extent to which they were affected by introduced diseases.

Clearly, the idea of a disease-free pre-contact America is not supported by the substantial evidence for infection. New directions in the study of ancient disease, stimulated by the new paradigm of emerging infectious disease, include greater attention to human-animal relationships (and the potential for cross-species transmission of infection) and consideration of how diseases and pathogens endemic to the Americas interacted with new micro-organisms introduced from Europe.

3

Contact and disease

The decimation and extinction of many indigenous peoples of the Americas is a matter of historical fact. The process was initiated by a cascade of changes that included ecological disruption through the importation of new plants and animals, including pathogens (Crosby 1986); interference with and subversion of the social order by missionaries, traders, and government officials; the arrival of settlers to farm the lands of people already shattered by epidemics and the persecution of resisting survivors; and social fragmentation and reorganization as surviving groups coalesced on the margins of European settlement (Upton 1977:133).

The relative influence of each of these processes, either alone or in combination, on the size and demographic structure of Aboriginal populations varied from time to time and from place to place. Evaluating the nature and extent of depopulation and the local, regional, and hemispheric factors that explain the phenomenon continues to be one of the major thrusts of inquiry into the post-contact period. Since the 1970s, particular weight has been accorded to the role played by pathogens introduced from Europe and Africa in this process.

As we have seen in the last chapter, the presence of new pathogens and the absence of immunity to them are insufficient as the sole explanation for epidemics in the Americas or elsewhere. Epidemics occur when the complex relationship between human populations and their social and physical environment is altered, disrupted, or conducive to the flourishing of micro-organisms. The problem then becomes one of teasing out the social histories of Aboriginal populations and understanding how new opportunities were created for the transmission of infectious diseases through socio-ecological change resulting from

European contact. This includes determining the toll of lives taken by individual or successive epidemics on specific populations and regions, as well as evaluating how epidemics inhibited demographic recovery and set in motion dramatic changes in the social order. It is a difficult task, especially since the information available for addressing these questions is sparse, spotty, and often of disappointingly poor quality.

This chapter considers the main theories regarding the role of epidemics in the demographic transformation of Aboriginal populations in the post-contact Americas and describes aspects of health and disease from selected regions in Canada. We illustrate the complexity of the social and ecological changes that underlay population declines in Canada and emphasize the new sociopolitical relationships that emerged with European contact and that engendered the fundamental conditions that allowed epidemics to flourish.

INTRODUCED DISEASES AND DEMOGRAPHIC DECLINE

Few researchers doubt that diseases of European origin figured prominently in the post-contact history of Aboriginal communities. From the seventeenth century onward, smallpox, measles, influenza, dysentery, diphtheria, typhus, yellow fever, whooping cough, tuberculosis, syphilis, and various unidentifiable 'fevers' caused illness and death as they spread from person to person and from village to village. Many of these are considered to have been 'virgin soil epidemics,' epidemics characterized by unusually high mortality in all age categories. Such a pattern of mortality occurs either because the disease is new or because it has not been present in a population for so long that individuals with antibodies to it have died and community immunity (called 'herd immunity' in the epidemiological literature) has been lost. A similar phenomenon can be observed today with emerging and resurging infectious diseases such as tuberculosis, HIV/AIDS, and hantavirus.

Although introduced diseases are recognized to have been a severely destructive feature of the post-contact experience of Aboriginal people, an intense debate swirls around the issue of the *extent* to which epidemics per se shaped the post-contact demography and history of the Americas (Trigger 1985:354). Indeed, the controversy about the depopulation of Aboriginal societies has come to turn on this question. This has generated a large literature in which records of epidemics have been compiled, routes of disease spread plotted, and evaluations made of their impact on indigenous societies.[1]

Some scholars accord extraordinary importance to the role of epidemics in post-contact disruption and population decrease. Russell Thornton asserts, for example, that 'Without doubt, the single most important factor in American Indian population decline was an increased death rate due to diseases introduced from the Eastern hemisphere' (Thornton 1987:44). Alfred Crosby maintains, 'It was their germs, not these imperialists themselves, for all their brutality and callousness, that were chiefly responsible for sweeping aside the indigenes and opening the Neo-Europes to demographic takeover' (Crosby 1986:196). The fundamental problem is how to fill in the picture with quantitative detail (Johansson 1982:139).

Scholars who embrace the idea that infectious diseases introduced from Europe were primarily responsible for the destruction of Aboriginal societies often argue that infectious diseases reached many groups well before Europeans themselves did (Dobyns 1966, 1983). Accordingly, they contend that even the earliest population counts must be gross underestimates (e.g., Cook 1973; Miller 1976; Upton 1977). Consequently, they derive high contact population size estimates through the application of depopulation ratios as high as 25:1 (Dobyns 1983) to the earliest recorded figures. This encourages the impression that even the most casual European contact resulted in immediate, catastrophic mortality, well before there were any written records to document it (Ramenofsky 1987:1).[2] Another related aspect of this point of view is the implication that the Aboriginal populations declined continuously from the early sixteenth century onward until a nadir, or minimum number, was reached, after which they rebounded, stabilized, or became extinct (Meister 1976:161).

An alternative interpretation of the history of the Americas takes the position that introduced disease was not a significant agent of depopulation early in the post-contact period (e.g., Helm 1980). Advocates of this reading of the evidence argue that severe population declines occurred later in a slower and more insidious fashion (Johansson 1982:140) after sustained and intense European contact. This perspective conveys the impression that populations did not dwindle continuously from the time of contact but declined later in concert with Aboriginal-European interaction that resulted in dramatic sociodemographic change. Scholars who espouse this point of view therefore tend to consider early censuses not simply as depictions of relics of much larger populations already depleted by epidemics but as reasonable starting points for developing representations of regional population sizes (Mooney 1928; Kroeber 1934). Kroeber, for instance, was well aware that Indian populations had dwindled by the twentieth century but attributed that decline to warfare, changes in subsistence patterns through intense European-Aboriginal interaction, and lack of political organization, rather than to the effects of disease (Kroeber 1925, cited in Ramenofsky 1987:9). Helm (1980) explored the capacity of Dene hunting tribes in subarctic Canada to sustain their population size in the face of introduced disease and concluded that selective female infanticide in the first half of the nineteenth century had a greater effect on mortality than introduced disease at that time.

In any event, the discourse on demographic change resulting from European contact is essentially couched in terms of these catastrophist or gradualist theories, with proponents of each arguing through the literature about the effects of disease on the population history of specific groups (e.g., Helm 1980 vs Krech 1983a, 1983b; Snow and Lanphear 1987 vs Dobyns 1983, 1989). Since the late 1970s, the catastrophist view that introduced diseases were the primary agents of demographic change has tended to dominate thinking about post-contact history (Johansson 1982:140–1). Recognition of the importance of epidemiological research was boosted by the coincidental publication of William McNeill's (1976) influential book, *Plagues and Peoples*, William Denevan's (1976) textbook, *The Native Population of the Americas in 1492*, and a special symposium on the topic at the 1976 meeting of the American Society for Ethnohistory (Dobyns 1976). Trigger (1985:234) observes that since then it has become fashionable to question conservative population estimates. For central Mexico, for example, contact population estimates have soared from 2 million people to 25 million during this period (Henige 1990:170). In less dramatic fashion, estimates of Huron numbers prior to the seventeenth-century epidemics have increased from 16,000–22,500 to 25,000–32,000 (Trigger 1985:233–5).

ESTIMATES OF POPULATION SIZE AT CONTACT

Given these very different visions and ways of interpreting the evidence, it is not surprising that contact population estimates for North America (what is now Canada, the continental United States, and Mexico) cover an extraordinarily wide range. While most seem to hover between 1 to 2 million people, Dobyns's (1966) figure of 9.8 million, which he subsequently doubled to 18 million (Dobyns 1983), is substantially higher than the rest, as is Thornton's (1987:32) figure of 7 million.[3]

Over and above the differences in philosophical and theoretical orientation among researchers, Ubelaker (1992:170–2) notes that much of the variation in population estimates stems from disagreements about the geographical expanse of various regions in North America and from the disparate methodologies and sources of data used by the estimators. It bears recalling, however, that most historical demographic reconstructions stand or fall on the observations of a relatively small number of explorers, missionaries, physicians, traders, or government officials. A great deal of attention is therefore normally paid to evaluating the accuracy of recorded counts and comments and to determining whether they are tainted by intentional or accidental bias (W.G. Ross 1977:1–3; Ubelaker 1988:289; Boyd 1999).

The amount of *reliable* information on population counts, birth rates, mortality rates, migration rates, and disease episodes varies from region to region and from time to time. During the late fifteenth and early sixteenth centuries, when fishermen and explorers plied the northeastern waters along the Atlantic coast of Canada, there is virtually no historical documentation of Aboriginal people, diseases, or epidemics. In fact, the series of outbreaks that swept through the Montagnais, Algonquins, and Hurons of the St Lawrence and Ottawa Valleys between 1734 and 1741 are among the best documented early historic epidemics in the northeast (Trigger 1985:229–97). Unfortunately, the early explorers showed more interested in charting the coastline or recording and retrieving the available resources, including occasional human souvenirs to take back to Europe, than in commenting on Aboriginal life (Carlson et al. 1992:145–6). But this hundred-year lacuna means that we can only speculate about the demographic results of Aboriginal-European interaction and the effects of epidemics during this period. And to complicate matters further, it would appear that health and nutrition in the Western hemisphere declined prior to European contact, the deterioration dating from about 7,500 years ago (Steckel and Rose 2002c:565). How existing indigenous trends in health and disease may have interacted with new conditions introduced with contact remains a fascinating issue worthy of careful study.

Because of local and regional variability in the amount and quality of epidemiological and demographic information, researchers often look to complicated methods to circumvent the weaknesses in the primary source data. It is becoming more common to combine ethnohistoric and archaeological evidence, experiments with projective techniques, Monte Carlo simulations, mathematical models, and model life table comparisons. These adjust as much as possible for errors in the initial observations and for distortions in the data due to sampling error and generate a range of possible demographic scenarios from as many sources as possible.[4] For instance, a comprehensive health index has been developed that combines measures of the length of life with skeletal and dental indicators of the physical health of populations (Steckel, Sciulli, and Rose 2002).

Even the best methods, however, cannot compensate for the initial assumptions upon which they are built. Estimates of population sizes for the Americas are influenced, moreover, by the biases of scholars themselves (Borah 1976). The figures reflect the investigators' views on the density and complexity of pre-contact societies and the perception of the health of pre-contact indigenous North Americans. We have already seen, for example, that serious diseases with the capacity to erupt into epidemic form were present in the Americas prior to AD 1492. But because of the widespread assumption that infectious disease was not an important feature of pre-contact life, there have been few attempts to evaluate the extent to which extant infectious disease loads might have influenced the experience of introduced, post-contact disease (Herring 1992:154; see Molto 1999 for an exception). The new paradigm of emerging infectious disease, however, is beginning to change this perspective, as we saw in the previous chapter.

It is tempting to ignore these theoretical and methodological hornets' nests or to dismiss them as academic trivia. Yet these images have profound effects on the kinds of images projected in the literature about disease and the contact experience. Population estimates are important because they establish the baseline for all subsequent demographic estimates and for the construction of social histories (Johansson 1982:137). The larger the estimate of the initial population, the more devastating the impact of European contact is inferred to have been; the more conservative the estimate, the less demographically disruptive (Ramenofsky 1987:1). This helps to explain why the magnitude of the population estimates shifts with the political wind: conservative numbers typified the 1910s, liberal ones the 1920s, and so on (Ubelaker 1976). The most extravagant estimates date to the period between the 1960s and 1980s, emerging in concert with the shift in theoretical orientation towards appreciating and emphasizing the potential devastation of early contact epidemics (Ubelaker 1992:172).

Apparently, larger questions beyond the scope of the demographic data at hand are being discussed through the depopulation literature (Bruner 1986; Henige 1990), and estimates of Aboriginal population sizes and population dynamics remain incomplete, patchy (Ubelaker

1992:169), and speculative. This should caution researchers and students alike 'to establish what was, not what should have been' (Thornton 1987:36). The bleakest assessment waves all the estimates aside, claiming that the fundamental insufficiency of the evidence makes the endeavour no different from a guessing game comparable to deducing the number of elves in J.R.R. Tolkien's Middle-earth (Henige 1990:169). At the very least, most estimates are influenced by political and cultural biases and all deserve to be viewed with suspicion (Johansson 1982:137). It is perhaps worth recalling Romaniuk and Piché's (1972) caution that *reliable* estimates of demographic rates for Canada's Aboriginal people only begin to be available in the 1960s (see also Piché and George 1973).

POST-CONTACT CHANGES IN POPULATION SIZE

The most comprehensive reassessment of North American contact population figures was undertaken by Douglas Ubelaker (1988, 1992) of the Smithsonian Institution. To compensate for as many disparities as possible in the work of previous investigators, he based his study on forty-five articles submitted in 1976 for the Smithsonian's *Handbook of North American Indians* by scholars most familiar with primary sources. The new estimates subsume ethnohistorical, archaeological, and ecological factors, as well as the possible impact of early epidemics. After independently assembling each tribal estimate, he calculated regional totals, population densities, and the percentage of reduction in population size, to correspond with the ten culture areas included in the *Handbook*. With the exception of the Southeast, by Ubelaker's account, all appear to have reached their nadirs in the twentieth century, with population depletions ranging from a low of 53 per cent in the Arctic to extraordinary highs of 89 per cent for the Northwest Coast and 95 per cent for California (Ubelaker 1988:293). Figure 3 shows the estimated population decline in the six culture areas in Canada.

Which of the two post-contact scenarios discussed earlier best explains this phenomenon? The problem in selecting *either* explanation is illustrated by Carl Meister's (1976) comparison of the demographic history of five groups of Indians from the western United States. His findings for the Pueblo, Maricopa, and California Indian/Ute appear to conform to the catastrophist model, suggesting that introduced diseases took a major toll of mortality early in their contact experiences. On the other hand, the Navajo and Gila River Pima histories do not fit the model at all. The Navajo experienced a brief, ten-year period of popula-

Figure 3. Estimated decline in Aboriginal population in selected culture areas in North America

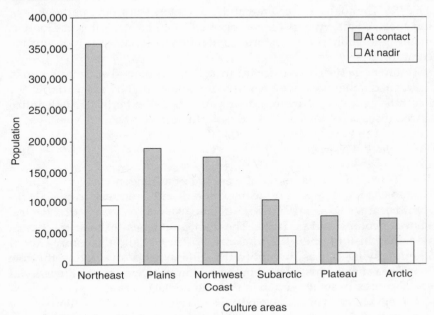

Culture areas

Source: Based on data from Ubelaker 1992

tion reduction between 1860 and 1870, but at the end of that decline their population was still several times larger than it was at the time of initial contact. The Gila River Pima show yet another pattern, with two periods of population decline separated by periods of population growth, evidence that they were able to recover from epidemics well before the introduction of European medicine. Meister suggests that the increase in Pima mortality in the latter half of the nineteenth century was more likely the result of their having been driven from their land than to a lack of immunity to diseases of European derivation (Meister 1976:162–5).

Meister's study shows that no single explanation can be expected to apply to every indigenous group. Variation in the phenomenon of contact was so great that it is fundamentally meaningless to try to fit each social history into a rigid category of experience. On a larger scale, the *Health and Nutrition in the Western Hemisphere* database confirms that the process of contact led to 'ethno-culturally diverse [demographic] systems with the merging of the Old and New World biospheres' (McCaa 2002:95). Demographic change and encounters with new pathogens of European origin involved a complicated, multifactorial process located in the particular social histories and interaction networks of specific communities.

To illustrate the complexity intrinsic to the contact-disease problem in the Canadian context, we turn to the evidence for the extinction of the Beothuk people of Newfoundland and to the experience with introduced diseases of the people of the Northwest Coast.

The Beothuk of Newfoundland

The Beothuk of Newfoundland were the first indigenous North Americans to encounter Mediterranean explorers and fishermen in the late fifteenth century (Upton 1977:133).[5] In just over 300 years, by 1829, the last known Beothuk had perished. The utter uniqueness of their tragedy in Canadian history (ibid. 1977; Pastore 1987, 1989) and the complexity of its underlying causes exemplify the difficulties of evaluating the role that disease may have played in their demise, as well as the diversity of social processes set in motion in the post-contact period.

Despite decades of archaeological and historical research, there are no firm and reliable estimates of Beothuk numbers at contact, which is generally defined as AD 1500. Archaeological reconstructions of the ecology of Newfoundland over the past 5,000 years show that while the island had the potential to support 'sizeable' human populations through its rich biome of marine and terrestrial resources,[6] many important food sources were available only on a seasonal basis and were subject to failures or periods of unavailability (Tuck and Pastore 1985:74). The fluctuating and precarious nature of the resource base meant that human populations were subject to recurrent booms and busts, as suggested by a record of at least three pre-Beothuk Aboriginal extinctions on the island, prior to the arrival of Europeans (Tuck and Pastore 1985:70–2).[7]

Upton's (1977:134) review of the published best guesses of Beothuk contact population size reveals an extraordinary range of 500 to 20,000 people, indicative of the poor quality of the information on this question. This is in keeping with what is known about the early contact period, which essentially consisted of sporadic coastal encounters between Beothuk and transient European fishermen. Any trade conducted between them was on a very small scale and so marginal in nature that it may have taken the form of a dumb barter, in which trade goods are left at a specific location and the trading parties do not meet (Pastore 1987:50).

As is the case elsewhere in the Americas (see Henige 1990), some of the early population estimates for Newfoundland are entirely without foundation, while others have an air of crypto-science because they are derived from climatic considerations and from assessments of the capacity of northeastern forests and coastlines to support the Beothuk hunter-gatherer lifestyle (see Upton 1977:134, especially note 2).[8] In fact, Beothuk contact population size will remain purely speculative until the unlikely event of a systematic archaeological survey of the entire Newfoundland coast and much of the interior (Pastore 1989:55). Even so, it is extremely difficult to estimate Aboriginal population sizes from archaeological evidence (Trigger 1985:231).

Population estimates for the mid-eighteenth century to the early nineteenth century fare little better, for most were 'based on casual contacts with Beothucks and mostly on heresay [sic]' (Marshall 1977:234). This is largely the result of the Beothuk strategy of withdrawal to the island's interior by the early seventeenth century (Upton 1977:135) and apparent decision not to engage in trade with Europeans (Pastore 1987:59). Furthermore, the fishery-based economy of Newfoundland and unusual settlement circumstances meant that there were no clergymen, traders, soldiers, or government agents (Upton 1977:153) – those who elsewhere recorded population estimates of Aboriginal peoples.

Whatever their numbers at contact, Marshall (1977:235) speculates that there could have been about 350 Beothuk in 1768, based on John Cartwright's map of their dwellings on the Exploits River, on the reckonings of planters in the area, and from the accounts of Shanawdithit, the last surviving Beothuk. By 1811, there were only 72, and they had dwindled to 13 by 1823. With the death of Shanawdithit in 1829, the Beothuk vanished. Without reliable population estimates, we cannot know how quickly their fate unfolded, and the magnitude of the decline and the speed of the death of a people does not diminish in any way the fundamental tragedy of that loss.

Despite the scarcity of demographic data, there is a growing body of opinion that a constellation of events and processes contributed to the Beothuk demise. Introduced diseases may have played a role, but there is so little evidence that it is impossible to do anything other than speculate about their impact. Smallpox was observed on the island from 1610 onward, but no major outbreaks were recorded. Although measles and other epidemics were sporadically noted among European immigrants, Marshall (1981:5) considers that the isolation of the Beothuk made the chances of transmission to them slim, except perhaps in the last fifty years or so, when contact increased.

Tuberculosis is the only disease to have been documented among the Beothuk. Three women were said to have been suffering from pulmonary consumption when captured by furriers in 1823 (Marshall 1981:6), 'which *they may have contracted prior to their capture*, and it must be *assumed* that this disease had taken its toll among the Beothucks' (italics mine) (Marshall 1977:236). Marshall speculates that from 1730 onward 'this disease played a significant role in the eventual demise of the Beothuk group' (Marshall 1981:7). Unfortunately, this quite plausible idea cannot be verified because there is no evidence with which to support or refute it. The argument is based on the single mention of tuberculosis in 1823, in conjunction with the estimated drop in Beothuk population from 350 in 1768 to 13 in 1823. It is also made with reference to the likelihood of increased contact between Beothuk bands as their territory shrank in the eighteenth century and more frequent contacts with Europeans, which together could have given rise to the high tuberculosis mortality rates recorded for Aboriginal groups here and elsewhere (ibid. 74–5).

Where Marshall's (1977, 1981) review of the literature suggests that introduced diseases became a more important determinant of Beothuk mortality after 1730, Upton (1977) focuses on their impact in the early contact period. Not only does he postulate that there was massive depopulation, he also suggests that epidemics may have been the stimulus behind the Beothuk avoidance of contact with Europeans between AD 1612 and 1750 (Upton 1977:135). Following Cook's (1973) analysis of the decline of seventeenth-century Amerindian groups in New England, he writes that, 'Presumably the first phase of contact had the same results in Newfoundland as elsewhere in the northeastern coastal region. European diseases had been introduced there by casual trade and there is no reason why the Beothuks should be exempt' (Upton 1977:138). This is a remarkable proposition given that many other features of Beothuk history stand in stark contrast to conditions elsewhere in the northeastern coastal region (Upton 1977:153) and in light of the lack of any supporting documentation (Marshall 1981:1).

Apart from the lack of evidence, there are other reasons for scepticism about massive initial depopulation of the Beothuk by introduced diseases. Marshall (1981) observes, for instance, that the sporadic encounters typical of the early contact period were not conducive to the transmission of acute community infections. Certainly the silent trade postulated by Pastore (1987:50) in the sixteenth and early seventeenth centuries lends support to this inference. On the other hand, if Basque whalers plying the Strait of Belle Isle in the mid-sixteenth to early seventeenth centuries employed the Beothuk in shore-based activities, there would have been greater opportunities for the transmission of pathogens (Pastore 1989:70).

Having estimated an initial Beothuk population of about 2,000 for AD 1500, Upton (1977:152) assumes 'a rapid loss of population as a result of first contact diseases followed by a period of recovery and stabilisation.' This is a good example of the depopulation-to-nadir model. He then conjectures that if this assumed depopulation occurred on a similar scale to that in New England, the Beothuk would have been reduced by disease to about 400 by the early seventeenth century (Upton 1977:137–8) and at an annual rate of 1.01 per cent from AD 1500 to 1811 (ibid. 152). Henige's observation is particularly apt here: 'It is all too easy to confuse the possible with the probable ... the notion that newly introduced diseases quick [sic] assumed epidemic (or "pandemic") proportions throughout the New World is, by its very nature, detached from any evidence' (Henige 1990:185). In the absence of documentation, it is tempting to begin with a story and locate the appropriate 'facts' within it (Bruner 1986:141–2).

Although it is not yet possible to resolve the extent of early cross-cultural contact or disease exchange, there is no doubt that the Beothuk opted for a pattern of avoidance of Europeans by the early seventeenth century, gradually withdrawing into the resource-poor interior of the island and disappearing from the written record until 1766 (Upton 1977:138). Whereas archaeological evidence indicates that the pre-contact Beothuk had a broad-based diet drawn from the seasonal exploitation of both marine and land resources, their displacement from the coastal regions by other ethnic groups meant that they were cut off from important foods, especially seal, and forced to rely on the relatively meagre resources of the interior. This strategy could not work in the long term, given the precarious nature and periodic failure of important staples such as caribou and the lack of fall-back foods, such as porcupine, deer, and moose (Tuck and Pastore 1985:73–6). With a hostile settler population preventing access to coastal marine resources (Marshall 1977:3), the necessary conditions for a subsistence crisis were created. This exclusion from resource-rich areas was probably the major factor in the decline of the Beothuk (Tuck 1976:76). The Beothuk world appears to have gradually become more tightly circumscribed as Europeans moved inland along the Exploits River and its tributaries to hunt for furs (Upton 1977:139). With the loss of contact with Labrador, which could have provided a refuge on the mainland, their fate was sealed (Pastore 1989:71).

The reasons for the Beothuk retreat inland remain unknown, but appear to have been closely associated with the growing exploitation of coastal resources by other ethnic groups and to increasingly hostile relations with them: 'Although the spread of permanent English settlement on the island may have been the most important factor denying the Beothuks access to vitally needed coastal resources, to that equation must now be added the Basque and Inuit presence in the Strait of Belle Isle, the Micmac use of the southern third of the island, and the French base at Placentia' (Pastore 1989:71). The Beothuk, moreover, never developed a full-blown fur trade with Europeans and, indeed, the seventeenth-century settlers to Newfoundland never became fur trappers (Pastore 1987:60). This gave rise to several important consequences. Because the Beothuk were interested in some European goods, a pattern of acquiring them through theft developed. This resulted in reprisals and killings of an unknown number of Beothuk by Europeans. The abhorrent killings of Beothuk have been popularized in the press as 'the people who were killed for fun' (Horwood 1959, cited in Pastore 1989:56).

Another consequence of the lack of cross-cultural trade was the absence of cultural brokers in the form of European traders, whose own economic interests would have been served by intervening with the settler population on behalf of the Beothuk (Upton 1977:153). In fact, in circumstances perhaps paralleled only by those of the Labrador Inuit (Pastore 1987:60), 'There was no missionary to plead for their souls, no trader anxious to barter for their furs, no soldier to arm and use them as auxiliaries in his wars, no government to restrain the settlers' (Upton 1977:153). It appears, then, that the Beothuk were not pushed to extinction by the effects of introduced diseases and epidemics. Rather, starvation from the loss of resource-rich territory and their marginalization into the impoverished Newfoundland interior led to their demise. Evidently, post-contact economic and sociopolitical relationships were the ultimate sources of the Beothuk's crisis and tragic disappearance.

The Northwest Coast

At the opposite end of the country, the people of the Northwest Coast began to encounter epidemics of pathogens introduced from Europe and Africa much later, as recently as 1774. Unlike the case of the

Beothuk, there is a substantial body of evidence that reveals some of the complexity of this new disease ecology.[9] Difficulties nonetheless remain in tracing the disease history of the region. For instance, despite the richness of the ethnohistoric record, neither the geographical origin (Mexico, the Great Plains, or Kamchatka) nor the date of the first smallpox epidemic (1769, 1774, 1775, 1779, or 1782) has been resolved (Boyd 1999).

To derive post-smallpox population estimates for the Northwest Coast, moreover, it has been necessary to work backwards from the earliest reliable figures (the 'anchor number') and then assume an across-the-board loss of one-third of the population from the first smallpox epidemics. Using this arithmetic, and setting aside the questionable validity of across-the-board mortality estimates, we can surmise that Northwest Coast populations may have been drastically reduced from about 183,000 to 37,000 people, or by about 80 per cent, during the first century of contact. The effects of depopulation were uneven, with estimates for the North Coast area suggesting a drop of 66 per cent between 1836 and 1880 compared to an astounding drop of 90 per cent for the lower Columbia area between 1805 and 1855 (Boyd 1999:21–38, 262–5).

Certainly the epidemiological and social context of contact on the Northwest coast was in no way comparable to that experienced by the Beothuk in AD 1500. By 1774 there were many more sources of infectious diseases, a more diverse disease ecology, and numerous routes by which epidemics could reach the region. Smallpox, influenza, mumps, dysentery, and meningitis arrived quickly in concert with the growth of trade within the region and with other areas, expansion of the Hudson's Bay Company, enhanced sea links, and the arrival of missionaries and migrants from the east. By 1835, Northwest Coast Aboriginal populations had all suffered major epidemics and can be said to have been incorporated into distant disease pools, a process described by William McNeill (1976:69ff) as the 'confluence of disease pools.'

Even so, there was a patchwork of effects, with populations in the south more severely depleted than those in the north (Boyd 1999:116). In fact, the disease profiles of various regions were sufficiently distinct to warrant delineation of six 'epidemic areas,' 'groups of geographically contiguous peoples who shared a common disease history' (ibid. 143–7).[10] In the south, where malaria ('fever and ague') became endemic, recovery from other acute epidemics was further compromised and depopulation was more severe than in the north. In addition to the chronic and debilitating effects of the disease itself, malaria suppresses fertility and increases infant and child mortality, with the result that 'most affected populations declined to near extinction' (ibid. 269). Here we see the synergistic and mutually enhancing negative effects of endemic and epidemic disease taking a persistent toll in mortality. In addition, the particular effects of endemic malaria are clear, the disease having consistently dealt a blow of 'heavy depopulation and minimal population and cultural survival' wherever it took hold in the Americas (ibid. 269). In northern areas where malaria failed to become endemic, epidemics were sporadic, occurring at wide enough intervals to allow populations to recover (ibid. 268–70).

Evidently, there was no single pattern of disease experience for the Northwest Coast but instead a mosaic of effects and responses, conditioned by local sociocultural, ecological, historical, and demographic contingencies, and by the mix of pathogens that became established in various parts of the region. Still, the available evidence suggests that Aboriginal populations in the region continued to decline into the twentieth century, reaching an estimated nadir of 22,605 people in 1929 (Kelm 1998:4).

TRADE AND EPIDEMICS

If the undeveloped trade relationship between the Beothuk and Europeans buffered the Beothuk from disease (but not from starvation), other areas where trade thrived were especially vulnerable to epidemics. Trade centres often became the nucleus for disease outbreaks and central points of diffusion of epidemics to the hinterland (Ray 1976; Dobyns 1983, 1992). This is because they represented points of convergence between Aboriginal people, Europeans, and their pathogens and created conditions conducive to the spread of infection. Trade centres also attracted long-distance Aboriginal trading partners who brought pathogens with them or acquired new ones at the trade centre, which, in turn, they unwittingly took with them on their return journey. Temporary and permanent settlers tended to cluster around the fringes of trade centres, typically resulting in higher population densities than characterized the surrounding areas. The higher the population density, the greater the chance that contagious diseases, either introduced or local, would spread quickly from person to person.

This is illustrated by the disease history of the central Canadian Subarctic. The establishment of Hudson's Bay and Northwest Company fur-trade posts in mainland Canada, for instance, not only stimulated significant relocations of Aboriginal peoples and restructured intergroup exchange networks (Ray 1974, 1996) but also set up novel patterns of Aboriginal-European contact and brought together widely separated disease pools. Exchange networks, centred on trading posts, created routes for the spread of contagion. Micro-organisms were conveyed alongside trade goods, enmeshing some regions in epidemics while others had little experience with them (see Dobyns 1983:12–13; Reff 1991:119–24; F.P. Hackett 2002).

Clearly, the reorganization of trade relationships and geographical distribution of Aboriginal groups along with alterations in intergroup contact attendant upon the fur trade were probably as significant for the disease history of the Americas as the introduction of foreign diseases per se. Examples from the post-1670 fur trade at York Factory and Norway House, both in present-day Manitoba, illustrate how economic and social change associated with trade centres influenced the transmission of epidemic diseases between communities and over long distances.

York Factory, established in 1714 at the mouth of the Hayes River, was one of the earliest posts on Hudson Bay and became the main port of entry for trade goods for western Canada. As the most important source of European cargo on the bay, York Factory housed a small European population of young Hudson's Bay Company (HBC) officers and servants and drew a far-flung network of Cree and Assiniboine from central and southern Manitoba and Saskatchewan (Ray 1974:72). HBC post journal records and Anglican Church of Canada death registrations from 1714 to 1801 show that European and Aboriginal people alike died from infectious diseases, including a protracted epidemic of influenza in 1717 and a devastating smallpox epidemic in 1782 (Ewart 1983).

By the nineteenth century, European physicians resided at the post, and causes of death were identified with greater precision, allowing Ewart (1983:573) to construct an unusually detailed profile of mortality (figure 4). Tuberculosis, influenza, and dysentery were the leading infectious diseases, and the presence of poliomyelitis, typhoid fever, and puerperal fever indicate that sanitary conditions at York Factory were less than ideal during this period. The detail provided by this compilation underlines the danger of relying solely on accounts of epidemics as a means of fleshing out disease profiles. Not only does a focus on epidemics stress the unusual and catastrophic; it also fails to reveal the presence of many serious afflictions, such as bronchitis and meningitis, which Ewart was able to identify at York Factory.

Arthur Ray (1976) was one of the first scholars to try to go beyond the construction of disease inventories to examine the spatial dynamics of

Figure 4. Distribution of deaths by cause at York Factory, 1801–1900

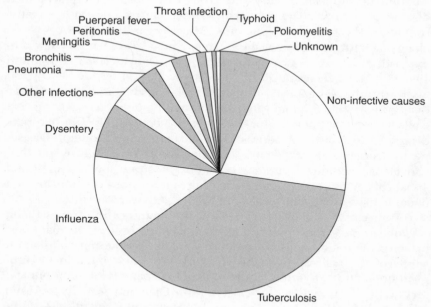

Source: Redrawn from data in Ewart 1983

epidemics of European origin and to assess the cumulative effects of a *sequence* of epidemics on Aboriginal people. His study focuses on the period between 1830 and 1850 in the western interior of Canada, a vast expanse of land that embraced present-day Saskatchewan, the Northwest Territories, Manitoba, and parts of northern Ontario. A series of major and minor epidemics of scarlet fever (1843), measles (1846–7), smallpox (1837), and influenza (1835, 1837, 1843, 1845, 1847, and 1850) affected the region during this time, with heavy tolls of mortality accompanying the 1835 influenza epidemic, the 1837 smallpox epidemic, and the 1846–7 measles outbreak. Because the post records do not contain precise information on the number of deaths or on the incidence of illness, the demographic consequences of these diseases cannot be evaluated. However, Ray's analysis of the origins, patterns of spread, and processes that fuelled their spread reveals that York Factory and Norway House were central to the movement of pathogens through the region.

Boat, canoe, and cart brigades linked these two posts to a large network of HBC posts throughout the western interior. Most of the traffic moved through this widespread exchange network during the summer months when open water made transport easier. The summer season was also marked by large-scale population shifts. Assiniboine, Cree, and Objiwa groups, for instance, spent the winters in the forested parts of the parkland, while summers were taken up with bison hunting and travel south to trade in the Missouri River valley. Any movement of people carries with it the potential concomitant movement of pathogens, with the result that summer eruptions were more likely to spread rapidly because of the larger encampments, increased visits to trading houses, and generally high volume of boat and canoe movement between districts that distinguished the season. Other aspects of social life nevertheless contributed to the way in which epidemics played out in communities. Changes in the way families congregated on the land as they managed different plant and animal resources during the seasonal round, for instance, altered the extent to which people came in contact with each other. During winter epidemics, fur-trapping communities were dispersed on the land in relatively small family trapping groups, and only in occasional contact with the posts, which were often the sources of epidemics. Families unlucky enough to be exposed to a virulent pathogen while visiting the post were likely to have been hard hit and, in some instances, wiped out during winter outbreaks (Herring and Sattenspiel 2003; Sattenspiel 2003).

Nine of the outbreaks identified by Ray (1976) in the HBC post journals struck two or more districts, spreading outward from trading centres. Both Norway House and York Factory experienced more epidemics than other less central posts, and the Norway House District endured ten different epidemics, making it the most unhealthy of all. Since the HBC boat brigades were primarily responsible for the transmission of both cargo and disease from one district to another, the vulnerability of the Norway House District is not startling. In view of its key position in the fur-trade network and frequent contact with locations to the west, northwest, northeast, and south (Fort Garry), it was exposed to pathogens from a wide geographical area (Ray 1976:156–7). Even as recently as the 1918–19 influenza pandemic, Norway House continued to be a central source of infection and point of diffusion for infectious disease in the region (Herring 1994).

But boat brigades and trade routes were not the only means by which diseases spread. In the case of the 1780–2 smallpox epidemic, information gleaned from post journals and scrutinized from the perspective of epidemiologic principles led Decker (1988:18–24) to conclude that Indians, travelling overland or by river from their camps for the purpose of trade or to obtain aid, brought the dreaded 'red death' to York Factory and Cumberland House. Through a variety of means, therefore, diseases moved with people from near populations to more distant peripheral populations, expanding disease frontiers in the process (F.P. Hackett 2002:9).

Building on Ray's work, Decker (1989) studied a series of epidemics that struck the northern plains between 1774 and 1839, tracing the pattern of transmission and calculating mortality rates for each. How devastating was this series of smallpox, measles, influenza, and whooping cough epidemics, and did they depopulate the people of the northern plains?

Before addressing this question, it is essential to recognize that all epidemics do not necessarily result in depopulation. Epidemics are outbreaks of disease that produce excessive morbidity or mortality compared to the norm for that population and are typically sporadic and short term. They are generally followed by a return to pre-epidemic mortality levels and age structure. Populations experiencing depopulating epidemics continue to be susceptible to the infectious disease and experience recurrent bouts of it, along with high mortality in selective age categories. Under these circumstances, the age structure of the population is fundamentally changed through the experience of recurrent epidemics, and this, in turn, may affect the population's ability to reproduce itself (Palkovich 1981:71). It is worth recalling, too, that endemic diseases, such as malaria in the southern portions of the Northwest Coast, can also fuel the depopulation process.

Bearing these differences in mind, it appears that of the four epidemics, only smallpox fulfilled the criteria for a depopulating epidemic in the northern plains. Smallpox is also distinctive because of its enhanced capacity to spread, relative to other diseases. Its ability to survive in a dried state on corpses and inanimate objects for long periods of time, and its long period of infectivity, lasting from the onset of its typical rash to the peeling of the last scars, allowed it to move explosively and inexorably over long distances.

The smallpox epidemic of 1781–2 was the first severe epidemic recorded in the Subarctic. Decker (1989:221) speculates that the depopulation of the region observed between 1774 and 1839 resulted from depletion of the adult cohort during the 1781–2 smallpox epidemic, which reduced the number of marriages and births in the subsequent generation. It appears that all the Plains groups recovered from the devastation nonetheless and that a demographic turning point was reached around 1820. Significantly, 'no group experienced a continual steady decline in population, despite the fact that nine major epidemics swept through the Plains within two generations' (Decker 1989:220). The demographic resurgence of the Plains Cree was aided in the 1830s by the absorption of entire extended families of Woodland Cree, who migrated to the plains in the wake of disease and resource depletion (ibid. 225). As McGrath (1991:418–19) emphasizes, social responses are instrumental in determining an epidemic's course and impact. Evidently, a complex configuration of social, ecological, and disease features were influencing the decline and subsequent recovery of northern Plains people at this time.

WIDENING DISEASE POOLS AND ENVIRONMENTAL DEPLETION

The expansion of disease pools within the Americas, which began in the seventeenth century in northeastern North America, intensified throughout the centuries. Whereas epidemics in the seventeenth and eighteenth centuries were essentially separate events, fuelled by pathogens arriving by ship from external sources in Europe, Africa, or the West Indies, regional disease systems eventually emerged in which epidemics flowed overland back and forth between the American, British, and French colonies (F.P. Hackett 2002:28–31). In other words, crowd diseases were able to continue circulating after they normally would have died out, to be carried to the interior and farther west by missionaries, traders, soldiers, and Aboriginal people who visited eastern settlements such as Montreal and Quebec City for the purposes of trade or political negotiations.

The growth of urban disease pools from the late seventeenth to the eighteenth centuries capacitated the spread and lengthened the reach of epidemics. F.P. Hackett (1991), for instance, links the 1819–20 measles epidemic in the Canadian Northwest to the establishment of an endemic measles focus in the urban centres of Baltimore, Philadelphia, and New York in the northeastern United States. By 1818, the combined populations of these three cities had surpassed the critical size necessary to maintain a constant supply of new susceptibles (F. Black 1966), and measles was carried westward from the Atlantic coast by small groups travelling along major transportation routes, through the upper Great Lakes, along the north shore of Lake Superior, and on into the Northwest. As Dobyns (1983) has emphasized, previously isolated Aboriginal groups were sometimes affected by outbreaks in distant locations, even in the absence of direct contact.

It appears that the first quarter of the nineteenth century constitutes a watershed in the disease history of the Northwest, after which epidemics other than smallpox began to strike Aboriginal peoples with greater frequency (Decker 1989; F.P. Hackett 1991, 2002). This widening of the infectious disease spectrum was closely connected to the westward expansion of the American frontier and to improvements in transportation efficiency. Together, these two developments opened up the Northwest to diseases characterized by shorter periods of infectivity and lower diffusion potential than smallpox, such as measles, influenza, and scarlet fever (F.P. Hackett 1991:140). Influenza, for instance, became the most frequent epidemic disease in the Petit Nord by 1830 (F.P. Hackett 2002:241).

At the same time, large and small game alike were being depleted in the Northwest, and declining fur harvests prompted the HBC to close many trading posts during the course of the nineteenth century. The important relationship between diet and disease is well known. Malnutrition and undernutrition can occur for many reasons, but whatever the cause, they increase susceptibility to infectious disease.[11] Places like Norway House were basically 'trapped out' by the mid-nineteenth century, making it necessary to travel long distances, as much as 300 miles, to hunt furs. Reports of scarcity and hunger in the HBC post journals are also quite frequent, but it is difficult to interpret their meaning or to connect them specifically to outbreaks of disease because 'starvation' has connotations beyond its literal definition (Black-Rogers 1986). In any event, the combined effects of the depletion of local resources, periodic hunger, and the introduction of more exogenous acute community infections at greater frequency must have increased the susceptibility to disease of Aboriginal people in the north and exacted a high toll of morbidity, if not mortality.

EPIDEMICS AND RESERVES

By the twentieth century, disease ecologies and epidemiological patterns that characterized the nineteenth century were in a process of transformation in many regions, as the transition from infectious to chronic diseases began to emerge (Young 1988a). At Moose Factory and in the Moose River region, for instance, epidemics of acute community infections typical of the nineteenth century, such as whooping cough, measles, and influenza, still occurred but with lower frequency and at longer intervals (Herring and Hoppa 1997). Crowded housing on reserves, the growing concentration of children in residential schools, and the virtual transformation of all aspects of social life attendant with the change 'from a portable home within an ecological range, to housing in sedentary settlements' (Preston 1986:245) meant that, among other transitions, twentieth-century mortality was no longer tightly tied to the seasons (Herring and Hoppa 1997). In places like Moose Factory, moreover, there was a reduction in life expectancy in the first half of the century that 'coincided with increased involvement of the Canadian Government in Aboriginal life, new development projects and increased penetration of non-natives into the northern economy' (Herring, Abonyi, and Hoppa 2003:306). The growing plague of tuberculosis contributed to this phenomenon.[12]

By the twentieth century, tuberculosis had become a major health problem both as a specific cause of death and as an underlying condition that reduced resistance to other infectious diseases (Stone 1926). The growing tuberculosis problem resulted in a tuberculosis death rate among Indians in the western provinces that was ten to twenty times higher than that for non-Aboriginal people (D.A. Stewart 1936:675). The prevalence of acute forms of the disease, the wide range of expressions of it, and extraordinarily high rates relative to other groups led some observers to conclude that North American Indians had a special susceptibility to tuberculosis because they lacked 'racial immunity' (McCarthy 1912:207). Some feared the complete extinction of Aboriginal North Americans (Hrdlicka 1908). As we shall see in chapter 7, the 'disappearing Indian' discourse became a powerful theme among medical and other authorities writing in the early twentieth century.[13]

Other scholars noted that the idea of unusual genetic susceptibility was simply an assumption rather than an established scientific fact (Wherrett 1965). It is now generally accepted that ethnic differences in susceptibility to tuberculosis can be explained in terms of how long and under what circumstances the population has experienced the epidemic, and the extent to which herd immunity has been acquired through experience with it (J. Bates 1982). A community's experience of a tuberculosis epidemic is intimately tied to local sanitary conditions. Deteriorating living conditions or the development of an environment conducive to the spread of tubercle bacilli can propel low, endemic rates into a full-blown epidemic. R. Ferguson's (1928) work in the Qu'Appelle Valley of Saskatchewan from the 1880s onward emphasized the importance of radical social, spiritual, and ecological disruptions that underlay the rising tuberculosis mortality rates. He asserts (1955:6) that tuberculosis became a serious problem among western Native populations only after they were settled on reserves. Relocation of Aboriginal people to reserves with minimal resources, where people lived in crowded houses, and where children were concentrated in boarding schools, essentially guaranteed their complete and rapid tuberculinization.

As Walker noted in 1909 (cited in Bryce 1909:282), increasing tuberculosis mortality on Canadian reserves in the early twentieth century was emblematic of 'the whole story of the passing of the Indian from the nomadic to the settled habits of life.' We would argue that this is simply another way of saying that the reserve system fuelled the epidemic. In turn, tuberculosis became a key element in the development of syndemic conditions at many reserves. A syndemic is 'a set of interactive and mutually enhancing epidemics involving disease interactions at the biological level that develop and are sustained in a community/population because of harmful social conditions and injurious social connections' (Singer and Clair 2003: 429). Basically, a syndemic refers to two or more epidemics that interact synergistically, thereby enhancing the biological effects that each has on the community and increasing a community's disease burden. Tuberculosis, for example, opens up already compromised immune systems and debilitated lungs to other respiratory infections, such as influenza. It may have played a key role in the long-term impact of the 1918 influenza pandemic (Noymer and Garenne 2003). Other respiratory infections, in turn, make existing tubercular disease worse.

By the mid-twentieth century, many reserves were impoverished. York Factory, erstwhile centre of the North American fur trade, essentially had been abandoned by the 1950s because the lack of a sustainable economy had prompted the Aboriginal population to migrate south to more prosperous locations. Medical parties in the 1930s and 1940s found worrying levels of malnutrition in many parts of the Canadian north (Honigmann 1948; Tisdall and Robertson 1948), including York Factory, as environmental degradation and increased competition for natural resources took a heavy toll (Beardy and Coutts 1996:xxi). Tuberculosis rates were propelled upward by these conditions and, in turn, exacerbated the effects of other outbreaks. Here we see how intertwined epidemics became the biological expression and emblem of declining social conditions on reserves in the twentieth century.

CONCLUSIONS

Infectious diseases, especially acute community infections introduced from Europe, struck Aboriginal communities in Canada from the time of contact, adding to the infectious disease load already present before contact. The opportunities for the transmission of diseases of European derivation varied extensively, as did the effects they had on each community, and both of these were conditioned by the time of contact (early vs late). Over and above the distinctive features of the pathogens themselves (which include the severity of symptoms, ease of transmission, and capacity to induce immunity), the social circumstances surrounding the encounter with pathogens are of paramount importance. Similarly, the mix of pathogens and the order in which they struck varied substantially. No single depopulation model can explain all cases; the social history of each Aboriginal community must be evaluated to determine the extent to which infectious disease debilitated and depleted it.

Aboriginal communities in closer and more intense contact with European settlements were at greater risk of contracting introduced diseases than more peripheral communities, or than those that chose not to become entangled in social and economic relationships with European groups. The Beothuk case shows, however, that strategies of avoidance brought their own survival risks, especially when there was no viable hinterland to which to escape.

As the larger sociodemographic and political fabric of the North American continent changed during the post-contact period, and as diseases common to urban centres increasingly expanded into the periphery, the capacity for diseases to afflict Aboriginal communities was enhanced. Late-contact regions, such as the Northwest Coast, encountered a wider range of pathogens from many more sources than was the case for the early-contact Beothuk. In light of the poor quality of most early population estimates in Canada, it is difficult to evaluate the demographic consequences of these differing epidemiologic transformations. Ewers (1973:104) observed thirty years ago that 'the long range effects of successive epidemics on the populations of particular tribes have not been sufficiently studied.' It is also unlikely that scholars will be able to determine with any degree of precision or certainty the extent to which Aboriginal populations in Canada (or elsewhere) declined, or to specify the impact made by infectious diseases in this process, in isolation from the social and economic circumstances that allowed the diseases to thrive.

The inescapable conclusion, however, is that across the continent, regional and local developments all contributed to the increasing ease of spread of infectious diseases, indigenous and introduced to Aboriginal communities in Canada. The growth of North American cities in the nineteenth century through immigration and natural increase created population densities necessary to support acute community infections in endemic form. Increasingly extensive and numerous trade and transportation routes opened up previously isolated parts of the country to the movement of pathogens, old and new. The escalating speed of travel made possible by the invention of the steam engine allowed infectious diseases with short incubation periods, such as influenza, to diffuse more widely along waterways, and later via road and railway routes. Poor living conditions on reserves, coupled with the marginalization of Aboriginal people from political and economic power, ensured that chronic infections, such as tuberculosis, took hold and contributed to syndemic conditions.

By the twentieth century, the infectious disease load in many Aboriginal communities was high. It is against this backdrop of persistently high infection rates that yet another epidemiological profile began to emerge, the subject of the next chapter.

4

Aboriginal peoples and the health transition

In the last two chapters we have had a glimpse of the likely circumstances surrounding the health of Aboriginal people in Canada from before the arrival of Europeans. While an idealized, disease-free paradise was unlikely ever to have existed, there is sufficient documentary evidence to suggest that a series of epidemics and famines of varying extent, severity, and duration affected different regions at different times subsequent to contact. We have also seen that a major epidemic disease – tuberculosis – remained largely out of control well into the middle of the twentieth century.

In this chapter, we review the pattern of health and disease of Aboriginal people from the end of the Second World War to the early twenty-first century. During this period most infectious diseases were increasingly brought under control, but they are by no means eradicated. Many infectious diseases remain at a persistently higher level than for the rest of the Canadian population, especially in some pockets across the country, and fresh epidemic outbreaks, albeit of short duration and geographically localized, continue to occur. New emergent infections, such as HIV and AIDS, pose threats to Aboriginal communities as well as to the Canadian population at large. Concurrently, there has been a shift to the so-called chronic, non-communicable diseases such as heart disease, diabetes, hypertension, and obesity, which have become major health problems. An even more alarming trend is the new epidemic of injuries – both intentional and unintentional – including suicide, violence, and traffic accidents.

The shift from infectious to chronic diseases has been experienced by most populations at different times of their history. It is referred to as the 'epidemiologic transition' or 'health transition,' referring to long-term temporal changes in the pattern of health and disease in populations (T.K. Young 1988a). Aboriginal people within developed countries began the transition much later than the rest of the population, but as we shall see in this chapter, they have overtaken them in certain respects.

A CONVERGING PERSPECTIVE ON HEALTH

Since the first edition of this book, the 'determinants of health model' has been embraced by health researchers in a number of disciplines. It provides a useful framework for understanding the impact especially of current social and economic conditions on Aboriginal health (e.g., Wilson and Rosenberg 2002). Although the number and classification of health determinants vary according to the authors, they usually can be grouped into genetic susceptibility; the physical environment; personal lifestyles and behaviours; and social, economic, and cultural factors. Such determinants interact with one another and are interrelated in a complex causal web, and they influence health status throughout the life course from the perinatal period to senescence (T.K. Young 2005). We have touched on several of these throughout the book already.

Interestingly, in recent years there has been a convergence in thinking on the concept of health between Western-trained biomedical scientists and Aboriginal health specialists. What is usually referred to as a 'holistic' framework in many Aboriginal health programs is similar in many ways to the health determinants model. The general model of the 'Medicine Wheel,' found today throughout many different parts of Aboriginal Canada, has been developed to explain health determinants in a manner that reflects Aboriginal world views. While specific Medicine Wheel models vary from place to place, they commonly consist of four quadrants representing the four directions, which in the health context can be used to indicate different dimensions of health, such as the physical, mental, emotional, and spiritual.

This general framework has been applied to specific communities in a manner that renders it particularly compatible with local cultural exigencies. Figure 5 depicts one such model, in both Cree-Ojibwa syllabics and English, which was adopted by the Sioux Lookout First Nations Health Authority in the mid-1990s to guide its regional planning activities. We believe that the convergence between contemporary biomedical and Aboriginal models of health represents a positive step towards better research and programming.

Figure 5. Holistic model of health adopted by the Sioux Lookout First Nations
Health Authority

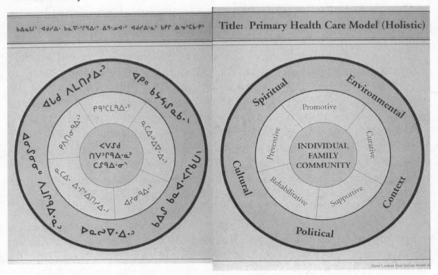

Source: Pamphlet produced by Sioux Lookout First Nations Health Authority, circa 1995

MEASURING THE HEALTH OF ABORIGINAL PEOPLES

The preceding chapters indicate the difficulty in reconstructing the state
of health of Aboriginal people before contact and in the early years after
contact. With the expansion of health care services to Aboriginal communities across the country since the beginning of the twentieth century, the
quantity and quality of health data have improved, especially since the
1950s. Even so, many important gaps and deficiencies still exist today.
Furthermore, not all groups of Aboriginal people are equally well represented in surveys and studies. In general, First Nations people, particularly those residing on reserves, and Inuit in the northern territories, are
best documented. The least is known about non-status Indians and Métis,
particularly those residing in urban areas (T.K. Young 2003). In 1991 the
Native Council of Canada, the national organization of non-status Indians, decried the lack of health data relating to this group of Aboriginal
people, a lack that rendered invisible their serious health problems, particularly among those residing off reserve and in urban areas. The council

saw a clear link between the lack of health information and the lack of policy and cultural sensitivity on the part of governments (Wigmore and McCue 1991). Since then the situation has improved, with the availability of large national surveys that include off-reserve and urban Aboriginal people (see below).

Among the health indicators, life expectancy, which is based entirely on the mortality experience of the population, is frequently used in international comparisons. Substantial gains have been recorded in the Aboriginal population of Canada. The life expectancy at birth of the Inuit in the Northwest Territories more than doubled between 1941–50 and 1978–82, when it reached sixty-six years (Robitaille and Choinière 1985). In 1999–2001, Nunavut reported an average of sixty-nine years (Nunavut Department of Health and Social Services 2004). The steady increase among First Nations and the narrowing of the gap with Canadians nationally between 1960 and 2000 is shown in figure 6. In 2000 the life expectancy at birth of First Nations men was seven years shorter than for Canadians nationally; the deficit was five years among women.

The major contribution to the reduced life expectancy at birth among Aboriginal people has been their higher infant mortality rate. Substantial gains have also been made in the post-Second World War years (figure 7). By the first decade of the twenty-first century, the First Nations rate (6.4/1,000 live births) has almost converged with the Canadian national rate (5.4/1,000 live births) (Health Canada 2003c). The decline has been steepest among the Inuit, although their infant mortality rate still remains higher than the First Nations rate and is about three times the Canadian national rate (Nunavut Department of Health and Social Services 2004).

Figure 8 shows how First Nations and Inuit, if they were separate countries, would rank among all the countries in the world in terms of the infant mortality rate. While the comment that the Canadian Aboriginal population constitutes a 'Third World in our backyard' is frequently made, this is no longer true, at least when infant mortality rate is used as an indicator. The Inuit rate would put it alongside some eastern-European countries and the more developed Asian and Latin American countries.

There have been many studies on the causes of mortality and morbidity, regionally and nationally (Mao et al. 1986, 1992). In general, Aboriginal people suffer from an excess of injuries and most categories of health problems, with the exception of cancer (figure 9). Since the 1950s, while the overall mortality from all causes has shown a steady

Figure 6. Life expectancy at birth among First Nations and all Canadians, 1960–2000

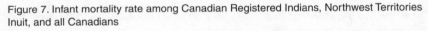

Sources: Norris 1990; DIAND 2002, *Basic Departmental Data*

Figure 7. Infant mortality rate among Canadian Registered Indians, Northwest Territories Inuit, and all Canadians

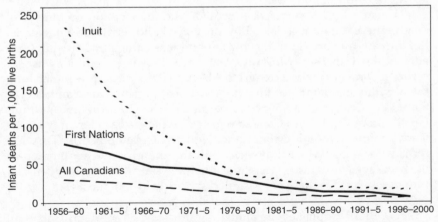

Sources: Updated from first edition with data from Health Canada, Indian and Northern Affairs Canada, Statistics Canada, and Nunavut Department of Health and Social Services
Note: Inuit data refer to Northwest Territories Inuit prior to 1990 and the total population of Nunavut after 1995.

Figure 8. International comparison of infant mortality rates

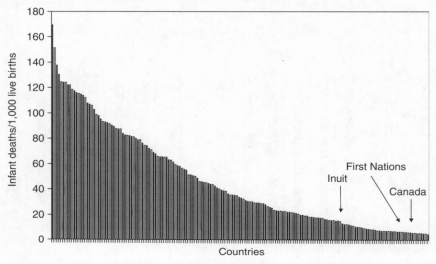

Source: Data from *World Health Report* (WHO 2000)

decline, the relative importance of chronic diseases and injuries has grown (figure 10).

In Canada, death certificates provide the information on causes of death. These data are collected by provincial and territorial vital statistics bureaus and are centrally collated and maintained by Statistics Canada as the Canadian Mortality Database. However, ethnicity is not recorded, and attributing deaths to Aboriginal people requires matching them with some listing of known Aboriginal persons, for example, the Status Verification System (SVS) operated by the First Nations and Inuit Health Branch of Health Canada (FNIHB), which is based mainly on the Department of Indian Affairs and Nothern Development's (DIAND) Indian Register. (When done electronically the procedure is known as data linkage.) It is also possible to identify deaths among residents of Indian reserves, as these are assigned specific codes in most (but not all) provinces.

The FNIHB publishes an annual health status report on Canadian First Nations, based on reports submitted by the regions. There is tremendous variation in terms of the source of the data, the extent of coverage, and the ability to distinguish on- and off-reserve residence status.

Figure 9. Ratio of age-standardized mortality rates by selected causes, First Nations versus Canada, 1999–2000

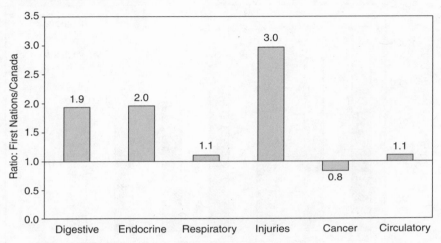

Source: FNIHB, Health Information and Analysis Division, 2004
Note: Ratios >1.0 indicate an excess risk of mortality among First Nations; ratios <1.0 indicate a lower risk among First Nations, relative to the Canadian national population

Regions in western Canada rely on data transmitted from the provincial vital statistics agencies and include all First Nations members, both on and off reserve. Other regions (Atlantic, Quebec, and Ontario) collate reports collected by nursing stations and health centres and cover only First Nations clients living in reserves served by FNIHB.

In order to compute the rates of various health events, an accurate count of the size of the Aboriginal population is critical. For First Nations, there are two sources of population data: the Indian Register operated by DIAND and the census conducted by Statistics Canada. The census, since it is based on self-report of ethnic origin, is the only source of information on non-status Indians, Métis, and Inuit. There are problems associated with both of these sources. Late reporting of births and deaths to the Indian Register has been documented. Non-cooperation of a large number of First Nations with Statistics Canada since the 1980s has resulted in incomplete enumeration. In 1981, only 6 bands were not enumerated. In 1986, 136 bands with an estimated 45,000 residents were incompletely enumerated. In 1991, the number of bands not participating in the census declined to 78, representing approximately 38,000

Figure 10. Change in crude mortality rate by cause, First Nations, 1950–2000

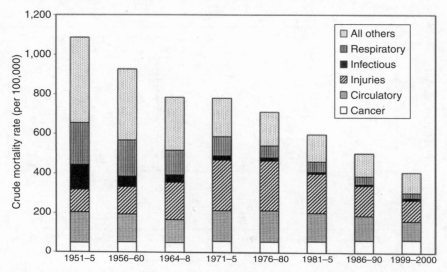

Sources: Updated from first edition; 1999–2000 data from FNIHB, Health Information and Analysis Division 2004. Data are not available for all years.

Aboriginal persons. This number remained relatively stable for successive censuses. Viewed nationally, this number accounted for less than 5 per cent of the total Aboriginal population. However, for specific regions or cultural and linguistic groups (e.g., Iroquoian speakers in Ontario and Quebec), the proportion of the undercount would be considerably higher.

Because the census's determination of ethnic status is based on self-identification, it can be influenced by the respondents' social experience and cultural ties. Failure to identify with any of the Aboriginal categories, particularly for non-status Indians and Métis, will significantly affect the population count of those with Aboriginal ancestry. On the other hand, heightened cultural pride and perceived benefits (e.g., entitlements to government services, land claims settlements) may increase the number of self-identified Aboriginal Canadians.

Data collection and processing procedures may not be comparable from census to census – for example, those relating to the number and labelling of Aboriginal categories, the reporting of multiple origins/

Figure 11. Impact of Bill C-31 on First Nations population

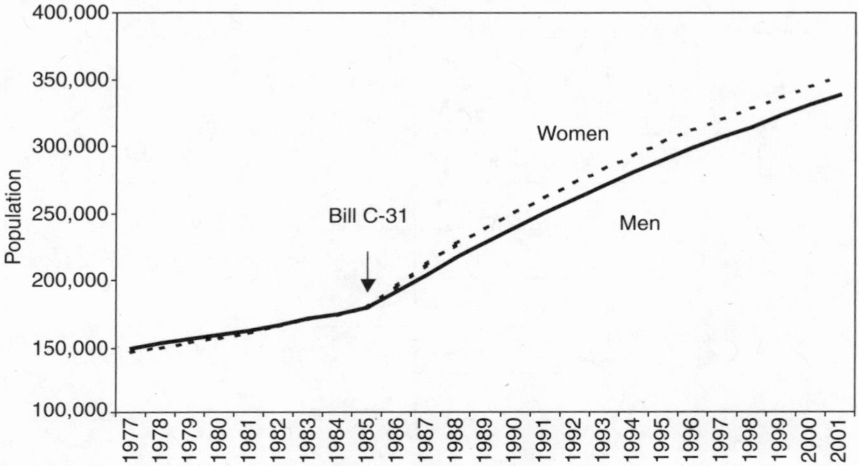

Source: DIAND 2002, Basic Departmental Data

mixed heritage, the inclusion of reserve residence and legal status in the definition of Indian status, and differences between information obtained by self-enumeration (since 1971) and by enumerators. (For a historical review of ethnic origin data in Canadian censuses from 1871 to 1986, see Kralt [1990].)

The passage of Bill C-31, An Act to Amend the Indian Act, in 1985, which restored Indian status and band membership rights to a large number of Indians (particularly women), has had a significant impact on the First Nations population. By 1990 the registered First Nations population was estimated to have increased by 19 per cent over and above population growth due to natural increase (DIAND 1990). Because the law affected mainly women, the population increase among First Nations women has outstripped that of men (figure 11).

The age-sex structure of the Aboriginal population differs substantially from that of Canadians nationally, and resembles that of many developing countries today, and that of Canada over 100 years ago (figure 12). In the 2001 census, only 19 per cent of Canadians were aged under fifteen years, compared to 39 per cent of Inuit, 35 per cent of First Nations, and 29 per cent of the Métis population. The proportion of the elderly, those aged sixty-five and above, accounted for 12 per cent of the

Figure 12. Age-sex pyramid of Canadian population, 2001 census

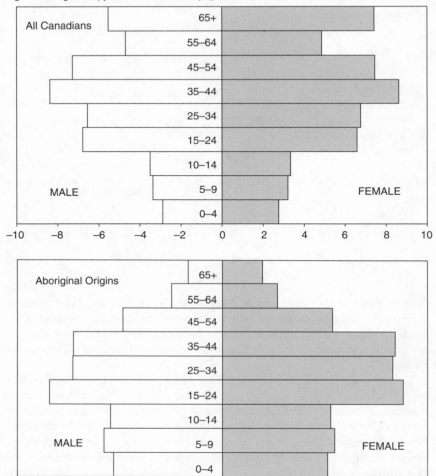

Source: Statistics Canada 2003

Canadian population, but only 3 per cent of the Inuit and 4 per cent of the First Nations and Métis populations. The wider, though constricted, base composed of those under fifteen years of age reflects fertility decline since the 1980s and earlier.

The pattern of mortality provides only a partial picture of the health status of a population. Most diseases, after all, do not result in death. The existence of universal health insurance in all Canadian provinces and territories, all of which maintain databases of all hospital and physician care utilization, can potentially provide a source of data on morbidity. However, ethnic identification is not available, although special identifiers of status First Nations people are provided in the western provinces. Where such data are available, higher hospital admission rates tend to be evident among the First Nations population compared to the total provincial population, and the morbidity pattern for different disease categories parallels the pattern for mortality. It should be cautioned that health service utilization data do not reflect entirely the burden of illness in a population. Many other factors, particularly those relating to access to health care facilities and the practice styles of health care providers may account for differential use.

The only way to 'capture' information on health conditions that do not result in any kind of formal contact with the health care system is to ask people directly about them. Health surveys solicit the participants' subjective judgment of their health and/or recall of past health events. They provide an opportunity to inquire about health behaviours, practices, attitudes, and beliefs. Health surveys are therefore important sources of data on the prevalence of diseases and their risk factors. One should, of course, recognize the limitations of surveys that are based on self-reports, which are subject to many sources of error.

While there have been many large, national health surveys since the 1970s, most have specifically excluded the northern territories and reserves. A rare exception is the Nutrition Canada Survey, conducted during 1970–2, which had a separate Indian sample selected from twenty-nine bands across the country (n = 1,808) and an Inuit sample from four communities in the Northwest Territories (n = 346). This survey provides a wealth of health and nutritional data collected through interviews, physical measurements, and laboratory tests. The Health and Activity Limitation Survey of 1986, which provides a national perspective on the prevalence of disabilities, did sample the Northwest Territories and Indian reserves. While Canada's Health Promotion Survey of 1985 also excluded reserves, it did include the two northern territories.

It is possible for off-reserve Aboriginal people to be sampled in national health surveys. Beginning in the mid-1990s, the series of National Population Health Surveys (NPHS) and Canadian Community Health Surveys (CCHS) included questions on both 'ethnicity' (with categories for 'North American Indians,' 'Métis,' and 'Inuit') and 'race' (with a category for 'Aboriginal peoples of North America') based on self-identification. The NPHS of 1994–5, for example, includes 28 Inuit, 855 Métis, and 1,821 Indians. The CCHS of 2000–1 includes 4,216 Indians, 1,497 Métis, and 827 Inuit, which add up to more than the 3,898 individuals who categorized themselves as 'Aboriginal' in response to the 'race' question. Tjepkema (2002) analysed the health status and common chronic conditions of Aboriginal respondents to the CCHS.

The Aboriginal Peoples Survey (APS) conducted in 1991 rectified some of the deficiencies in survey data on a national scale. As a 'post-censal' survey, it was conducted by Statistics Canada shortly after the 1991 census and made use of census data in selecting its sample. The target population of the APS comprises all individuals who reported Aboriginal origins and/or reported being a registered Indian under the Indian Act in the 1991 census. It should be noted that the seventy-eight Indian reserves/settlements (estimated to comprise 38,000 individuals) that did not take part in the 1991 census were therefore not included in the APS. Further attrition occurred, with an additional 181 Indian reserves (representing 20,000 individuals) and 14 other Aboriginal communities (2,000 inhabitants) refusing to take part in the APS (Statistics Canada 1993a).

In 2001, Statistics Canada conducted another Aboriginal Peoples Survey (APS-2), which included 123 First Nations communities, 53 Inuit communities, 8 Métis settlements, 35 communities with high Aboriginal population, and 9 urban areas. The First Nations participation was especially poor, with less than 15 per cent of communities that participated in the 2001 census also participating in APS-2, representing 44 per cent of the self-identified Aboriginal population. Note that the census itself also did not achieve full enumeration, with some 30 reserves 'incompletely enumerated.' Statistics Canada cautioned against generalizing the on-reserve data in APS-2 to the on-reserve population nationally. Some data relating to the non-reserve population have been released (Statistics Canada 2003).

The First Nations and Inuit Regional Health Survey (FNIRHS) is a First Nations- and Inuit-controlled health interview survey conducted during 1997 in nine regions (B.C., Alberta, Saskatchewan, Manitoba, Ontario, Quebec, Nova Scotia, New Brunswick, and Labrador). While each region designed its own survey questions, a set of national core questions was included in each regional survey. The total sample nationally was 9,870 respondents. Various regional reports have been published (e.g., MacMillan et al. 2003 from Ontario) as well as a national report with chapters devoted to specific topics (NAHO 2004a).

A second wave of the FNIRHS was coordinated by the National Aboriginal Health Organization (NAHO) in 2002–3. FNIRHS-2 consists of three national surveys (adults 18+, adolescents 12–17 years, and children 0–11 years), using computer-assisted survey techniques. These national surveys address a comprehensive range of health status, health care, and health determinants measures. In addition, there are also regional modules with varying size and contents. Some preliminary data on First Nations adults (n = 10,888) were released in September 2004 (NAHO 2004b).

For many specific diseases and health conditions, special disease registers and surveys, usually covering a particular community or region, have been conducted over the years. In the rest of the chapter, some of these studies will be reviewed. Since most health problems tend to be studied only once in one location, a historical narrative is rarely possible. It should be noted that 'infectious' is used here to refer to a disease caused by micro-organisms such as bacteria or viruses. Not all infectious diseases are 'contagious' in the non-technical sense of the word, meaning easily passed from person to person. Chronic diseases represent a mixed group of diseases usually characterized by slow, insidious onset and are not caused by micro-organisms.[1] The term 'injuries' has, by and large, replaced 'accidents' in the prevention literature to highlight the health impact on the person and the existence of preventable factors in their causation.

THE DECLINE AND PERSISTENCE OF INFECTIOUS DISEASES

The success of immunization programs has reduced the epidemiological significance of diseases such as measles, rubella, mumps, poliomyelitis, tetanus, and diphtheria in Aboriginal communities. As late as the 1950s, virgin-soil epidemics of these diseases still occurred in some areas in the Arctic – for example, in the Yukon during the construction of the Alaska Highway by the U.S. Military during the Second World War (Marchand 1943). In Chesterfield Inlet, Northwest Territories, 8 per cent of the Inuit population contracted polio from non-Aboriginal workers stationed in Churchill, Manitoba, and 2 per cent of the population died (Adamson et al. 1949). In 1952, a measles epidemic swept through Baffin Island, Northwest Territories, and the Ungava peninsula in northern Quebec, afflicting 99 per cent of the population, between 2 per cent and 7 per cent of whom

Figure 13. Trend in incidence of tuberculosis among Canadian Inuit, First Nations, and all Canadians

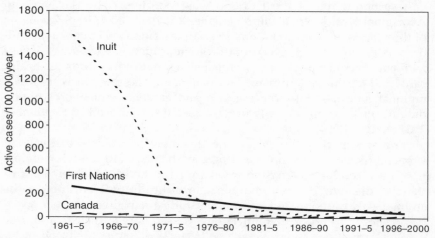

Sources: Updated from first edition; data since 1990 from *Tuberculosis in Canada 2002* (Public Health Agency of Canada 2004b)

died. This epidemic was traced to Inuit visitors to the Armed Forces base at Goose Bay, Labrador (Peart and Nagler 1954).

Tuberculosis (TB)

The availability of effective anti-tuberculosis therapy and the large-scale control efforts of the 1950s resulted in a steep decline in tuberculosis mortality. Despite such improvements, however, the disparity between Aboriginal people and Canadians nationally remains great. Figure 13 shows the decline in the incidence of new cases among Canadian First Nations, Inuit, and the national population from 1961 to 2000. If the Canadian national rate is further disaggregated into the Canadian-born and the foreign-born, the disparity between the Aboriginal and the non-Aboriginal Canadian-born rate is even greater. The average incidence for 1997 to 2001 for the non-Aboriginal Canadian-born is 1.4/100,000/year; by comparison the non-Aboriginal, foreign-born rate is 21/100,000/year; while those of First Nations and Inuit are substantially higher, at 37 and 62/100,000/year, respectively (Public Health Agency of Canada 2004b).

Tuberculosis is potentially a completely treatable disease, and a variety of efficacious drugs are available. The emergence of strains of *Mycobacteria* that are resistant to currently available anti-tuberculosis drugs in some populations, particularly among transient, homeless people, is cause for concern. The former practice of prolonged hospital treatment, often at centres far removed from the home community, imposed severe personal hardship and family disruption among Aboriginal patients and has been generally superseded since the 1970s by shorter courses of intermittent and supervised therapy. A key informant survey in thirty-one Indian reserves in British Columbia revealed a widespread belief that tuberculosis was a disease of the past and little knowledge of recent improvements in treatment. There was also substantial resentment towards, and mistrust of, non-Aboriginal health professionals (Jenkins 1977). Successful therapy requires not only individual responsibility but also the existence of a continuing source of care, as well as commitment and sensitivity among the health care staff providing the treatment.

In terms of prevention, Aboriginal people are one of the few groups in Canada that receive the BCG (Bacille-Calmette-Guérin) vaccine at birth. One of the early field trials of this vaccine, conducted among Indian infants in Saskatchewan during the 1930s, found it to be highly protective, in the 80 per cent range (Ferguson and Sime 1949). In the 1980s, studies conducted among First Nations in Manitoba (Young and Hershfield 1986) and Alberta (Houston et al. 1990) still showed that the vaccine had a protective effect of at least 60 per cent. Mass prophylaxis with the drug isoniazid (or INH) was also tested among the Inuit in various circumpolar regions, including Frobisher Bay, Northwest Territories (Dorken et al. 1984). A study from British Columbia indicated that directly observed preventive therapy (DOPT) resulted in a higher compliance at six and twelve months than the traditional self-administered delivery method (Heal et al. 1998). An investigation of an outbreak among the Mistassini Cree in Quebec during the early 1990s showed that the disease occurred even among individuals who had previously received some – but incomplete – isoniazid prophylaxis. The decline in compliance with the year-long course of preventive treatment was associated with a shift of responsibility from indigenous Community Health Representatives (CHRs) to the better qualified, but non-indigenous, nurses (Rideout and Menzies 1994).

These studies are examples of situations where the high burden of illness among Aboriginal communities has led to their being selected as sites for intervention trials. The results of such studies have broader national and international implications and applications beyond the individual communities where they originally took place.

Gastro-enteritis

Other infectious diseases that strike particularly hard at Aboriginal communities include pneumonia, meningitis, and gastro-enteritis. In 1991, a large outbreak of gastro-enteritis occurred in the Keewatin region of the Northwest Territories. It was traced to food contaminated by the toxin-producing micro-organism *Escherichia coli* 0157:H7. Reputedly the largest such outbreak ever reported, there were 521 cases during the six–month course of the epidemic, among which twenty-two people developed and two people died from the serious complication called haemolytic uremic syndrome, which may lead to kidney failure (Rowe et al. 1998; Ogborn et al. 1998).

While in the long term the improvement of community infrastructure such as water supply and sanitation will reduce or eliminate the health impact of diarrhoeal diseases, individual-based efforts directed at encouraging breastfeeding can be effective. The protective effect of breastfeeding against diarrhoeal disease has been demonstrated among Indian infants in northern Manitoba (Ellestad-Sayed et al. 1979), likely the result of the transfer of protective antibodies from the mother to the infant in breast milk. In communities without access to clean water, breastfeeding avoids the use of contaminated water in the preparation of infant formula.

Acquired Immunodeficiency Syndrome (AIDS)

Although solid statistical data on a provincial or national basis are lacking, sexually transmitted diseases such as gonorrhoea and chlamydia are important health problems in Aboriginal communities. In urban areas, the situation is likely to be far more serious, because of the social circumstances associated with city living, including the sex trade and drug abuse.

The new epidemic of acquired immunodeficiency syndrome (AIDS) had by mid-2003 resulted in about 19,000 reported cases in Canada. Of these, 3 per cent were of Aboriginal origin, according to data available from the Public Health Agency of Canada (2004a), roughly corresponding to their share of the Canadian population. Despite the relatively small number of Aboriginal AIDS cases, the potentially explosive situation has

been recognized by Aboriginal political leaders, health care professionals, and the federal government. The number of Aboriginal cases may
indeed be misleadingly low, as reporting of ethnic identity is available for
only about 85 per cent of AIDS cases. Furthermore, the situation has deteriorated: the proportion of Aboriginal cases among all cases in Canada
was 1.3 per cent prior to 1991, and steadily increased, reaching a high of
13 per cent in 2002, among cases for whom ethnicity was known. Aboriginal cases differ in significant respects from non-Aboriginal cases: the
proportion of women among Aboriginal cases was much higher (25 per
cent vs 9 per cent); and the proportion of intravenous drug users was 38
per cent among Aboriginal cases, compared to 7 per cent among non-
Aboriginal cases.

The proportion of the Aboriginal population infected by the AIDS virus
(called human immunodeficiency virus, or HIV), demonstrable in a blood
test but without the signs and symptoms of the disease, is simply not
known, as there is no systematic sampling and testing of the population.
Based on data collected from a variety of sources by the Public Health
Agency of Canada (2004a), Aboriginal people are over-represented
among individuals who tested positive for HIV and for whom ethnicity
was known, increasing from 19 per cent in 1998 to 24 per cent in 2002.

A few local studies attempted to examine the natural history of HIV
infection. In Vancouver, among injection drug users (IDUs) who were
initially HIV-negative, Aboriginal IDUs were becoming HIV-positive
(referred to as sero-conversion) at twice the rate of non-Aboriginal IDUs.
Those who had frequent injection of cocaine, with or without heroin, and
those who went on binges were found to be significantly more likely to
sero-convert (Craib et al. 2003).

A study of Aboriginal knowledge, attitudes, and practices related to
AIDS in eleven Indian reserves across Ontario provided some data on the
extent of at-risk behaviour. While 40 per cent of men and just under 20 per
cent of women reported having multiple sexual partners, only 1 per cent
reported intravenous drug use. However, some 80 per cent of respondents reported unprotected sexual intercourse at least some of the time
(Myers et al. 1993). It should be emphasized that local attitudes and practices can be expected to vary widely, resulting in differences in the prob-
ability of disease transmission, case-finding, reporting, and treatment.

A Joint National Committee on Aboriginal AIDS Education and Prevention, consisting of all key 'stakeholders,' was established in 1989 and
embarked on a public education program across the country. Since then
other community-based organizations have been established, such as the

Canadian Aboriginal AIDS Network (CAAN). In 2001 the National Aboriginal Council on HIV/AIDS (NACHA) was created to increase collaboration among, and consultation with, Aboriginal communities, and to advise the federal government on the development of a National Aboriginal HIV/AIDS Strategy. It is clear that any education and prevention strategy should be holistic and rooted in Aboriginal culture and traditions. It must also empower communities and individuals, provide equity of access to services, be sensitive to different views of sexuality, and be tolerant of those who are infected. An important stumbling block in the prevention and control of HIV/AIDS is the reluctance of communities to admit the existence of the problem or the prevalence of risk behaviours related to sexual practices and intravenous drug abuse. There have also been cases of communities resorting to ostracism and expulsion of infected individuals and the banning of sex education in schools. On the other hand, there are also courageous Aboriginal persons with AIDS who travel across the country to increase awareness, promote safe sex, and plead for tolerance.

Sexual behaviour is relevant for health because of its association not only with the occurrence of AIDS and other sexually transmitted diseases but also with unplanned pregnancies and their associated psychosocial problems. Having multiple sexual partners is also known to promote the acquisition of the human papillomavirus, certain subtypes of which cause cancer of the cervix in women.

EMERGENCE OF CHRONIC DISEASES

Over the past several decades infectious diseases have been supplanted by chronic, non-communicable diseases and injuries as the predominant causes of mortality and morbidity affecting Aboriginal people. The division of diseases into 'infectious' and 'chronic' is entirely arbitrary. Indeed, certain chronic diseases, those labelled by some researchers as 'diseases of modernization' or 'Western diseases,' are of particular interest because of their ability to serve as a 'barometer' of lifestyle and social change. We shall look in more detail at such chronic diseases as cancer, heart disease, stroke, hypertension, and diabetes.

Cancer

Most studies of cancer mortality and incidence indicate that, among Aboriginal people as a group, cancer is still less of a problem than it is among Canadians nationally, with the exception of certain specific types.

While all Canadian provinces have had population-based cancer registries for some time, data on the number of cancer cases among Aboriginal people are not readily available. Statistics Canada does not report or collect cancer statistics by ethnic status. It is possible to determine cancer incidence/mortality for members of First Nations from some provincial registries through data linkage with the Status Verification System population registry or based on residence on a reserve. A Canadian Inuit cancer registry, comprising cases from the Northwest Territories, Nunavik, and Labrador, was established as part of an international, circumpolar review of cancer among Inuit (Gaudette et al. 1996). This registry is not being maintained or updated, although the Northwest Territories and Nunavut both maintain cancer registries.

In the 1970s, data from British Columbia (Gallagher and Elwood 1979), northwestern Ontario (Young and Frank 1983), and Manitoba (T.K. Young and Choi 1985) all showed a lower incidence when all cancer sites are combined. There are, however, a few sites in which Aboriginal people are at an increased risk compared to the national rate: kidney in men and gallbladder and cervix in women. The risks of cancer of the breast, colon, lungs, and prostate are lower in the Aboriginal relative to the non-Aboriginal population, although they are still among the commonest cancers within the Aboriginal population. A study conducted in Ontario during the period 1968 to 1991 continues to show the same pattern (Marrett and Chaudhry 2003).

The Inuit pattern has generally been different from that of First Nations people. They are at extremely high risk for several cancers that are very rare in other populations: nasopharyngeal, salivary gland, and esophageal cancer (Gaudette et al. 1993). These have been called 'traditional' Inuit cancers. Since the 1970s, there has been a decline in the proportion of these traditional cancers relative to those cancers more commonly found in non-Inuit society such as lung, cervix, colon, and breast (Schaefer et al. 1975; Hildes and Schaefer 1984).

Time trend data are available for only a few groups. An overall increase in cancer from all sites combined was observed among the Inuit of both sexes in the Northwest Territories between 1970 and 1984 (Gaudette et al. 1991), Saskatchewan First Nations between 1967 and 1986 (Gillis et al. 1991), and Ontario First Nations between 1968 and 1991 (Marrett and Chaudhry 2003). Much of the increase in cancer incidence among these groups is accounted for by cancer of the lung, breast, and colon. The rising trend continues to be observed in Ontario (unpublished data presented by Marrett at the First Nations Cancer Research and Surveillance Workshop, Ottawa, September 2003).

While many consider cancer as a 'mystery' disease, many risk factors – preventable either by individual or societal means – have been known for some time. One of the most important of such risk factors is cigarette smoking, responsible for lung and a host of other cancers, not to mention other diseases of the heart and respiratory tract, and harmful effects on the fetus. The high prevalence of smoking among Aboriginal people in Canada has been consistently demonstrated in national surveys (see below).

Cancer may be prevented by reducing the prevalence of risk factors (called primary prevention) and by early detection, or screening. In terms of primary prevention, educational efforts directed at behavioural changes in smoking, alcohol consumption, sexual activity (in terms of delaying onset, limiting the number of sexual partners, and protection from sexually transmitted diseases), and perhaps diet (e.g., reducing the percentage of energy derived from fats; increasing fibre, fresh fruits, and green vegetables; and maintaining energy balance) could bring about a reduced incidence of some cancers.

Many strategies for the early detection of cancer exist, but the effectiveness of all of them has not been demonstrated. The Pap smear for cervical cancer and manual examination and mammography for breast cancer are two of the few for which the evidence is strong.

Several studies from British Columbia, where there is a computerized Pap smear registry, have shown a lower coverage among Aboriginal women (Hislop et al. 1992; Calam et al. 1992). The Santé Québec surveys among the Inuit in Nunavik (Jetté 1994) and the James Bay Cree (Daveluy et al. 1994) found that the Inuit had a higher Pap smear participation rate than Quebec women, whereas the Cree had a lower rate. The higher rate among the Inuit can be attributed to the existence of an organized program of tracking and recall. Among Cree women who stated that they had never had a Pap test, 83 per cent said that no one had ever suggested the test. With regard to breast self-examination and examination by a health professional, both Aboriginal groups fared worse than the provincial population.

A study in Manitoba compared the participation rate for Pap smear screening between First Nations and non-First Nations women in the province using provincial health care databases. While First Nations women were at higher risk for cervical cancer, they were less likely to have had at least one Pap smear in the preceding three years, with the exception of those aged fifteen to nineteen (T.K. Young, Kliewer, et al. 2000).

In interviews with British Columbia Cancer Agency researchers (Deschamps et al. 1992; Hislop et al. 1996), Aboriginal women mentioned that they were not comfortable talking about Pap smears, even among family and friends. Many women reported having been screened because of pregnancy, and some confused the test with testing for sexually transmitted infections, while others thought it was necessary for obtaining oral contraceptives. On the whole, they were embarrassed and uncomfortable both psychologically and physically, particularly when dealing with male physicians. Clearly, cultural factors must be taken into account in any program to promote cancer screening among Aboriginal people.

Cardiovascular diseases (CVD)

This is a heterogeneous group of diseases of the heart and blood vessels. Within the context of 'diseases of modernization,' it is primarily ischaemic heart disease (IHD) (or 'heart attacks') that is of particular interest. However, data are often available only for the broader category of CVD as a whole, which also includes cerebrovascular disease (or stroke). In populations undergoing the transition from a high to a low rate of infectious diseases, it is well recognized that rheumatic heart disease, which has an infectious etiology, tends to decline, while IHD increases as a result of socio-economic and lifestyle changes.

National studies of mortality among residents of First Nations communities in the 1970s and 1980s show that the female IHD and stroke mortality rate was higher than for all Canadians, while among males, the stroke rate but not the IHD rate was higher (Mao et al. 1986; Mao et al. 1992). In 1999–2000, the age-standardized mortality rate (ASMR, i.e., mortality rate statistically adjusted to account for the much younger Aboriginal population) of all cardiovascular diseases among First Nations was slightly higher than that of all Canadians. The ASMR for IHD is not significantly different between First Nations and Canada, but for stroke, the ASMR was 1.7 times higher for men and 1.4 times higher for women in the First Nations population (Health Canada 2003c).

The rising trend in IHD during the period 1981 to 1997 was demonstrated among forty-one First Nations communities in Ontario, based on the provincial hospital admission statistics. For the First Nations popu-

Figure 14. Age-specific hospital separation rate for cardiovascular diseases, First Nations (1997) and Canada (2000)

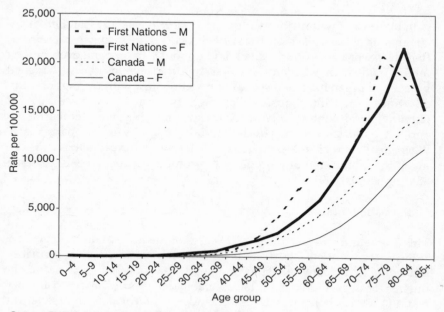

Source: FNIHB, Health Information and Analysis Division 2004
Note: First Nations data are for 1997 from British Columbia, Saskatchewan, and Manitoba; Canadian data from 2000. 'Separation' refers to discharge from hospital, whether dead or alive.

lation, the hospital admission rate increased from <80/10,000/year in the early 1980s to over 150 in the mid-1990s, compared to a declining trend for the overall provincial (as well as the northern Ontario) population (Shah et al. 2000).

Figure 14 shows the age-specific hospitalization rate for all cardiovascular diseases in the late 1990s. It is clear that in the older ages, the First Nations rate, for both sexes, exceeds the Canadian rate in the same age groups.

A lower incidence of IHD among the Inuit has been recognized for some time, based on mortality and hospitalization studies (e.g., T.K. Young, Moffatt, and O'Neal 1993), although diagnostic accuracy is a major problem affecting the validity of the conclusion (Bjerregaard, Young, and Hegele 2003). Analysis of death certificates from Nunavut in the 1990s shows a lower risk of death (Statistics Canada 2004). While myocardial infarction mortality in Canada has been steadily declining, the trend for Nunavut, when smoothing out the variation due to the small population, was sloping upward during the same decade.

Among the risk factors for ischaemic heart disease are hypertension, high plasma cholesterol, diabetes, and obesity. These can also be considered 'diseases,' and they themselves have risk factors, such as physical inactivity and poor diet.

Hypertension

Data on self-reported history of hypertension or high blood pressure are available from most health surveys. According to the FNIRHS, 18 per cent of respondents reported having been diagnosed with high blood pressure. At each age-sex group, the prevalence is higher among First Nations than among all Canadians. When age is adjusted for, the First Nations prevalence is 2.8 and 2.5 times higher than that among Canadian men and women respectively.

Surveys involving actual blood-pressure measurement have been conducted in several regional groups – for example, in northwestern Ontario (T.K. Young 1991), northern Quebec (Thouez et al. 1990), and the Six Nations Territory (Anand et al. 2001). A survey of more than 700 Ojibwa and Cree in northern Ontario and Manitoba in the 1980s showed higher mean diastolic blood pressure (BP) in all age-sex groups compared to Canadians nationally, while for systolic BP, the level was lower above the age of forty-five (T.K. Young 1991). In the Keewatin region of the Northwest Territories, the prevalence of hypertension (defined as diastolic BP ≥90 or on treatment) among the Inuit was lower than among Manitobans in all age-sex groups except men aged twenty-five to forty-four (T.K. Young, Moffatt, and O'Neil 1993). In an international circumpolar review of blood pressure among the Inuit, substantial regional variation was found, although mean levels tend to be lower than in European populations (Bjerregaard et al. 2003).

Plasma lipids

The level of various lipids (or fats) circulating in the blood is strongly associated with the risk of developing cardiovascular disease. Cholesterol and triglycerides are commonly measured plasma lipids. Some fraction of cholesterol is actually protective – this is the high-density

lipoprotein (HDL) cholesterol, commonly referred to as the 'good cholesterol.' Low-density lipoprotein (LDL), on the other hand, is the 'bad
cholesterol.'

There have been no national level studies of various lipids among
Aboriginal people since the Nutrition Canada Survey of the early 1970s
(DNHW 1975a, 1975b), which provided some data on serum cholesterol
and triglycerides for twenty-nine First Nations across the country and
four Inuit communities in the Northwest Territories. The proportion of
people classified as at high risk was lower among First Nations and
Inuit than among Canadians in general, except for First Nations men
aged fifty-five and above.

In the Six Nations Territory, a mixed pattern was found with respect to
the lipid profile. There was no significant difference in mean total and
LDL-cholesterol, while the mean triglycerides was higher and HDL-cholesterol lower, indicating higher cardiovascular risk (Anand et al. 2001).

Among the Inuit in the Keewatin region, the mean total cholesterol
was not different from that in Manitoba, although the level of triglycerides was lower and that of HDL-cholesterol (which has a protective
effect) was higher than in Manitoba, except for women aged twenty-five
to forty-four (T.K. Young, Nikitin, et al. 1995).

Most public health authorities advocate primary prevention to reduce
the prevalence of multiple risk factors. While smoking cessation, cholesterol reduction, control of hypertension, maintenance of ideal body
weight, and regular exercise all appear to reduce the risk of heart disease substantially, the effectiveness of currently available strategies to
modify personal behaviour and lifestyle is variable. While there are scattered efforts by health professionals in individual communities to influence lifestyle, few primary prevention trials have been attempted and
evaluated in an Aboriginal population.

Effective strategies for behavioural change must be directed at both the
individual level through education and at the social level through such
actions as protecting traditional subsistence activities, ensuring the availability of foods at affordable prices, and promoting the marketing of
appropriate foods. Such strategies are likely to be more effective if they
are community-based rather than driven by non-Aboriginal initiatives.

Health professionals within the Western biomedical tradition generally lack an understanding of or interest in Aboriginal concepts of disease causation, manifestation, and treatment. Working among the
Ojibwa in southern Manitoba, Garro (1988) found that the cultural
model of hypertension can be at odds with the prevalent biomedical

view on the chronicity of the illness and the importance of 'compliance' with treatment. At the time of her study, hypertension was conceived by the Ojibwa as episodic in nature, accompanied by perceptible symptoms, with treatment needed only when symptoms were present. Thus, hypertension control is complex, involving considerably more than recalling patients for blood pressure checks and pill counts. Investigation of local understandings and meanings ascribed to symptoms and conditions needs to be part of any health care intervention program.

Diabetes

Of all the chronic diseases, diabetes (more specifically, non-insulin-dependent or type 2 diabetes) has achieved particular prominence because of its high prevalence among most Aboriginal groups studied (e.g., Bobet 1997; Aboriginal Diabetes Initiative 2000; T.K. Young, Reading, et al. 2000). Particularly high prevalence has been detected among the Cree-Ojibwa (T.K. Young, McIntyre, et al. 1985; Harris, Gittelsohn, et al. 2005), Mohawk (Montour et al. 1989), Oneida (Evers et al 1987), and Algonquin (Delisle and Ekoé 1993). Some groups, such as the Inuit and Dene, appear to be at lower risk for the disease (T.K. Young, Schraer, et al. 1992; Szathmary and Holt 1983). In Manitoba, a trend towards earlier onset of NIDDM during the young teen years has been observed (Dean et al. 1998).

The burden of diabetes can be determined on the basis of self-reports. As figure 15 shows, the prevalence of diabetes among First Nations people has increased between 1991 and 1997 and also exceeds the rate for all Canadians in all age-sex groups.

The APS of 1991 remains the only source of information on the prevalence of self-reported diabetes of all three groups of Aboriginal people in Canada – First Nations, Inuit, and Métis (figure 16). It can be seen that the prevalence of diabetes among Inuit is lower than in both the First Nations and Métis populations.

Provincial databases of hospitalizations and physician visits can also be used to generate estimates of cases of diabetes among Canadians. For Aboriginal people (more specifically First Nations), this type of information is only available from several western provinces. In Manitoba, a rising trend in prevalence throughout the 1990s has been observed (Green et al. 2003).

The extent of geographical variation in diabetes prevalence among Aboriginal Canadians was demonstrated in a national review of diag-

Figure 15. Age-sex-specific prevalence of self-reported diabetes, First Nations (1991, 1997) and Canada (1994)

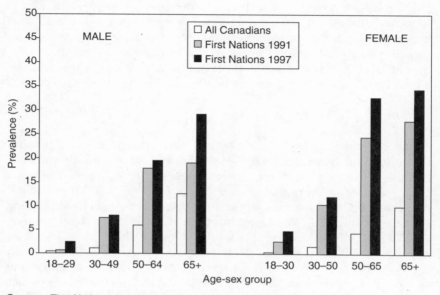

Sources: First Nations data from APS-1 and FNRHS-1; Canadian data from the NPHS-1994

nosed cases (T.K. Young, Szathmary, Evers, and Wheatley 1990). The lowest rates were observed in the Northwest Territories while the highest can be found in the Atlantic region. In comparison to Canadians nationally, the prevalence of diabetes in Aboriginal people was higher in all regions except British Columbia, the Yukon, and the Northwest Territories. In other regions, Aboriginal rates were two to five times higher than in all other Canadians.

The prevalence of diabetes also varied according to language family and culture area, and was lower in more northern latitudes, western longitudes, and in geographically remote regions, suggestive of an interaction between genetic susceptibility and environmental factors in accounting for the observed spatial distribution of diabetes. Language affiliation can be used as a proxy measure of genetic relationship between groups, since genetic distances (i.e., summary statistical measures based on a variety of genetic markers) between language families

Figure 16. Prevalence of self-reported diabetes among First Nations, Métis, and Inuit, 1991

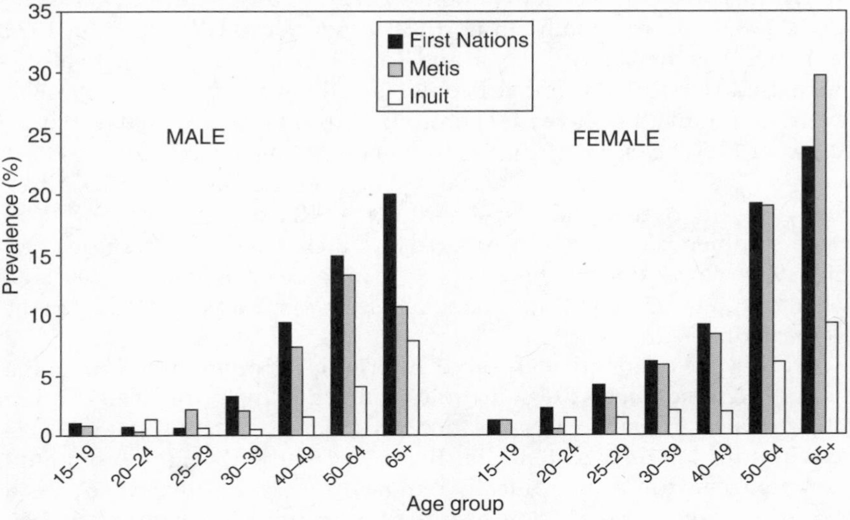

Sources: APS-1; figure adapted from Bruce et al. 2003

are larger than genetic distances within language families. Culture area reflects the subsistence pattern before European contact and is useful in some regions as an indicator of the baseline from which sociocultural changes proceeded after contact. Longitude and latitude, within certain regional groups, provide a rough measure of the intensity and duration of non-Aboriginal influences. Such differences are also reflected in the degree of geographical isolation and proximity to urban areas.

Diabetes is an example of a chronic disease with a multifactorial etiology. To date, epidemiological evidence of varying consistency has implicated heredity, obesity, physical activity, diet, and metabolic factors as potential risk factors.

Diabetes is of public health importance primarily because of its association with various acute and chronic long-term complications affecting the heart and circulation, the eyes, the kidneys, and the peripheral nerves, leading to heart attacks, stroke, blindness, kidney failure, and amputations (Macaulay, Montour, and Adelson 1988).

Aboriginal people suffer more than Canadians generally from chronic renal failure, which may ultimately lead to end-stage renal disease

(ESRD), a condition that requires dialysis and/or kidney transplantation to ensure survival. Data both nationally (T.K. Young, Kaufert, McKenzie, et al. 1989) and regionally, in northeastern Ontario (Wilson et al. 1992) and in Saskatchewan (R.F. Dyck and Tan 1994), have shown several-fold increased risk for Aboriginal people, and the rate of ESRD in the First Nations population increased throughout the 1980s and 1990s. Not all cases of ESRD can be attributed to diabetes, which accounts for 41 per cent of the cases (R.F. Dyck 2001). The clinical outcome also differs between Aboriginal and non-Aboriginal ESRD patients. Among those who commenced dialysis in Alberta, Saskatchewan, and Manitoba during 1990–2000, Aboriginal patients were more likely to die and less likely to undergo transplantation (Tonelli et al. 2004). The explanation for this observation is not clear.

Health professionals who serve Aboriginal people with chronic diseases such as diabetes are sometimes confronted with the need to adapt their treatment plans and education programs to the culture and social environment of their patients. Furthermore, many Aboriginal communities are located in geographically remote areas with little or no access to the specialized services often required for the optimal treatment of these complex diseases. It is difficult for many health professionals to appreciate fully the impact of these diseases and their treatment on individual patients and their families. Individuals with diabetes are expected to modify their lifestyle drastically and follow a complex regimen of rules relating to diet, physical activity, medications, self-monitoring, and self-care, on a daily basis, for the rest of their lives. It is no wonder that compliance with prescribed treatment plans is generally low. It is important for non-Aboriginal health care professionals to understand how Aboriginal people interpret their illness experience and respond to treatment regimens, and to respect the logic and rationality of another system of thought. Furthermore, many communities lack the infrastructure to support people who need to participate in exercise programs. Also, the high cost of healthy foods, especially in northern communities, often puts them beyond the means of many families (Abonyi 2001).

As diabetes is considered to be a 'new' disease that has rapidly increased in magnitude and extent, Aboriginal people have little previous collective experience of it, and the cultural response is still evolving (Hagey 1984; Garro and Lang 1994). Some ethnographic research on Aboriginal cultural understanding of diabetes has been conducted in an Ojibwa community in southern Manitoba (Garro 1995, 1996), among the James Bay Cree (Boston et al. 1997; Abonyi 2001), among Cape Breton

Mi'kmaq (Travers 1995), and in a multicultural urban setting (Waldram, Whiting, et al. 2000). Chapter 9 presents a further discussion of this work.

The Canadian Diabetes Association's *Clinical Practice Guidelines* contains a section on Aboriginal people. It recommends that 'there must be recognition of, respect for, and sensitivity regarding the unique language, culture and geographic issues as they relate to diabetes care and education in Aboriginal communities' (Canadian Diabetes Association 2003).

Data from Australia and Hawaii indicate that adopting traditional lifestyles can have beneficial effects on metabolic control in diabetes patients. In Canada, an attempt to replicate such studies was conducted among the James Bay Cree. Diabetes patients who spent three months in the bush were compared to those who stayed in the village. Bush living was found to have only limited effects on a variety of indices (body weight, plasma glucose, glycated haemoglobin, and blood pressure). While bush dwellers became more active, they also brought along large quantities of store-bought foods for sustenance (Robinson et al. 1995). The relatively short duration of the study may not be sufficient to result in any observable change in metabolic indicators.

In the late 1990s, Health Canada in consultation with Aboriginal organizations developed the Aboriginal Diabetes Initiative (ADI), and began funding many community-based diabetes prevention/health promotion projects across Canada. Predating the ADI are several projects: for example, in Kahnawake, Quebec (Macaulay et al. 1997), Sandy Lake, Ontario (Gittelsohn et al. 1996), and Okanagan, British Columbia (Daniel et al. 1999). These projects, with intervention sites in schools, stores, and the community at large, respect Aboriginal cultures, traditions, and learning styles, and have achieved a high degree of community support and awareness. A project focusing on physical activity and directed at gestational diabetes was initiated in Saskatoon (R.F. Dyck and Cassidy 1995).

The Sandy Lake and Kahnawake projects shared many commonalities but also differed in terms of the community-researcher partnership, the approaches and types of interventions used, and their impact (Macaulay et al. 2003). There are now successful models from two types of communities – one highly urbanized and the other remote and air-accessible only – that Aboriginal communities can adapt to suit their local circumstances. The National Aboriginal Diabetes Association, formed in the mid-1990s, has organized annual conferences where community-based projects are showcased and where front-line diabetes workers can share their experiences.

Figure 17. Prevalence of overweight (BMI 25.0–29.9) and obesity (BMI ≥ 30), First Nations and all Canadians, 2002–2003

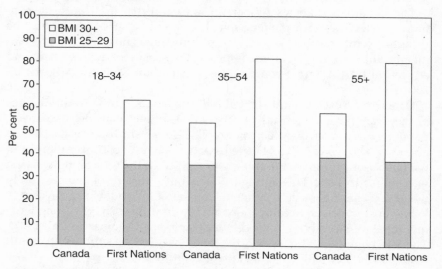

Sources: FNRHS-2 and CCHS, reported in NAHO 2004b

Obesity

Concurrent with the emergence of the diabetes epidemic in the latter half of the twentieth century is an increase in the prevalence of obesity, a strong risk factor for diabetes, as well as other diseases such as cardiovascular diseases and some cancers. Yet, only a few decades ago, many Aboriginal communities were still hovering on the brink of starvation, with deficient energy and nutrient intakes (Vivian et al. 1948; P.E. Moore et al. 1946).

Data based on self-reported height and weight, from which the body mass index (BMI) can be computed, are available from national surveys such as the APS and FNIRHS.[2] Figure 17 provides the most recent data from FNIRHS-2, showing that the proportion of all First Nations individuals with a BMI of twenty-five and above exceeds 80 per cent in some age groups and is even higher than that of Canadians nationally, among whom the obesity epidemic is also a concern.

BMI provides a measure of overall obesity. Increasingly, it is a central or abdominal fat distribution that is recognized as the important predictor of obesity-related diseases. Limited data (e.g., from the Cree-Ojibwa of northwestern Ontario and from the Six Nations Territory) do indicate that obesity among Aboriginal people is predominantly of the central type, characterized by a high waist-to-hip ratio (T.K. Young and Seven-huysen 1989; Anand et al. 2001).

Of increasing concern in recent years is the rise of obesity among children, which has been demonstrated in a variety of locations, including the Cree-Ojibwa in northern Manitoba (T.K. Young, Dean, et al. 2000) and northwestern Ontario (Hanley et al. 2000), the Mohawks of Kahnawake (Potvin et al. 1999), and among the James Bay Cree (Bernard et al. 1995). Childhood obesity is clearly associated with the amount of physical activity. Excessive television watching has been shown to be more prevalent among obese children in most studies (Horn et al. 2001; Hanley et al. 2000; Bernard et al. 1995). Fibre consumption and measures of overall diet quality have also been found to be significant factors in some studies (Hanley et al. 2000; Bernard et al. 1995).

Among the Inuit, skinfold thickness data collected by Schaefer (1977) in various parts of the central and eastern Arctic during the 1960s revealed a generally lean population. According to Rode and Shephard (1992), who have monitored residents of Igloolik over two decades, substantial increase in subcutaneous fat has occurred since 1970, accompanied by a decline in physical fitness and muscular strength. In the 1990s, high levels of BMI have been reported from the Inuit, although the obesity in this population is associated with a lower lipid risk profile than among either First Nations or Euro-Canadians (T.K. Young 1996a).

INJURIES AND VIOLENCE

Among the most serious health problems affecting Aboriginal people in the decades since the end of the Second World War, particularly the younger age groups, are injuries sustained as a result of accidents and violence. Injuries account for about one-quarter of all First Nations deaths, compared to less than 10 per cent in the Canadian population (figure 18). As shown earlier in this chapter (figure 10), the age-standardized mortality rate for injuries is three times higher among First Nations than among other Canadians.

Motor vehicle accidents

In the 1990s, motor vehicle accidents were the highest ranking cause of injury deaths among First Nations in British Columbia (24 per cent), closely followed by accidental poisoning (22 per cent) and suicide (20

Figure 18. Distribution of causes of death, First Nations and Canada, 2000

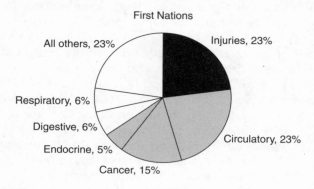

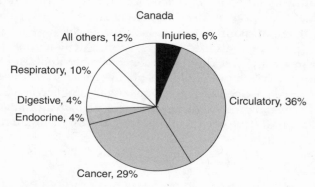

Source: FNIHB, Health Information and Analysis Division 2004

per cent) (Health Canada 2001). In many remote Aboriginal communities, where roads and motor vehicles are few, the risk of mortality from motor vehicle accidents may be lower than for the national population. On the other hand, the risk of death from other transport accidents (e.g., railway, boats, and snowmobiles), where these are the chief means of transportation, can be extremely high (Hislop et al. 1987).

Fires

The quality of housing in First Nations communities is responsible for the excessive risk of fire-related injuries. During the 1990s, the age-standardized injury mortality rate among British Columbia First Nations was eight times the provincial rate. In Manitoba, the hospitalization rate for burns was four times higher in the First Nations population (Health Canada 2001). A review by DIAND attributed the causes of 18 per cent of on-reserve house fires to heating equipment, 14 per cent to arson, 13 per cent to electrical installation, 11 per cent to child-related factors, 7 per cent to smoking, and 6 per cent to the burning of grass and trash (DIAND 1989).

Many factors are responsible for the high number of residential fires in Aboriginal communities. These can be examined from the perspectives of the person, the agent, and the environment. Personal factors include behaviours such as smoking, drinking, leaving children unattended, and having suicidal intent. The agents responsible for the fires may be candles, oil burners, woodstoves, electrical appliances, and faulty wiring in the dwelling. The presence in the physical environment of unsecured combustible materials, buildings with blocked exits, nonfunctional fire extinguishers, and inflammable clothing and mattresses and a lack of piped water in the homes contribute to injuries from fires. Contributing factors from the social environment are largely attributable to poverty (leading to disconnected electricity for non-payment of bills), alcoholism, lack of fire protection service in the community, nonadherence to building codes, and lack of child care and mental health programs (Friesen 1985).

Drowning

Because of the proximity of many Aboriginal communities to bodies of water, drowning is also an important cause of injury deaths. According to data collected by the Canadian Red Cross Society, the drowning rate during the 1990s for Aboriginal people ranged from twice (in Quebec) to ten times (in the Northwest Territories and Yukon) the national rate (Health Canada 2001).

Suicide

Acts of violence are intimately related to the mental health of individuals and the social health of the community. Such violent acts may be self-inflicted or directed at others, and often result in suicide and homicide.

The devastating impact of suicide on the victims' families and communities was vividly and movingly recounted in testimonies to the Royal Commission on Aboriginal Peoples, which produced a special report on suicide entitled *Choosing Life* (RCAP 1995). The document also reviewed various known risk factors for suicide, including

- psychobiological factors – pre-existing mental illness (e.g., depression, anxiety disorders, schizophrenia), personality disorders, cognitive style (e.g., negative and rigid thinking);
- life history of situational factors – early childhood trauma, current dysfunctional family, substance abuse, conflict with authority, absence of spiritual commitment;
- socio-economic factors – unemployment, poverty;
- culture stress – loss of confidence in understanding life (norms, values, and beliefs that were taught to them within their original cultures).

The pattern of suicide has been described in various regional studies. In Manitoba, a review of coroner's records during 1988 to 1994 revealed a mean age of twenty-seven years among First Nations suicides, compared to a much older forty-five years among non-First Nations suicides. Blood alcohol levels at the time of death were twice as high in First Nations as in non-First Nations victims. First Nations victims, however, were less likely to have sought psychiatric help (Malchy et al. 1997).

Among the Inuit in Nunavik, seventy-one cases were recorded between 1982 and 1996, of which 55 per cent were by hanging and 30 per cent from gunshot. About a third of the victims had had some contact with the health care system in the month prior to death, about five times the rate for those who did not commit suicide, even allowing for the higher likelihood of psychiatric diagnoses among suicide victims. This observation points to potential preventive intervention by health care workers if they could identify the suicidal risk status of those seeking their help (Boothroyd et al. 2001).

Aboriginal homicide victims are distributed evenly in all ages, whereas for suicide the highest risk is among young adult males, with a relatively low rate beyond age forty-five (figure 19). One characteristic of adolescent suicides is their tendency to occur in epidemics, or space-time clusters (C.A. Ross and Davis 1986). It is also noteworthy that suicides occur in Aboriginal children, both boys and girls, under the age of fifteen.

Suicide mortality represents only the tip of the epidemiological 'iceberg.' For every successful suicide, there are many more suicide attempts (also called parasuicide). These may or may not result in any contact with the health and social service system, and their true magnitude is thus difficult to estimate. In a survey of Inuit youths aged fourteen to twenty-five

Figure 19. Age-specific suicide rate, First Nations and Canada, 1989–1993

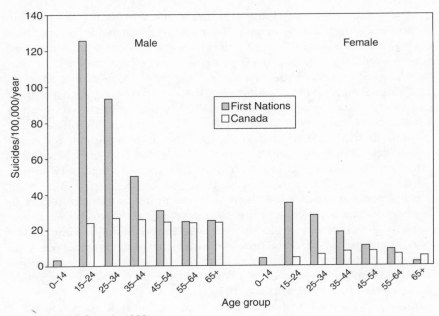

Source: Health Canada 1996

in Nunavik, it was found that 34 per cent had a previous suicide attempt; while 43 per cent had entertained thoughts of suicide in the past (Kirmayer et al. 1996).

Family violence

One particular form of violence that has received increasing attention in recent years is the abuse and neglect of children. Accurate data are extremely difficult to obtain, and media reports of flagrant cases do not reflect the true scope of the problem. In the Aboriginal Peoples Survey of 1991, 39 per cent of respondents reported that family violence was a concern in their community. Many Aboriginal leaders are convinced that physical, sexual, and psychological abuse of children in residential schools, an increasing number of cases of which are brought to public attention, may have produced a generation of adults who in turn inflict violence on their own children, spouses, and elders.

Homicide

A study conducted among inmates incarcerated for criminal homicide in British Columbia in the mid-1970s involved extensive record reviews and standardized psychiatric interviews of twenty-two Aboriginal inmates and a group of Euro-Canadians matched on the basis of sentence, age at first homicide, and IQ (Jilek and Roy 1976). While Aboriginal peoples were over-represented in the prison system, manslaughter charges far exceeded capital murders. The typical homicide committed by an Aboriginal person was directed against another Aboriginal, usually female and a relative of the offender. The non-Aboriginal victim of a homicidal Aboriginal, on the other hand, tended to be male and a stranger. The Aboriginal homicide offenders generally had only limited education, were occupationally unskilled, and had a past history of alcohol abuse, but were less likely than the non-Aboriginal offender to show evidence of psychiatric illness or sexual deviance. In terms of personality development, a lack of exposure to traditional Indian culture was associated with early onset of antisocial behaviour. Those who showed a positive identification with their Aboriginal heritage, however, were more likely to benefit from education and therapy provided in the institutions (Jilek and Roy 1976).

Many Aboriginal people recognize that the interrelated problems of self-inflicted and interpersonal violence (including child and spouse abuse) can only be resolved through a healing process undertaken by the communities themselves. The re-establishment of individual and community self-esteem requires overcoming the denial of embarrassing and/or painful community problems on the one hand, and emphasizing and enhancing positive traditional values and customs on the other. In British Columbia, spiritual leaders involved their young people in the revived Spirit Dance ceremony where they found a renewed Aboriginal identity and cultural pride (Jilek 1982a, 1982b). In northern Saskatchewan, one project aimed to empower abused Aboriginal women by developing mutual support networks (Dickson 1989). Various resource guides and training manuals to assist communities have been developed by the Nechi Institute of Alberta (Martens et al. 1988) and Les Femmes Autochtones du Québec (Lamoureux 1991). A landmark conference entitled 'Healing Our Spirit Worldwide' brought together in Edmonton in 1992 Aboriginal groups from around the world who shared their experiences in healing the wounds of violence and substance abuse.

Community-wide healing projects are emerging that seek to detail and remediate the harm caused by alcohol and substance abuse, in conjunction with other related factors such as residential schools and other substitute-care experiences. The Anishinabe community of Hollow Water, Manitoba, for instance, has become renowned for its community-wide effort to deal with alcohol and substance abuse and their connection to sexual abuse by employing both treatment and restorative justice programs (Four Directions International 2002). Aboriginal women in particular have long complained about their victimization and were often silenced; the once-taboo topic of domestic and family violence is now openly addressed and researched (Proulx and Perrault 2000; Aboriginal Healing Foundation 2003). Further, condemnation of Canada's record in protecting Aboriginal women from violence by Amnesty International has exposed this as a problem of major proportions, one that can no longer be hidden (Amnesty International 2003).

ALCOHOL AND SUBSTANCE ABUSE

Alcohol and substance abuse have been found to be contributing factors in a high proportion of violent acts. Substance abuse includes gasoline sniffing, which is particularly prevalent among Aboriginal children and adolescents in some areas, with results ranging from acute intoxication to long-term neurological disorders, even death. In some communities in northern Manitoba in the 1970s, between 50 per cent and 100 per cent of children and adolescents were believed to be current and recent 'sniffers' (Boeckx et al. 1977). In one Indian reserve in northwestern Ontario, 25 per cent of children five to fifteen years of age, or 10 per cent of the total population, were identified as sniffers (Remington and Hoffman 1984). Early in 1993, a group of Innu children in Davis Inlet, Labrador, were recorded on amateur video sniffing gasoline in an unheated shack. The film was broadcast on national television, and substantial media attention and public outcry ensued. Entire families were airlifted across the country to undergo treatment and rehabilitation at Poundmaker's Lodge in Alberta, an Aboriginal-operated centre. After six months, the children returned with their counsellors, accompanied again by much media fanfare. Unfortunately, the causes of the substance abuse, which are rooted in the poverty and despair of the community, remained unchanged – within months, most of the children had reverted to their gasoline sniffing.

In a survey in an Ojibwa community in eastern Manitoba, it was found that adults and school pupils who participated in hobbies were less likely to use alcohol. Young people who reported good family relationships were also less likely to use alcohol and marijuana (Longclaws et al. 1980).

A literature review of solvent abuse in a variety of populations concluded that parental alcohol abuse was the most significant determinant of gasoline sniffing (Barnes 1979). The author proposed a causal model that listed four environmental risk factors – low social assets, acculturative stress, parental drug use, and peer/sibling influence – mediated through a filter of 'psychological vulnerability' consisting of learned helplessness and alienation (Barnes 1979).

The approach to alcohol and drug abuse in most health jurisdictions is one of treatment and rehabilitation (whether residential, outpatient, or 'community-based') of those who have demonstrated a problem. Some programs are operated by Aboriginal agencies, a notable example being Poundmaker's Lodge in Alberta, as mentioned above. Both in terms of professional manpower and facilities, the demand for Aboriginal-controlled and culturally sensitive programs far exceeds the supply. There are instances also of successfully transforming non-Aboriginal solutions such as Alcoholics Anonymous into Aboriginal revival movements (Jilek-Aall 1981).

Nationally, the Medical Services Branch of Health and Welfare Canada developed the National Native Alcohol and Drug Abuse Program as a pilot project in 1975, and this became a permanent program in 1982. Contributions are given to communities for prevention programs, inpatient and outpatient treatment services, and construction of facilities, training, and research.

Prohibition is a systemic approach to alcohol abuse that has a long tradition in many societies. In Canada, various amendments to the Indian Act prohibited the possession and use of alcohol by Indians until 1963 (J.A. Price 1975). According to Price, prohibition created a new class of legal offences, stimulated conflict with the police, led to financial exploitation by middlemen and 'bootleggers,' reinforced the pattern of binge drinking, and prevented the development of internal social controls. Yet beneficial effects of prohibition have also been observed. In an Inuit community, O'Neil (1985) observed over a four-year period that alcohol prohibition had contributed to an increase in family integrity and respect between generations, an increase in youthful interest in traditional values and lifestyles, and a decrease in aggressive behaviours and abuse of other substances. Enforcement of the by-law was through local social pressure without resort to the externally imposed law-enforcement and justice systems. To be sure, clandestine drinking occurred, but it was tolerated as long as it remained private and did not result in disruptive behaviours in public. The supply difficulty meant that even habitual heavy drinkers had to reduce their consumption level substantially (O'Neil 1985).

Physical training has been identified as a potential means of enhancing Aboriginal adolescents' self-image and reducing drug and alcohol abuse. In an Algonquin community in northwestern Quebec, Scott and Myers (1988) studied the impact of assigning students aged twelve to eighteen to a twenty-four–week fitness program designed to enhance aerobic capacity, flexibility, and strength. Alcohol and drug use remained stable in the intervention group but increased among controls. Scores of self-esteem and body image did not change in either group, while physical 'self-efficacy' (perceived physical ability and self-confidence) did increase over time in the intervention group (Scott and Myers 1988).

Whether alcohol abuse or alcoholism has any genetic basis has been the subject of much controversy, particularly its policy implications among Aboriginal people. Reed (1985) enumerated nine categories of alcohol response where ethnic differences have been shown to occur: consumption rate, absorption rate from the digestive tract, metabolism rate, prevalence of variants of the enzymes alcohol dehydrogenase (ADH) and acetaldehyde dehydrogenase (ALDH), alcohol sensitivity, cardiovascular changes, psychological changes, and alcohol abuse. Of these, he concluded that enzyme differences were very probably due to single genes, while rates of absorption and metabolism were likely under the control of many genes.

The speed with which alcohol is absorbed from the stomach can be measured by the time it takes to reach peak blood alcohol concentration (BAC) after a test drink. Once absorbed into the blood stream, alcohol is metabolized in the liver first to acetaldehyde (catalysed by the enzyme ADH), and ultimately to acetate (catalysed by the enzyme ALDH).

A study in Alberta (Fenna et al. 1971) compared Euro-Canadian volunteers with Inuit and Indian hospital patients and found that, when administered alcohol intravenously, both Aboriginal groups had *slower* rates of disappearance of blood alcohol. This differential response persisted even after stratifying for the history of usual alcohol consumption (categorized as light, moderate, and heavy drinkers). This study gave credibility to the impression that Aboriginal drinkers took a longer time to 'sober up.'

Methodological problems were identified in the Fenna study (Leiber 1972), however, and subsequent studies tended to be inconclusive or suggestive of no biological susceptibility (e.g., Wolff 1973; Bennion and Li

1976), and some of which actually showed the opposite trend. In their comparative study of Euro-Canadians, Chinese, and Ojibwa Indians, Reed and colleagues (1976) showed that, in tandem with the fastest decline in blood ethanol concentration among the three groups, the Ojibwa Indians, at various times after the ingestion of ethanol, also showed the highest levels of acetaldehyde, the metabolic by-product of alcohol believed to be responsible for such symptoms of intolerance as facial flushing.

Alcohol studies among Aboriginal people remain controversial. Indeed, it was necessary as recently as 1987 for Fisher, among others, to point out that the notion of pristine Aboriginal 'races' in the twentieth century is fallacious. Considerable intermarriage among different Aboriginal groups and with non-Aboriginal people has altered gene pools considerably, making it virtually impossible to establish population boundaries for the purposes of these types of alcohol studies (Fisher 1987). Other researchers have argued that social deprivation and poverty (L.E. Dyck 1986) are better predictors of alcoholism and related health and behavioural problems. Levy and Kunitz (1974) provide still another possible perspective. They argue that drinking behaviour is learned, and hence is 'cultural.' Furthermore, they state that 'this, in turn, is largely determined by the ecological adaptation of the tribe in question.' In rejecting anomie theory, they offer that 'drinking behaviour is mainly a reflection of traditional forms of social organization and cultural values ...' In other words, the way people drink is determined by their culture and social organization, which, in effect, predate the introduction of alcohol. Alcohol simply fits into the existing cultural pattern. This explanation is tantalizing, for it allows for the fact that studies have frequently shown differences in drinking behaviour across cultures. Nevertheless, 'the biological explanation maintains its strongest existence in the realm of folk belief' (May 1984:15), with the potential to serve as an explanation for individual problems with alcohol abuse for Aboriginal and non-Aboriginal people who accept the idea. Waldram (2004) provides a more extensive review of the various theories concerning Aboriginal people and alcohol.

That so few imaginative treatment and prevention programs have emerged from all of this theorizing has frustrated many, including Native American scholar Gerald Vizenor, who has written,

The view that tribal people have a predisposition or genetic weakness to alcohol is a racist response to a serious national problem. The notion that tribal people drink to relive their past memories as warriors will neither explain nor mend the broken figures who blunder drunk and backslide through cigarette smoke from one generation to the next. Separations from tribal traditions through marriage or acculturation do not explain the behavior associated with drunkenness. Tribal cultures are diverse and those individuals who are studied at the bar, or on the streets, are unique, alive and troubled, not entities from museums or the notebooks of culture cultists. (Vizenor 1990:307–8)

The best approach to understanding the issue, therefore, involves setting aside biological and cultural explanations and dealing with it from a public health perspective, all the while acknowledging the simple fact that it is a minority of Aboriginal people who exhibit alcohol-related problems.

HUMAN BIOLOGY AND GENETIC SUSCEPTIBILITY

The preceding sections described the major patterns and trends of health problems. In this and subsequent sections, we shall discuss various determinants of health and how they influence the distribution of health and disease in the Aboriginal population.

Diseases ultimately originate from structural and functional derangements – biological in nature – in the human body at the molecular, cellular, tissue, organ, and organism levels. Human biology as a health determinant has traditionally encompassed studies into the genetic contributions to specific diseases and physiological adaptations to the environment; in the Canadian context, these are primarily cold related.

Genetic susceptibility plays some role in the causation of many diseases. The diseases that are most prevalent today, such as diabetes and heart disease, however, are complex, multifactorial, and polygenic. They are not the result of a single gene or a single mutation but are controlled by the action of many different genes. These genes interact among themselves, and also with environmental factors, to produce the clinical features of the disease. Since the late 1990s, much research has been conducted into the genetics of diabetes, cardiovascular diseases, and lipid abnormalities in Aboriginal populations, especially the Oji-Cree of Sandy Lake, Ontario (e.g., Hegele, Connelly, et al. 1997; Hegele, Sun, et al. 1999), and the Inuit in the Kivalliq region of Nunavut (e.g., Hegele, Young, and Connelly 1997). A new variant of the gene encoding the hepatic nuclear factor-1α, believed to be unique to the Oji-Cree, was discovered. Called S319, the gene is present in 20 per cent of the diabetic subjects, twice its frequency among non-diabetic subjects (Hegele, Cao, et al. 1999; Triggs-Raine et al. 2002).

The 'thrifty genotype' is often invoked to explain why diabetes is so prevalent today in many Aboriginal populations around the world (Neel et al. 1998). The hypothesis states that, in times of food shortage, the thrifty genotype enables an individual to produce insulin rapidly in response to rising blood glucose levels, facilitating the storage of glucose in the form of triglycerides in fat cells. With the assurance of a continuous and ample food supply, this quick 'trigger' in releasing insulin results in excessive levels of circulating insulin and glucose, and ultimately leads to obesity and diabetes.

Critics of the theory (Szathmary 1990, 1994; Ritenbaugh and Goodby 1989) note that it assumes a nutritional environment in which carbohydrate intake exceeds daily energy requirements. The early occupants of North America lived in an arctic/subarctic environment on a protein and fat-based diet with few carbohydrates. Alternative pathways to provide energy (e.g., through enhanced gluconeogenesis and free fatty acid release) may have been favoured by natural selection. At any rate, the thrifty gene is more of a theoretical construct than any specific region of the human genome. The idea, however, has also taken on significance for Aboriginal identity (Abonyi 2001).

The pattern of genetic markers among Canadian Aboriginal groups is by no means clear. Various 'deleterious' (or harmful) genes that have been shown to be markers for atherosclerosis and diabetes in other populations occur in higher frequency in Aboriginal populations, while the reverse is true for others. The Inuit also differ from the Oji-Cree in the frequencies of these genes. It should be emphasized that the genetic contributions to different diseases are variable. A genetic predisposition to certain diseases does not mean a 'death sentence,' as there are lifestyle and environmental changes that can modify the action of the gene, or prevent its expression altogether. While not modifiable, genetic risks can be identified through screening and can be useful tools in the control of the disease. Again, extensive intermarriage between Aboriginal and non-Aboriginal populations means that genetic risks will likely vary considerably from group to group.

THE PHYSICAL ENVIRONMENT

As a health determinant, 'environment' is usually discussed in contradistinction to 'genetics' or 'biology' and encompasses all that is external to the human body, while the 'physical' environment is distinguished from the 'social' when referring to physical, chemical, and biological hazards – whether of natural or human origin – that may occur in the air, water, soil, and food and affect health adversely.

Housing and sanitation

Environmental health issues affecting Aboriginal people can be considered to be composed of both the 'old' and the 'new.' The 'old' refers to the 'visible' environment such as housing and sanitation. There is nothing scientifically new in these quarters: the health effects of inadequate housing and sanitation have long been well recognized and the means to control them available. Yet in Aboriginal communities, although substantial progress has been made over the years, survey after survey has indicated that such community infrastructure continues to lag behind that provided for the rest of the population. DIAND's Capital Asset Management System conducts annual surveys and rates the adequacy of housing ('not requiring major or minor renovations'), water supply ('presence of piped, community well, trucked delivery systems'), and sewage disposal ('presence of piped, community/individual septic field/tank'). In 2000 the adequacy ratings were 56 per cent, 98 per cent, and 95 per cent for housing, water, and sewage, respectively, up from 44 per cent, 86 per cent, and 80 per cent recorded a decade earlier (DIAND 2002).

The association between community infrastructure and infectious diseases is particularly striking. A study in Manitoba in the mid-1990s showed that the incidence and hospitalization rates for shigellosis, a diarrhoeal disease, were twenty-nine and twelve times higher, respectively, in First Nations communities than the rest of the province. The incidence rate varied according to community infrastructure for sanitation and housing: it was four to seven times higher in communities where the average household density was four or more persons per house; three to six times higher in communities without a piped water delivery system; and twice as high in communities without sewage systems (Rosenberg et al. 1997). A study of tuberculosis among First Nations nationally found that the incidence of the disease was associated with housing density, degree of isolation, and income levels (Clark et al. 2002).

Contaminants

The 'new' environmental threats are largely 'invisible.' These come in the form of contamination of the traditional food of the people with chemical substances such as PCBs (polychlorinated biphenyls), tox-aphenes, pesticides, and heavy metals that are transported over long distances as well as produced through industrial and mining activities closer to home. The health effects of contaminants are subtle and very difficult to detect. Health risks also need to be balanced with potential benefits in terms of employment and economic development, both of which are desired and needed by many Aboriginal communities. Risk management and communication are important functions of the public health system, and they involve not just environmental scientists and government regulatory agencies but also the communities that are directly and indirectly affected.

Certain cancers are associated with radiation and chemical contaminants present in the physical environment. Air pollution has a major impact on chronic respiratory diseases. Aboriginal people engaged in industrial occupations would be exposed to the same occupational hazards as their non-Aboriginal co-workers. For Canadian Aboriginal people, extensive data are available for methylmercury in First Nations communities (Wheatley and Paradis 1996), and for organochlorines (e.g., PCBs, toxaphenes, and chlordane) and heavy metals in Inuit communities in Nunavik, Nunavut, and the Northwest Territories. Such contaminants are transported to the Arctic by ocean and atmospheric currents and then are biomagnified in the food chain, and high levels have been found in traditional foods and body tissues (Dewailly, Ayotte, et al. 2001a; Van Oostdam et al. 1999; Chan et al. 1997). Of particular concern is the prenatal exposure of infants as well as the presence of contaminants in the breast milk (Muckle et al. 2001; Ayotte et al. 1996). The presence of contaminants in breast milk and traditional foods, however, needs to be weighed against the health-promoting and disease-preventing benefits of such diets.

Community perception of the magnitude of the hazards posed by contaminants varies. In a study of Inuit women in the central Arctic, Egan (1999) found that in their eyes, the issue of contaminants, while important, paled beside many more pressing social problems.

PERSONAL BEHAVIOURS AND LIFESTYLES

Many personal behaviours or lifestyles are associated with the development of a variety of diseases. Of particular importance are such individual behaviours as smoking, diet, alcohol use, physical activity, and sexual behaviour. The modification of such behaviours has become the mainstay of current efforts in health promotion.

Figure 20. Prevalence of smoking, First Nations and all Canadians, 2002

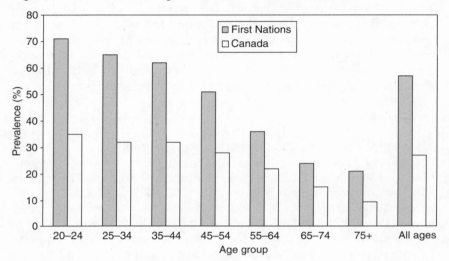

Sources: First Nations data from FNRHS 2002/03 (NAHO 2004b); Canadian data from CCHS 2000/01

Smoking

The high prevalence of smoking among Aboriginal people is well recognized (Millar 1992; Reading 1996). What is particularly of concern is the even higher rate of smoking among adolescents: in a 2002 survey of school students in the Northwest Territories, 36 per cent of Aboriginal children between the ages of ten and seventeen were current smokers, compared to only 13 per cent of non-Aboriginal children (Northwest Territories 2004).

The Aboriginal Peoples Survey provides national estimates of smoking prevalence among the different Aboriginal groups. The most recently available data are from FNIRHS-2 and the Canadian Community Health Surveys (figure 20) and show that the prevalence of smoking among First Nations people exceeds that for all Canadians in all age groups.

Any discussion of smoking among Aboriginal people must recognize that tobacco was an indigenous plant in the Americas – the introduction of tobacco to Europe in the seventeenth century was part of the 'Columbian Exchange.' Health promotion efforts directed at smoking cessation and prevention must also acknowledge the important ceremonial role of tobacco in many Aboriginal cultures that continue to the present time. There is, however, a clear distinction between the ceremonial offering and smoking of tobacco and the addiction to manufactured cigarettes and other commercial tobacco products. The high prevalence of smoking in all Aboriginal groups raises concerns about potential future epidemics of smoking-related diseases, such as cancers and cardiovascular diseases, which are already on the rise in the Aboriginal population.

Diet and nutrition

Many studies have been conducted to assess the composition and nutrient value of Aboriginal diets as well as the nutritional status of the population. The only national study that included Aboriginal communities was the Nutrition Canada Survey of 1972 (DNHW 1975a, 1975b). The scope of this survey, which included a twenty-four-hour dietary recall, anthropometry, clinical examination, and biochemical tests of serum samples, has not been duplicated since. More recent dietary surveys have been conducted in selected communities in the Arctic and Subarctic (reviewed in Kuhnlein and Receveur 1996).

Polyunsaturated fatty acids (PUFAs), especially the long-chain omega-3 fatty acids such as eicosapentaenoic acid (EPA) and docosahexaenoic acid (DHA), have been found to be protective against ischaemic heart disease. Various studies have been done in Canadian Aboriginal populations showing a high intake of PUFAs, for example, among the Inuit (Innis and Kuhnlein 1987; T.K. Young, Gerrard, and O'Neil 1999; Dewailly, Blanchet, et al. 2001), consuming caribou and various marine mammals, and the Tsimshian on Vancouver Island, with a salmon-rich diet (Bates et al. 1985).

Among dietary factors that have been implicated in the causation of cancer is animal fat for colorectal and breast cancer. On the other hand, vitamin A and its precursor, the beta-carotenoids, are protective for lung cancer, while fibre reduces the risk of colorectal cancer. The Aboriginal diet in the Arctic and Subarctic traditionally contains few leafy green vegetables rich in vitamin A. First Nations in the Eastern Woodlands and St Lawrence valley were horticulturalists who cultivated vegetables, including several varieties of corn, beans, and squash (Health Canada 1994). The store-bought diet that has replaced the Aboriginal diet in many locations tends to be high in saturated fat but low in vitamin A and fibre content.

Few studies have been done in Canada examining the association of specific dietary factors with the presence of chronic diseases. Research in Sandy Lake, Ontario, has shown that impaired glucose tolerance and diabetes are associated with reduced fibre intake (Wolever et al. 1997) and also with the consumption of 'junk foods' and a 'fatty' method of food preparation (Gittelsohn et al. 1998).

Diet and nutrition are sensitive to the effects of sociocultural changes, which are reflected in the changing proportions of store-bought foods and foods obtained from the land. The botanical characteristics and nutrient values of Aboriginal plant foods are extensively described and catalogued in the monograph by Kuhnlein and Turner (1991). The high cost of store-bought foods and inadequate income from employment and social assistance have meant that the nutritional value of the land foods cannot be matched and compensated in full. Exchanging a traditional for a 'modern' diet high in fats, particularly saturated fatty acids, would have a detrimental impact on the risk of chronic diseases. Nationally, Aboriginal people who still obtain most of their meat and fish from hunting and fishing are in the minority (about 10 per cent), according to APS-1, although the proportion is considerably higher among the Inuit, about 28 per cent (Statistics Canada 1993b).

Infant nutrition, especially breastfeeding, has important health implications, including for childhood obesity, which also predisposes to adult chronic diseases. Surveys have generally shown a decline in breastfeeding among First Nations mothers in recent decades (Martens and Young 1997).

Physical activity

Many Aboriginal people, particularly elders, recall times when most activities of daily living involved vigorous physical exertion. The decline in physical activity often accompanies the transition to a more sedentary lifestyle. Few survey data on participation in leisure-time physical activity were available for Aboriginal people, until the Aboriginal Peoples Survey, which shows that 54 per cent of Aboriginal adults nationally participate in leisure-time physical activity (Statistics Canada 1993b). However, survey questions on exercises may not be relevant to people who still spend a significant portion of their time living on the land.

There is some evidence of the benefits of physical activity. In Sandy Lake, total (leisure and occupational) physical activity measured by questionnaire and physical fitness (maximal oxygen uptake) were associated with fasting insulin levels, independent of obesity (Kriska et al.

2001). Among children, television viewing of more than five hours per day was associated with obesity (Hanley et al. 2000).

SOCIO-ECONOMIC, CULTURAL, AND POLITICAL FACTORS

The relationship between socio-economic conditions and health status is well recognized. A consistent phenomenon is the social gradient across different measures of health outcomes, whether mortality or morbidity, and applicable both to individual diseases and when all causes are combined. This gradient has persisted despite major improvements in the health and wealth of many populations. For some diseases, the association with socio-economic status has actually reversed over time. Many chronic diseases, such as diabetes and ischaemic heart disease, were once identified as 'diseases of affluence.' They are now more likely to affect lower socio-economic status groups, at least within developed countries.

Several socio-economic indicators of Aboriginal people are presented in chapter 1. Some evidence linking socio-economic status with chronic disease among Aboriginal people in Canada is available. In FNIRHS-1, the prevalence of self-reported chronic diseases increased with decreasing level of completed schooling (figure 21).

A study on the prevalence of diabetes in Winnipeg neighbourhoods found that diabetes is not evenly distributed in the city but varies according to measures of socio-economic status and environmental quality, and is concentrated particularly in the core area where there is a high proportion of Aboriginal residents (Green et al. 2002). In the Six Nations Territory, both the prevalence of ischaemic heart disease (based on medical history and the presence of electrocardiographic abnormalities) and the presence of three or more cardiovascular risk factors increase with decreasing income levels. Moreover, within each income category, the prevalence of heart disease and risk factors is still higher in the First Nations group than in a Euro-Canadian comparison group (Anand et al. 2001).

While most studies of suicide tend to focus on risk factors at the individual level, a different methodological approach was taken by a team from British Columbia, who found substantial variation in the suicide rate among British Columbia's 200 First Nations. They investigated community-level determinants (i.e., using each First Nation as a 'case'), and hypothesized that 'cultural continuity' protects a community from suicide. Cultural continuity was measured from six attributes: involved with land claims; engaged in self-government; operated their own edu-

Figure 21. Association between education and a history of chronic disease,
First Nations, 1997

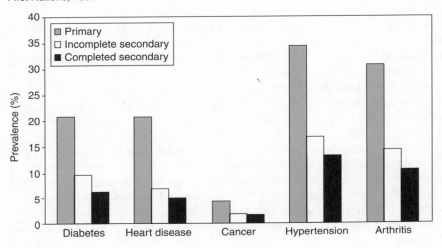

Source: FNRHS-1

cation, health care, and police and/or fire services; and provided cultural
facilities. Communities where one or more of these practices or activities
occurred had lower suicide rates than those without them. When all six
factors were present, the suicide rate was nil, compared to 138/100,000
among communities where none of these factors were present. They concluded that when communities make a collective effort to control their
affairs, suicides are less likely to occur (Chandler and Lalonde 1998). This
study is further discussed and critiqued in chapter 10.

   The concept of 'social capital,' well known to sociologists, is now often
applied in health research to explain why some communities or populations are healthier than others, as well as possessing attributes such as
less crime and more democracy. Social capital includes such features of
social organization as social relationships, social networks, social norms
and values, the extent of interpersonal trust between citizens, and the
norms of reciprocity and sharing of resources. Increasingly, the lack of
social capital has been shown to be associated with poor health status,
even after other socio-economic factors have been adjusted for. Some
research has begun in Canada to investigate if the concept can be defined
and measured in First Nations communities (White et al. 2000). A group

in Manitoba (Mignone 2003) produced a guide to measure social capital by capturing three dimensions:

- bonding – the relations between individuals within a First Nations community;
- bridging – ties with other First Nations communities or other communities (e.g., nearby towns); and
- linkage – the connections between a First Nations community and institutions (e.g., government ministries, public utilities, private corporations).

It is proposed that policy decisions, whether made by governments, corporations, or First Nations leadership, should be evaluated in terms of how, intentionally or unintentionally, they weaken or strengthen First Nations communities and, consequently, affect the health and well-being of their populations (Mignone 2003).

While social and economic factors seem to influence health in Aboriginal and non-Aboriginal populations, there is evidence that the attachment of Aboriginal people to their culture is also an important health determinant. Based on data from the Aboriginal Peoples Survey of 1991, measures such as participation in traditional activities and spending time on the land have been found to be independently associated with self-rated health (Wilson and Rosenberg 2002). More refined and nuanced analyses of cultural attachment beyond those available from national surveys are needed and may yet provide a uniquely Aboriginal framework to understanding health determinants.

A LIFE-COURSE PERSPECTIVE

The life-course approach focuses on exposure to a variety of health determinants throughout different life stages, from gestation, through childhood and early adulthood, to midlife.

It is increasingly recognized that many diseases that manifest themselves in adulthood have their origin in early childhood and prenatal life, probably mediated through fetal and infant nutrition. Substantial evidence has now been accumulated relating to the early-life origins of diabetes, cardiovascular diseases, cancer, mental illness, and neurocognitive development.

The health of pregnant women has an important impact on both the immediate health outcomes around delivery and on the later health of offspring. In a study in Edmonton, a group of pregnant women were recruited at their first prenatal visit and followed through to delivery. Known risk factors for adverse pregnancy outcome were more common among Aboriginal than non-Aboriginal women in the cohort, such as a previous history of premature births, smoking, poor nutrition, and vaginal infections (Wenman et al. 2004).

Unlike the situation in many marginalized minority populations (e.g., African Americans), low-birth-weight births are not common in the First Nations population of Canada. Low birth weight (LBW) is defined as birth weight less than 2,500 grams. In Canada the proportion of LBW births among all births is about 6 per cent in both the Aboriginal and non-Aboriginal populations. On the other hand, high birth weight (or macrosomia), defined as birth weight equal to or above 4,000 grams, is much more common in the First Nations population (22 per cent) than among Canadians nationally (12 per cent) (Health Canada 2003c).

One explanation of the high frequency of high birth weight is the presence of diabetes among the mothers (Caulfield et al. 1998). Surveys in northern Ontario and Quebec have shown that diabetes during pregnancy is prevalent among First Nations women (Harris, Caulfield, et al. 1997; Rodriguez et al. 1999; Godwin et al. 1999). Diabetes during pregnancy has been shown to be a strong risk factor for type-2 diabetes in Aboriginal children in Manitoba. An important finding from this study was that breastfeeding during infancy can reduce the risk of diabetes, providing further evidence of the health benefits of breastfeeding as a method of infant nutrition (T.K. Young, Martens, et al. 2002).

During infancy and childhood, Aboriginal children are at risk for a variety of health and nutritional problems. Anaemia is common among First Nations infants, often as a result of iron deficiency, which can lead to psychomotor impairment. In a survey in the James Bay region, anaemia was detected in 32 per cent of nine-month-old Cree infants, compared to only 8 per cent among a group of urban non-Aboriginal Canadian infants using the same diagnostic criteria (Willows, Morel, and Gray-Donald 2000). Among Inuit infants in Nunavik, about a quarter had iron-deficiency anaemia by six months of age. While breastfeeding should be encouraged in the first year of life, infants should also be introduced to iron-rich foods such as meat and iron-fortified cereals (Willows, Dewailly, and Gray-Donald 2000). There is also a link between poverty and iron-deficiency anaemia (Herring, Abonyi, and Hoppa 2003), reinforcing the view that health care interventions should not be implemented in isolation from the social and economic context.

As an individual ages, he or she is at risk for different health problems. Table 1 summarizes the various common health problems affect-

TABLE 1
Significant health problems associated with different stages of the life course among Aboriginal people

	Infants (<1)	Children (1–14)	Adolescents/ Young Adults (15–24)	Adults (25–64)	Elderly Adults (65+)
Infectious diseases	* acute respiratory infections * meningitis * gastro-enteritis	* acute respiratory infections * meningitis * gastro-enteritis	* sexually transmitted diseases	* tuberculosis	* pneumonia/influenza
Chronic diseases			* diabetes	* diabetes * gallbladder disease * cirrhosis	* diabetes * cancers * heart disease * stroke
Injuries	* accidents	* accidents * child abuse	* suicide * violence	* accidents * violence	
Other	* immaturity * birth-associated * congenital defects * SIDS	* congenital defects			

Note: 'Significant' refers to health problems where the risks of mortality and/or morbidity among Aboriginal people are higher than among other Canadians. Some conditions are also included for their importance to the Aboriginal population, even though their risks relative to other Canadians may not be substantially different.

ing different age groups, many of which have already been discussed in preceding sections. While health programs need to be targeted at the most vulnerable groups, it should also be recognized that many health problems extend throughout the entire life course.

CONCLUSION

This chapter presents an overview of the pattern of health and disease of Aboriginal people in Canada and some of the key determinants that influence its emergence. It is clear that health is multidimensional and is the product of a complex interplay of biological, behavioural, environmental, socio-economic, and cultural factors. The distribution of such factors or determinants differs substantially between the Aboriginal population and other Canadians.

In the next several chapters we move from describing health status to a discussion of health care. The nature and availability of health care services are also important factors in understanding the patterns of health and disease among Aboriginal Canadians, from the pre-contact period to the present.

5

Medical traditions in Aboriginal cultures

Previous chapters have described in some detail what is known about the state of Aboriginal health prior to contact and in the post-contact years up to contemporary times. Like all peoples, Aboriginal North Americans had complex and diverse medical and healing traditions to deal with the health problems that affected them.[1] Similarly, they had knowledge of those practices designed to ensure health and well-being. These traditions not only predated European contact, they also developed as they adapted to the environmental, economic, and political changes wrought by Europeans. The intent of this chapter is to survey elements of these traditions, including theories of disease and illness, treatment approaches, and the range of medical practitioners and healers. It is not possible to be comprehensive in this examination;[2] rather, the emphasis will be on describing some elements of selected medical traditions of the past that have relevance today. A later chapter (chapter 9) will examine the context of traditional medicine in the contemporary world.

HISTORICAL IMAGES OF ABORIGINAL HEALING

Most of the data on the Aboriginal medical traditions of the past are derived from accounts by European and Euro-Canadian traders, missionaries, physicians, and government personnel, as well as scholars such as anthropologists. Two points need to be made about this. First, there was a time when many details of Aboriginal medical practice were considered communal knowledge and freely provided to inquisitive outsiders, to the point where some have been allowed to witness and document various healing activities. By the end of the first quarter of the twentieth century, there appears to have been a shift in this attitude of

Aboriginal healers, and a period commenced in which the traditions went underground, shielded from the watchful eye of government administrators, missionaries, and legal authorities. A degree of cautious openness regarding healing began to emerge beginning in the 1980s, and today Aboriginal healing services are again available to a wide audience. Second, it can be said that most early observers of Aboriginal healing traditions retained an obvious bias in their writing. Aboriginal healing traditions were often seen as primitive, fraudulent, and even harmful; the healers as charlatans; and the patients as superstitious and ignorant. Healers were often labelled 'conjurers,' 'jugglers,' or 'magicians,' and their healing activities were often described as 'performances,' underscoring their highly visible and dramatic nature. Yet, close examination of these texts often reveals a grudging acknowledgment that many elements of Aboriginal medical practice did, indeed, work.

Writing in 1795, explorer Samuel Hearne described Dene-speaking healers as 'conjurers' who 'pretend to perform great cures' using techniques that involved 'laughing, spitting, and ... uttering a heap of unintelligible jargon.' Yet Hearne was also moved to write, 'I have often admired the great pains these jugglers take to deceive their credulous countrymen, while at the same time they are indefatigably industrious and persevering in their efforts to relieve them' (Glover 1958:123–4). Like many European observers, Hearne was hard pressed to explain, in his own rational way, some of the 'tricks' the healers used. In one instance, he watched a healer swallow a bayonet as part of a healing ceremony, and when queried by the Indians admitted he was not close enough to detect the 'deception.' He did note, however, that the patient subsequently recovered (ibid.:125–6). Similarly, trader Andrew Graham wrote that 'Their conjurors pretend to great skill in the medieval way; and by an abstemious regime accompanied with superstitious rites, effect such an alteration in the habit of body and mind of the patient that sometimes is of real service' (Williams 1969:230). Finally, even representatives of the Canadian government from time to time were forced to acknowledge the efficacy of Aboriginal medical practice, as did Dr George Orton, medical officer for Manitoba, in 1891, writing that the healers 'who by experience in the use of vegetables and other remedies in the treatment of wounds and disease handed down from generation to generation doubtless have been the means of saving many lives and relieving much suffering' (cited in Lux 2001:85).

George Nelson was a trader with the Hudson's Bay Company in northern Saskatchewan in 1823. A devout Christian, he took an avid interest in the religious and healing traditions of the Cree, and his journal represents one of the best published sources on Aboriginal healing (Brown and Brightman 1988). Amazingly, Nelson actually seemed to be converted after observing many so-called 'performances' by 'conjurers.' For instance, in describing a ceremony known as the 'shaking tent' (to be described in detail later in this chapter), he wrote, 'I have almost entirely converted myself from these foolish ideas of Ghosts and hobgoblins, but I assure you in truth that I more than once felt very uneasy' (ibid.:104). At the conclusion of the shaking tent ceremony, Nelson was humbled: 'I am fully convinced, as much so as that I am in existence, that Spirits of some kind did really and virtually enter [the shaking tent], some truly terrific, but others again quite of a different character. I cannot enter into a detail by comparisons from ancient and more modern history, but I found the consonance, analogy, resemblance, affinity, or whatever it may be termed so great, so conspicuous that I verily believe I shall never forget the impressions of that evening' (ibid.:106–7).

The unmistakable air of superiority that Europeans felt towards Aboriginal medicine is clear even from the following passage written in 1886, despite the author's attempts to be sympathetic:

The false and mistaken notions as to the principles and practice of medicine which prevailed among our forefathers are recalled by some of those in vogue among the red-man; and while, in the light of our own superior knowledge, we may be disposed to laugh at their primitive ideas, we are reminded that many – perhaps the majority – of the doctrines once taught among our own people were absurd enough. (Bell 1886:456–7)

Unflattering statements about Aboriginal medicine continued on through the twentieth century. A medical doctor writing in 1923 described his frustration with the 'interference from medicine men who chanted weird songs over the sick, removed imaginary fish bones from various parts of their bodies, pocketed evil spirits, and in other ways negated the work of the physician and made them despise the white man's medicine' (Shaw 1923:659). In his 1934 history of medicine in Canada, Bull (1934:19) began by describing the 'conjurer' or 'witch doctor' and 'his bag of tricks,' but was brought to admit nevertheless that 'these horrific-looking medicine men were not entirely without practical knowledge.' Likewise, P.E. Moore (1946:141), director of the then newly created Indian and Northern Health Services, stated that, 'The medicine men undoubtedly played on the superstitions of the natives, but they also possessed some knowledge of the use of herbs and native medicine.' American ethnologist Francis Densmore in 1929 described a Chippewa (Ojibwa) healer's actions as follows: 'he startled, amazed, terrified, and stimulated the sick person, and it is not impossible that in some cases the excited nervous condition produced an apparent or even real improvement in his condition' (1929:45). Even Canada's foremost anthropologist and academic 'expert' on Aboriginal peoples, Diamond Jenness (1972:387), sceptically referred to the 'medicine-men' and 'their supposed powers.'

There is no need to prolong this discussion. It is clear that Europeans have often viewed Aboriginal medical traditions through biased eyes. Even where forced to admit that success in treating patients was not uncommon, they were nonetheless unable to see traditional medicine for what it really was: sets of coherent beliefs and practices – in other words, knowledge – that were well integrated within Aboriginal societies and that served important social and religious as well as medical functions.

DISEASE THEORY

Aboriginal medical systems, like all such systems throughout the world, are built upon coherent, rational understandings of the universe and people's place within it. 'Rationality' must be understood to be a culture-specific notion; one culture's rational thought is not necessarily the same as another's. Indeed, the rational thought that underlies scientific inquiry and biomedical practice is but one type of thought. Inherent in any group's medical system are ideas about how disease is caused, what one can do to avoid the disease, and what types of treatment are called for.

In general, Aboriginal people in Canada saw disease as the product of both natural and supernatural occurrences.[3] It is not the case, as some authors (e.g., Beardsley 1941:486; Balikci 1963:384; McKennan 1965:79; Grinnell 1972:281; Hultkrantz 1992:1) have suggested, that they believed disease was caused only by supernatural intervention; Aboriginal people understood disease causation that was devoid of any spiritual or supernatural significance. For instance, while not having knowledge of the existence of bacteria, they were cognizant of the need and means to reduce infection in wounds. Much of the use of plant and herbal medicines, to be discussed shortly, was based on a disease theory of natural causation. Certainly the greatest attention throughout the literature has been on the understanding of and types of treatment for disease caused by or otherwise related to supernatural forces. In order to understand this, it is essential first to realize that Aboriginal terms that have subsequently been translated into English as 'medicine' actually refer to a much broader phenomenon than drugs or the practice of healing. Generally, these Aboriginal terms referred to a kind of 'power' in a spiritual sense, something that was influential on the lives of people, that was difficult to fully know or understand, and that therefore required certain preventive, propitiating, and/or prophylactic activities to occur. Hence, 'medicine' was fully within the realm of what we would call the religious, and many healers were also involved in religious activities. It is not possible to separate much of Aboriginal 'medicine' from 'religion' as Euro-Canadians would understand these terms.

One of the more comprehensive examinations of the role of disease in the world view of an Aboriginal people is Hallowell's (1963) study of the Ojibwa of the Berens River area of Manitoba. According to Hallowell, the terms 'natural' and 'supernatural' are not even appropriate for describing the components of their world view; instead of such a dichotomy, he suggests that there existed 'a basic metaphysical unity in the ground of being' (Hallowell 1963:267). Their world consisted of human beings ('anishanabek' in Hallowell's lexicon) and 'other-than-human beings.' One class of these latter beings were the 'pawaganak,' or 'dream visitors,' a term synonymous with 'grandfathers.' The pawaganak are willing to share some 'power' and knowledge with human beings if the humans behave in a socially prescribed manner, and in so doing serve to protect individuals and bring them good fortune. Both the ability to heal and the ability to protect oneself from disease or illness were predicated upon the assistance of these other-than-human beings. However, those individuals with stronger than normal power could actually use it to cause illness. Most Aboriginal healing traditions recognized that the power to heal also entailed the power to cause harm, illness, and misfortune to befall a particular victim (this is often referred to today as 'bad medicine'). Such activity was not, however, socially acceptable, and represented a heightened example of disreputable and amoral behaviour that was invariably punished. Within this world view, minor illnesses such as colds, headaches, and digestive disorders were not likely to arouse anxiety, and were treated with herbal remedies. Serious illness, in contrast, was viewed as a penalty for a prior transgression of the moral order and therefore required the assistance of a specialized healer. Such transgressions could involve only human beings, or they could involve a breach in the relationship between human beings and the other-than-human beings. The cause of illness is sought within the web of interpersonal relations involving both sets of beings; hence, both the occurrence of disease and its treatment serve to reinforce the social and moral order of Ojibwa society, an important function in a society where informal mechanisms of maintaining the moral order were the norm. Indeed, confession by individuals, detailing breaches of the order that they had committed in the past, was an essential ingredient of treatment.

In general, then, the Ojibwa case underscores a principle common to Aboriginal healing systems, and one found throughout the globe among many disparate peoples: the world is seen as a place in which harmony and balance exist between and among human beings and other spiritual or 'other-than-human' entities, and serious illness is indicative of a disruption in this balance (see Clements 1932 for an early articulation of this idea globally). Hence, the restoration of balance or harmony appears central to much Aboriginal healing and has led to the development of the idea of 'holism' as a central tenet of Aboriginal healing philosophy. In the late twentieth century, as treatments of Aboriginal philosophy have multiplied – fuelled in part by the 'New Age' movement in North America – it has been argued that Aboriginal peoples did not make a significant distinction between mind and body, what science would call somatic disorders and disorders of the psyche (e.g., Jilek-Aall 1976; Lewis 1980; Trimble et al. 1984; Silver and Wilson 1988; C.M. Fleming 1992; Hughes 1996:136). Accordingly, notions of 'sanity' and 'insanity' were not strictly defined, as in the case of the biomedical tradition, and the mind, body, and spirit were seen as an integrated whole. We are not so certain that the holism thesis is as sound as some commentators would have us believe, however, as there is also ample evidence that Aboriginal medical epistemologies harboured complex notions of the mind as separate from the body (e.g., Kaplan and Johnson 1964:207; Briggs 1970; Levy, Neutra, and Parker 1987; Kirmayer, Fletcher, et al. 1997; Waldram 2004). At the very least, as we do so frequently throughout this book, we would caution against overgeneralizing and romanticizing in the absence of sound empirical evidence.

Part of the problem Euro-Canadians have had with understanding these elements of Aboriginal healing traditions can be found in both the cognitive and the linguistic realms. For instance, Trimble and colleagues (1984:201) have suggested that in the Lakota language 'mental health' translates as *being* in a state of well-being, *not a state* of well-being, an important but elusive distinction. Even the term 'medicine' itself is fraught with ambiguous meanings, from group to group and through time. It can be taken to mean medical practice as biomedicine would understand it, but it also refers to elements of the spiritual realm, particularly in reference to spiritual power of some sort. Manson and colleagues (1996:275) noted a similar problem with the labelling of healing ceremonies, using that expression 'probably because that was the best available metaphor by which non-Natives could describe and understand ... what was happening.' 'These ceremonies greatly exceed that which is commonly understood as healing by the biomedical perspective,' they concluded.

It is possible to identify a small number of generally applicable theories of disease causation, many of which have been identified more globally in a pioneering work by Forrest Clements (1932). These would include spirit intrusion, object intrusion, soul loss, and sorcery or 'bad medicine.'

Spirit intrusion refers to the possibility of malevolent spirits or ghosts inhabiting the body. Object intrusion is similar, in that some object has entered the body and is causing illness. The object may not be something intrinsically pathogenic; upon extraction it is frequently demonstrated to have been a piece of hair, bone, wood, or some other benign substance (Ritzenthaler 1963:316). Soul loss involves the loss of one's soul or spirit from the body, which must then be recaptured (McKennan 1965:79). Soul loss was fairly common among the Indians of the Northwest Coast (Trimble et al. 1984:206). 'Bad medicine,' as noted above, involved the practice of sorcery or witchcraft, in which a malevolent healer, usually at the request of another individual, undertakes to cause illness or bad luck to befall an unaware victim. Soul loss could occur with bad medicine when, for instance, a malevolent shaman abducted a victim's soul at night (Hallowell 1942:61). The symptomatology for each of these problems varied somewhat from group to group, and included both somatic and psychological changes. Lethargy, anorexia, changes in emotional status or behaviour, and overt physical conditions such as tremors or palsy-like symptoms were common. Non-physical complaints might include the inability to attract a lover, or poor luck in hunting. In some cases, the symptoms of whatever type could actually be experienced by someone other than the individual who had caused the problem by breaching the moral order. So, for instance, since children were usually not viewed as being fully socialized into the normative order, serious illness among them was viewed as the product of a transgression by an adult.

As one can see, each of these types of disease causation implies a fairly direct intervention of spiritual or supernatural agents; these are not diseases as biomedicine would recognize them, although in recent years the psychological dimension of these problems has been recognized. Unlike biomedical approaches, however, Aboriginal medical systems may have been more concerned with delineating the etiology of the problem, since in so doing the type of treatment required became obvious. And since the cause invariably involved a breach of the normative order, repairs to the moral fabric of society became central to healing activities. Indeed, the communal nature of Aboriginal healing is in marked contrast to the more circumspect practices of biomedicine.

HEALERS AND MEDICAL PRACTICES

There were a great many types of healers and medical practitioners among the Aboriginal peoples of Canada. While there has been a general acceptance of the appellation 'medicine man/woman' in recent years to describe these individuals, such a term is somewhat meaningless in that it glosses over very important distinctions between the types of healers, their knowledge and skills, and how they acquired the authority or 'power' to heal.

It is first essential to emphasize that there existed among Aboriginal peoples a 'popular' sector of medicine (see Kleinman 1980) wherein certain knowledge regarding the maintenance of health and the treatment of illness or trauma was extant. As in any society, what we might call 'home management' of illness was common. Individuals tended to possess a generic knowledge of medicinal plants and what amounted to 'first aid' techniques, and applied this knowledge when necessary. The ability to do this did not represent the product of specialized training, which separates treatment within the popular sector from that of the 'folk sector,' where we find non-professional medical specialists of varying types. Generic medical knowledge was simply passed on through the generations as part of the necessary cultural heritage of the group (Lux 2001).

Hultkrantz (1992:17–18) has suggested that there are basically three types of healers: herbalists, 'medicine men,' and shamans. The difference between them, it would seem from Hultkrantz, is the degree to which spiritual assistance is required in the healing. The herbalists employ various botanical substances, often in combination, with which they treat a wide variety of disorders, including dressing wounds. Their knowledge is gained largely through experience and tradition handed down to them by older herbalists. The term 'medicine man' denotes a healer 'who has supernatural sanction to make a person well and who follows supernatural dictates in his curing activities' (ibid.:18). The 'shaman,' according to Hultkrantz, is an individual with the ability to fall into deep trance or 'ecstasy' and undertake spirit flight or summon spirits to counsel him. The distinction by Hultkrantz is somewhat arbitrary, for he notes that 'The ordinary medicine man may certainly heal the sick while in a light trance, but he does not sink down into the deep trance that is necessary for making contact with the supernatural world' (ibid.:19). The reality of healing may be much more complex than Hultkrantz suggests.

Andrew Graham (Williams 1969), in his observations along Hudson Bay in the late eighteenth century, distinguished between the 'conjurers' or 'jugglers,' who were directly involved with spiritual powers, and the 'tuckathin, or doctors' among the Cree who were highly knowledgeable herbalists. He also described 'itinerant druggists' who came up from the south every year to barter roots and herbs. The literature suggests that some Aboriginal groups had greater knowledge of plant medicines than others, and that borrowing or trading often took place. For instance, D. Smith (1973:21) states that the Chipewyan 'have freely borrowed root medicines from the Cree ... and are quick to give the Cree credit as the "inventors."' Jenness (1938:73) suggests that the Plains Indians in general had a 'scanty' knowledge of herbal remedies, and groups such as the Sarcee borrowed from the Cree, 'who seemed to know the mysterious virtues of every plant and shrub.' It would not be correct to suggest that herbalists always lacked spiritual assistance in their work, or that other healers were excluded from the use of herbs, for neither is true. Herbalists and other healers could even obtain knowledge of particular combinations through spiritual assistance.

It is virtually impossible to present a coherent and comprehensive discussion of the many botanical medicines that are known to have been used by Aboriginal peoples. There are many sources on this topic, of which the most useful are Hutchens (1973), Hellson (1974), Arnason and colleagues (1981), Ford (1981), Leighton (1985), and Moerman (1986, 1998). There have been relatively few pharmacological studies of these plants, and hence much of their value may well have been lost to time. Nevertheless, the testament to their efficacy can be found in two basic facts. First, the earliest fur traders, missionaries, and settlers often turned to the Aboriginal herbalists for treatment (Vogel 1970:111–23); and second, more than 170 drugs that have been or still are listed in the *Pharmacopoeia of the United States of America* owe their origin to Aboriginal usage (Vogel 1970:267). Various Aboriginal groups were able to prevent scurvy by brewing tea from spruce bark (rich in vitamin C); they were able to reduce pain by using willow extract, which contains salicin (similar to the product 'aspirin'); they had various kinds of anaesthetics, emetics, diuretics, and medicines that could induce labour or numb labour pains. Plant extracts also acted as antibiotics when applied to wounds. There is no doubt that the Aboriginal herbalists had a different understanding of how and why such plants worked in comparison to biomedicine; but clearly, through thousands of years of adaptation to their environments, and through experimentation, they had developed an impressive array of botanical medicines and preparation techniques. Perhaps only a minority of these have been made readily available to non-Aboriginal people, and many formulations have no doubt been lost as a result of the colonization of the Americas. Nevertheless, today one can typically find so-called Aboriginal herbal medical preparations available for sale in pharmacies across Canada as well as on direct-market websites.[4]

Beyond the herbalists is a variety of healers who, while they may still use botanical medicines in their healing, tend to rely more on spiritual activity. In this regard, the ability to contact spiritual entities to assist in diagnosis and treatment is essential, and the degree to which an individual can do this is a measure of the healer's standing within his or her society. As in all medical traditions, some practitioners were better than others, and their techniques included a number of inspirational, spiritually directed approaches plus pragmatic and learned techniques that no doubt required practice.

In the late eighteenth century, Andrew Graham described these shamans thus:

Jugglers or conjurers are very numerous amongst them [Cree]. They are generally men who are good hunters, and have a family; some of them are very clever at it. They are supposed to have intelligence with the Evil Spirit [actually the Creator], and by that means can procure anything to be done for the good or injury of others, foretell events, pacify the malignant spirit when he plagues them with misfortunes, and recover the sick. They have also several tricks of sleight hand; such as swallowing a string with a musket ball hanging to it; taking it directly out at the fundament; pretending to blow one another down; swallowing bears' claws, and vomiting them up; extracting them from wounds, or the breast, mouth etc. of a sick person; firing off a gun and ball to remain behind; and a thousand other pranks which make them be held in great esteem by the rest. (Williams 1969:161)

The notion that practitioners played tricks on their patients is rife in the historic literature. Techniques known today as 'sleight-of-hand' were particularly noted, including swallowing objects, making objects disappear, and undertaking 'surgery' in which objects were clearly removed from the body of the patient without any subsequent wound, suture, or scar. There is no question that such techniques were a part of healing, and some healers have, on occasion, even disclosed such practices. For instance, anthropologist David Mandelbaum (1979:162–3) relates that one of his informants, Fine-Day, a Plains Cree, was once shown how to take hot coals into his mouth by a healer, but could not bring himself to do it. Mandelbaum notes that, 'Officially, however, all these feats were performed in accordance with directions imparted in a vision' (ibid.: 163). Bell (1886:461) noted that some shamans who had become Christians had subsequently 'confessed that their former course had been all imposture.' Insofar as we are in a position to posit that some degree of deception was employed in treating patients, a number of logical reasons for this activity are evident. First, the ability to undertake apparently impossible feats no doubt served to impress upon the patient the degree of skill and spiritual power of the healer; it served as a kind of measure of competence. Second, there is also the likelihood that a placebo effect occurred as a result of such feats, in which some individuals subsequently recovered without the intervention of a pharmacological agent or surgical procedure. Samuel Hearne, writing in 1771, perfectly described the placebo effect among the northern Dene-speaking peoples:

Though the ordinary trick of these conjurers may be easily detected, and justly exploded, being no more than the tricks of common jugglers, yet the apparent good effect of their labours on the sick and diseased is not so easily accounted for. Perhaps the implicit confidence placed in them by the sick may, at times, leave the mind so perfectly at rest, as to cause the disorder to take a favourable turn; and a few successful cases are quite sufficient to establish the doctor's character and reputation. (Glover 1958:142)

As Moerman (1983, 2002) has indicated, the placebo effect is an essential ingredient of all medical traditions, including biomedicine with its highly visible system of healer validation (degrees on the wall, white laboratory coats, and stethoscopes, for instance) and the inclination for doctors to prescribe inappropriate medicines to help the patient feel that something is being done (such as prescribing antibiotics for viral infections). Clearly, Aboriginal healing traditions had developed a similar view towards the need to validate the healer's abilities and to empower the patient to heal himself or herself. Such validation is an integral, and essential, element of healing, whatever the culture.[5]

A common shamanistic method of healing has been referred to as 'sucking' or 'cupping,' and its practitioners are often referred to as 'sucking doctors.' This technique is called for particularly when it is believed that an object has entered the body and is causing a problem, or where an internal poison or body tissue is implicated. Most accounts suggest that a sucking horn or tube of some sort is used, although the healer may place his or her lips directly onto the flesh. By sucking and blowing, the healer removes the object, which is usually shown to the patient and the others attending. The ceremony involves prayer and singing, sometimes blowing on a whistle, all designed to summon the supernatural assistance required to locate and extract the object. Alexander Henry described an incident of sucking in 1763, likely among the Chippewa:

After singing for some time, the physician took one of the bones out of the bison: the bone was hollow; and one end being applied to the breast of the patient, he put the other into his mouth, in order to remove the disorder by suction. Having persevered in this as long as he thought proper, he suddenly seemed to force the bone into his mouth, and swallow it. He now acted the part of one suffering severe pain; but, presently finding relief, he made a long speech, and after this, returned to singing, and to the accompaniment of his rattle. With the latter, during his song, he struck his head, breast, sides and back; at the same time straining, as if to vomit forth the bone. Relinquishing this attempt, he applied himself to suction a second time, and with the second of the three bones; and this also he soon seemed to swallow. Upon its disappearance, he began to distort himself in the most frightful manner, using every gesture which could convey the idea of pain: at length, he succeeded, or pretended to succeed, in throwing up one of the bones. This was handed to the spectators, and strictly examined; but nothing remarkable could be discovered. Upon this, he went back to his song and rattle; and after some time threw up the second of the two bones. In the groove of this, the physician, upon examination, found, displayed to all present, a small white substance, resembling a piece of the quill of a feather. It was passed round the company, from one to the other; and declared, by the physician, to be the thing causing the disorder of his patient. (Henry 1976:120–1)

Mandelbaum's informant, Fine-Day, described a number of cases of sucking among the Plains Cree, and the similarities with Henry's account are striking. For instance, in the 1930s Fine-Day related the following incident:

All at once he drops his rattle and sucks at the sick man's temple. The thing was lodged in the back of the neck but he sucked it out through the temple. As soon as he got it he clapped his hand to his mouth and starts to reel backwards. His wife grabs the moccasins and hits him on the back with them. He straightens up and grabs the thing from off his tongue and holds it between his cupped palms. He shakes it and then gives it to me. I take it. It feels as though it is burning me. I shake all over. I feel it move between my fingers. I blow on it and soon it cools. I give it to my cousin. It burns him and he blows just as I did. We look at it later. It has a dragon fly's head with the wings folded back over the body. (Mandelbaum 1935)

Fine-Day also described Plains Cree sucking in a more general way:

Some doctors pass their hands over the sick person and hold him for a while. They lay their hands on him and feel where the sickness is and point it out. When they locate the spot, they take a buffalo horn, put some sweetgrass in it, put an ember on and clap it over the place. It sucks out the matter and has to be taken off sideways. You can see a yellow stuff in the horn after it is taken off.

Another important and widespread healing ceremony has been referred to in the literature as the 'shaking tent' or the 'conjuring lodge.' Similar to the sucking procedure discussed above, the shaking tent seems to have had a very broad geographical range in Canada, although most of the literature pertains to Subarctic and Plains hunting peoples. It has been identified among Montagnais (Flannery 1939), northern Cree (Preston 1975), Ojibwa and Saulteaux (Hallowell 1942), Plains Cree (Mandelbaum 1979), Blackfoot (Cooper 1944; Schaeffer 1969), Assiniboine (Cooper 1944), and no doubt many more. There are remarkable similarities in the description of the shaking tent rite. The best eyewitness accounts of this may be those of trader George Nelson, writing of the Cree in northern Saskatchewan in 1823 (Brown and Brightman 1988), and anthropologist Richard Preston (1975), writing of the James Bay Cree in the 1960s. Their descriptions are far too lengthy and detailed to recount here; however, some of the most common elements of the shaking tent can be presented.

The shaking tent ceremony had a variety of functions. Communion with the spiritual world was integral to all ceremonies, and through such contact the shaman, among other things, was able to predict the future (such as the weather, where game might be found, or that a sickness would soon arrive), locate lost objects, and diagnose the cause of illness. Characteristically, the shaking tent itself was a small, often conical lodge made of branches and skin covering, in which the shaman was seated or knelt. Frequently the shaman was bound hand and foot by his assistants before being placed in the lodge; sometimes he was gagged as well. Shortly after the commencement of the ceremony, with assistants and community members seated around the outside, the ropes that bound the shaman would be thrown out the door or the top of the tent. Then the sha-man would sing and invite his spirit helpers, and indeed any spirits, to enter the lodge. When they did so, the lodge would often shake violently back and forth. The people outside would then hear a succession of voices of the spirits as they entered and communicated with the shaman. These were not in the voice of the shaman, however, and sometimes were in a language unintelligible to those on the outside (often considered an ancient language). Some of the discussion in the tent was jovial, with the spirits and the shaman exchanging jokes (some quite bawdy), but the spirits also provided important information at the shaman's request. On occasion, an outside participant, such as the sick person, would be invited to enter the tent to see the spirits. Nelson (Brown and Brightman 1988:106) was provided such an opportunity and saw a variety of small lights. The existence of the spirits in the form of small lights has been reported by others who have witnessed the ceremony (e.g., Hallowell 1942),[6] although it is suggested that among other groups they appeared as hominoid figures or birds (Brown and Brightman 1988:152).

One of the functions of the shaking tent was to provide news of dis-tant relatives and events. Hallowell (1942:47) provided one example of this, in which an outside participant queried the spirits: 'The other Indian, who had left a brother sick with double pneumonia at the mouth of the river a few days previously and for whom there seemed no hope of recovery, wanted to know how the sick man was. The answer in this case was that he would recover. When we arrived at the mouth of the river he was up and walking about. And when I [Hallowell] arrived home at the end of the summer I found *mikinak's* [the spirit's] report concerning my father's health was not only judiciously phrased but quite true. He was no worse. Neither had he improved in health.'

As noted earlier, among the Ojibwa and many other Aboriginal groups, serious illness was often seen as the product of a transgression of the moral order of the society. Hallowell (1942:55–6) has described an incident in which the shaking tent was used to diagnose why a man was having problems passing urine. Ultimately, the spirits examined the issue by first questioning why the medicines offered by a previous healer for this complaint had not worked, adding 'Perhaps some of the old people did something wrong.' Subsequently, an older woman spoke up, admitting that, many years earlier, a group of youngsters and her had forced a sewing thimble onto a smaller boy's penis and then told him to go urinate. The boy responded that he couldn't, and that it hurt, and he began to cry. When the confession was over, the conjurer said, 'I thought there was something that stopped the medicine from working.'

While the shaking tent was a common feature of many Aboriginal medical traditions, even more common was the sweat lodge. Indeed, as Lopatin (1960) has demonstrated, a form of sweat bathing is common to many societies throughout the world, including other nordic areas such as Russia and Scandinavia. The function of the sweat lodge for North American Aboriginal peoples was multifaceted. It was used for purposes of prayer, to maintain health, and to address particular health problems or social concerns. It was also used as a precursor or conclusion to other religious and healing ceremonies. Among the specific health problems for which the sweat lodge was used, we find 'febrile symptoms, chronic rheumatism, headache, fast pulse, catarrh, and sore muscles' (Beardsley 1941:489), as well as more general colds and fevers (Ritzenthaler 1963:327); in general it was used as a panacea for most types of physical and mental health problems (Vogel 1970:256). Although both the structure of the lodge (although almost always made of willow) and the actual ceremony varied from group to group, Grinnell's (1972:282–3) description of the Blackfoot sweat lodge in the late 1800s is typical:

The sweat lodge is built in the shape of a rough hemisphere, three or four feet high and six or eight in diameter. The frame is usually of willow branches, and is covered with cowskins and robes. In the centre of the floor, a small hole is dug out, in which are to be placed red hot stones. Everything being ready, those who are to take the sweat remove their clothing and crowd into the lodge. The hot rocks are then handed in from the fire outside, and the cowskins pulled down to the ground to exclude any cold air. If a medicine pipe man is not at hand, the oldest person present begins to pray to the Sun, and at the same time sprinkles water on the hot rocks, and a dense steam rises, making the perspiration fairly drip from the body. Occasionally, if the heat becomes too intense, the covering is raised for a few minutes to admit a little air. The sweat bath lasts for a long time, often an hour or more, during which many prayers are offered, religious songs chanted, and several pipes smoked to the Sun.

The effect of the sweat lodge ceremony is to encompass the participants in complete darkness; sometimes only the soft glow of the heated rocks is noticeable. Some sweat lodge leaders will use a variety of herbs, either mixed into the water or sprinkled directly onto the rocks. On the prairies today, it is common to have four rounds, with the lodge being opened between each round for a brief period. And, unlike Grinnell's description, prayers today tend to be offered to the 'Creator' instead of the 'Sun.'

The therapeutic benefits of the sweat lodge have obviously been recognized widely, as evidenced by its global presence. Some of the early settlers to North America also participated in sweats with Indians. For instance, LeClercq wrote, 'The sweat-house ... is the great remedy of the Gaspesians; and it can be stated as a fact that a number of the French have also found therein a cure for chronic inflammations and sufferings which seem incurable in France'; and Denys wrote, 'Our Frenchmen make themselves sweat like them, and throw themselves into the water similarly, and are never incoded thereby' (cited in Bailey 1969:121).

Setting aside the religious significance of the sweat, a variety of explanations have been posited to explain its apparent therapeutic benefits. First, of course, is that the sweat acts as a placebo, empowering the mind to begin the healing process and opening the individual to subsequent treatment. The appeal to intervention by spiritual forces, based on the faith of the participants, is an integral part of this effect (Swartz 1988). This may well be the lesser of the effects, however. It is quite likely that the combination of sensory deprivation in some areas (lack of sight) combined with heightened sensory stimulation in others (the heat on the skin; smell of herbs) induces an 'altered state of consciousness,' which, among other things, facilitates the body's release of endorphin, a possible explanation that is not necessarily seen as being at odds with the understanding of traditional healers that it is the Creator who is doing the healing (Waldram 1997). Aboriginal sweat lodge participants have suggested to one of the authors (Waldram) that one must participate a few times before the mind is able to concentrate on prayer and ignore the intense heat and discomfort. Adair and colleagues (1969) have suggested that the sweat has a sedative effect, and Achterberg (1985) has suggested that the high temperature of the body in a sweat mimics that of the body during a fever, which may stimulate the body's natural reactions to toxins (and the high temperature may also kill heat-sensitive bacteria and viruses). David Young and colleagues (1988:84) have postulated that the steam releases salicylic acid from the willow branches of the lodge frame, a compound that is used today in various antiseptics and antineuralgic compounds, among other things.

THE MIDEWIWIN

The Midewiwin is a religious and healing movement that arose first among the Ojibwa in the 1800s, possibly as a reaction to the intrusion of Europeans and the disruption caused by their arrival. Subsequently, it spread to neighbouring Woodlands and Plains Indian groups, such as the Saulteaux, Plains Cree, and Dakota (as well as other groups on the American side of the border), where it was adopted in various forms. The Midewiwin is important because it represents an indigenous, hierarchical, religious and medical system with a well-defined structure. It is in contrast to the less structured, idiosyncratic approach of much Aboriginal healing in Canada.

The Midewiwin, sometimes referred to as the 'Grand Medicine Society,' was a society of individuals who came together periodically to perform various religious and healing ceremonies and to induct new members into the group (Vecsey 1983:179). It was built upon the foundations of traditional Ojibwa religion, as detailed earlier in this chapter. One of the major concerns of the Midewiwin was the maintenance of health, and the instruction of novices involved identifying and preparing botanical medicines. Other instruction involved ways to commune with the spiritual world to enhance individual power to heal; in a more general sense, the Midewiwin taught general principles of health maintenance, particularly as they pertained to the need for the individual to maintain harmony with the world and to refrain from breaking social norms or offending the pawaganak.

Members of the Midewiwin are often referred to as 'priests' in much of the literature, although this term fails to do justice to the broad role of these individuals within Ojibwa society. Individuals were initiated into the society, whereupon they were exposed to the knowledge of its members. A person could have a dream that he should enter the society, or he could fall ill and require the services of a Mide healer, which would result in his being initiated. There were at least four 'degrees' or levels of knowledge within the Midewiwin, with each higher level requiring the mastering of more complex knowledge and being rewarded with unique designations, such as furs and coloured scarves specific to the rank. Since illness was one means of entering the society, most community members attained at least the lowest rank. Rising further required one to apprentice with a teacher who acted as a sponsor or mentor, and the higher the rank aspired to, the greater the cost to the initiate (Ritzenthaler 1963:317–19).

The Midewiwin served to maintain social order as well as health. According to Densmore (1929:87), 'the ethics of the Midewiwin are simple but sound. They teach that rectitude of conduct produces length of life, and that evil inevitably reacts on the offender. Membership in the Midewiwin does not exempt a man from the consequences of his sins. Respect toward the Midewiwin is emphasized, and respect toward women is enjoined upon the men. Lying, stealing, and the use of liquor are strictly forbidden. The Mide is not without its means of punishing offenders. Those holding high degrees in the Midewiwin are familiar with the use of subtle poisons which may be used if necessary.'

Howard (1977:134) has hypothesized that the Midewiwin was a response to the general anxiety created among the Ojibwa as a result of the presence of so many shamans capable of causing illness and misfortune. In effect, through membership in the Midewiwin, these individuals were co-opted, and since almost everyone in the community was a member, the possibility of 'bad medicine' was greatly reduced.

It was once believed that the Midewiwin was on the verge of extinction and that it had ceased to function by the middle part of the twentieth century. However, like many other aspects of Aboriginal religion and healing, the pronouncements of its demise were incorrect. Quite likely, the Midewiwin went underground for many years; by the 1980s it had begun to resurface, particularly among the Saulteaux of Manitoba. Midewiwin ceremonies are currently held on an annual basis.

ANATOMICAL KNOWLEDGE AND SURGICAL PRACTICES

Virtually all the Aboriginal societies in what would become Canada were hunting peoples of some sort, and hence it is logical that some degree of anatomical knowledge would have been attained. The processing of meat and skins would afford ample opportunity to develop an understanding of the basic body organs and their functions. In some instances, deliberate autopsies of animals may have been carried out, as in the case of the Inuit in the western Arctic (Lucier et al. 1971:253). However, the extent to which pre-contact Aboriginal peoples understood human anatomy is, unfortunately, unknown. As well, despite claims by authors such as Bell (1886:534) that 'They never attempt any grave operation, although their general knowledge of anatomy is not to be despised,' there is little historical record of how that anatomical knowledge may have actually translated into surgical procedures.

For the most part, the surgical procedures that were documented tended to be relatively minor.[7] The treatment of wounds and trauma was certainly important, as both the palaeopathological and the historical records demonstrate. The Earl of Southesk (Southesk 1875:329), for instance, recorded two cases of gunshot wounds, one Indian and the other European, that were successfully treated by an Indian healer using herbal medicines. The frequent application of various botanical medicines on wounds suggests an understanding of the need to prevent infections; likewise, the use of tourniquets and bandages is also noteworthy.

Bloodletting of various forms was common. Morice (1900–1) described a number of different approaches used among the Dene to treat such ailments as headaches and general pains. His description of the surgery on the temporal artery is likely fairly common: 'This is slightly cut with as sharp an instrument as can be procured, and the blood is allowed to escape until a rich red colour has succeeded the dark hue of the first flow which is supposed to be the cause of the ailment. The wound is then compressed by the application of a piece of skin or of a green leaf, according to the season. The head is afterwards bandaged so as to ensure the speedy healing of the wound.' In general, only a little blood was ever allowed to escape.

Bone-setting was also important, and some Aboriginal groups had individuals with special skills in this area. Stone (1935:82–3) has written that 'their skill in the care of wounds, fractures and dislocations equalled and in some respects exceeded that of their white contemporary.' Typically, fractures and bones were set and splinted with wood, or tightly wrapped with reeds or other firm but flexible materials. The palaeopathological record demonstrates that many times these wounds healed effectively, although the record also suggests that limping or impaired function, combined with some degree of pain, likely plagued some individuals subsequent to injury.

Scarification was practised by many groups. Morice (1900–1) reports that the Dene would sometimes treat rheumatism, local aching, and sprains by scratching numerous lines on the affected limb with a sharp instrument, then applying herbs that acted as antibiotics. Vogel (1970:192) suggests that this was one of the commonest surgical practices among Aboriginal North Americans. Amputation was also known, in instances where limbs were crushed or where irreversible infections such as gangrene had set in.

The degree of sophistication of Aboriginal surgical practices is diffi-cult to ascertain. However, two examples demonstrate that at least some surgeons operated with great skill. Morice (1900–1) has described the manner in which Dene surgeons removed cataracts by carefully scrap-ing the surface of the eyeball with a sharp instrument. He reports that they were usually quite successful at this. Kidd (1946) has described cases of trepanation of skulls, as found in some British Columbia Indian remains. In these cases, surgical openings were made in the skull using some type of instrument, for reasons that still remain somewhat unclear. While Kidd postulates that patients may have sought the release of 'demons' enclosed within the skull, it is more likely that the theory behind the operation was not unlike that for bloodletting: some malig-nant influence contained within the body was causing problems and needed to be released. At any rate, Kidd (ibid.:514) notes that the sur-geons would have required great skill in carrying out the operation without killing the patient, and that the pain of the operation would have been so great that some kind of local anaesthetic would have been required, in addition to the ability to dress wounds.

In order to undertake surgery of various kinds, well-refined instru-ments would have been required. The archaeological record demon-strates that many stone and bone implements were fashioned for this purpose. For instance, bone was particularly useful for piercing and suturing (with animal sinew as stitching), and cutting instruments and awls were common. Certainly the technology that facilitated the manu-facturing of weapons and tools in general would have been applied to the creation of surgical implements, and much skill and practice would have been required to execute the surgery successfully (Fortuine 1985:36–41). Surgeons might also have been shamans, and highly skilled individuals no doubt gained renown as a result.

GENDER AND THE HEALING TRADITIONS

There exists a widespread belief, among both analysts and some Aborig-inal peoples, that the healing roles were primarily occupied by males. The ubiquitous term 'medicine man' is now part of the vocabulary of many people, both Aboriginal and non-Aboriginal. Part of the problem no doubt stems from a historical record that is based almost exclusively upon the observations of male traders, explorers, and missionaries. Not only were these observers largely unconcerned with female roles in Aboriginal societies, but also, by virtue of their gender, they were no doubt excluded from observing female activities and talking to females.

A close examination of the literature demonstrates that females did, indeed, occupy healing roles, although the poor state of the literature on this topic makes it impossible to determine whether there was a gender balance (e.g., Osgood 1931, 1936; Cruikshank 1979; Hultkrantz 1992).

A good example of the male bias in historical accounts is that of the Earl of Southesk (Southesk 1875:329), who wrote in 1859 of the Saulteaux and other northern Indians that certain herbs were 'known only to the medicine-men, – who are a sort of Masonic brotherhood, consisting of women as well as men ...' The contradiction of a brotherhood with female members was clearly lost on the Earl.

In the fieldnotes for his published study on *The Plains Cree* (1979), which are available at the Saskatchewan Archives Board in Regina, Mandelbaum recorded an incident in which his informant's uncle was unable to 'doctor' an ill young man:

They got an old woman to do it. I peeked in through a hole in the tipi. She was naked save for a breech clout. Her arms and legs were painted with horizontal lines. She made a big fire in the tipi. I watched her pick out of the fire something that looked like a section of gun barrel. It was red hot. All of a sudden it disappeared. She kept on rattling and soon reached around to her back and she had it again. One side was cool and she dropped it into a cup of water. The water steamed. She picked up a gun screw from the fire and did just the same thing, dropping it into another cup of water. Her husband was beating the drum. She blew all over the young man. She took the two pieces of metal out. They disappeared. Then she stood away from the sick man and sucked. The young man had to be held down so powerful was her sucking. (Mandelbaum 1935)

This account demonstrates that this medicine woman was fully versed in the techniques of sucking and sleight-of-hand. McLean (1889:27), in a late-nineteenth-century account, suggested that in some Aboriginal groups medicine women were particularly feared because of their power. And among the Inuit, evidence suggests that both males and female occupied shamanistic roles as 'angakkuq.' A survey of the literature has led Oosten (1986; see also Williamson 2000) to conclude that, as for Indians, ambiguity also exists with respect to the existence of specialized gender roles among the Inuit. Oosten (1986:128) concludes that 'The angakkuq has to cross the ideological boundaries between life and death, man and spirits, human beings and game to maintain or restore the religious quarter. From this point of view it may be that it is essential that his being a man or a woman is indifferent. When his soul leaves his body to explore the world of the dead or to recapture a lost soul his gender is no longer of importance. The soul itself is neither male nor female.'

Among some Northwest Coast groups, women also were able to assume healing roles, although it has been suggested that certain limitations were placed upon them. Kelm (1998) has suggested that young girls were often watched very closely to prevent premarital sexual relations, and that this made it more difficult for them to attain the necessary solitude to acquire the spiritual powers necessary to healing, usually through vision questing. A similar situation may have existed among some Plains groups, such as the Blackfoot, where women were more likely to obtain spiritual power through dreams than through vision quests (Lux 2001). Mature women, because of the spiritual power associated with menstruation, were sometimes considered too powerful to engage in healing and had to wait for menopause before becoming active (Kelm 1998).

There is, therefore, no concrete evidence in the literature that there were systematic gender limitations on any of the healing roles. Common knowledge today would suggest that women were more likely to be herbalists, and men shamans, but there is no real evidence to support this. If anything, it is possible that it was the men who were largely frozen out of at least one important medical role, that of midwife, and we are unaware of any evidence that suggests men had access to this role.

The overwhelming male bias in reports on Aboriginal medicine may be seen best, perhaps, in the almost total lack of details on childbirth practices, despite the fact that many non-Aboriginal women frequently availed themselves of the services of an Aboriginal midwife, at least in the early years before extensive biomedical services were available. Europeans seemed to have adopted the overly romantic notion that Aboriginal women experienced relatively painless, complication-free births, perhaps because the male writers generally were not witnesses to births (Lux 2001). Nevertheless, it is evident that some women were highly skilled birth attendants, and that a variety of surgical practices and herbal medicines could be called upon as needed.

THE ASSAULT ON ABORIGINAL HEALING TRADITIONS

The traditional medical systems of Canada's Aboriginal peoples were subjected to a variety of oppressive measures, particularly between 1880 and the mid-twentieth century. Undertaken by government and the churches (the latter with government support), for the most part these measures were not aimed at medical practices per se but rather at elements of Aboriginal spiritual and social life that were deemed by these agents to be prohibitive of assimilation. However, as noted previously in this chapter, Aboriginal medical systems were intertwined with other aspects of religion and culture, and hence an attack on the latter constituted an attack on the former. In this section, we will briefly detail the assault on two prominent Aboriginal traditions: the potlatch and the Sun Dance.

The potlatch was an integral part of the cultures of most Northwest Coast Indian societies. These societies were based on complex systems of status and rank, with 'chiefs and nobles' holding titles to large tracts of land in the name of their lineages or 'houses.' The potlatch ceremony was undertaken to signify ascension to a title by an individual, or any other change in the status quo that required witnesses (e.g., a high-status marriage, the raising of a carved pole). Potlatching was a means of validating individual status and responsibility. A key aspect of the potlatch was the distribution of wealth gathered by the potlatch sponsor and his supporters. Blankets and food items were popular 'give-aways' during the late nineteenth century. The ceremony served to redistribute wealth, and a family that appeared to impoverish itself at its own potlatch would benefit by being guests at others. The potlatch also enabled individuals and families to recount their histories and reaffirm their hereditary rights; hence, the potlatch served as an important institution reaffirming the oral tradition and history of the people (McMillan 1995).

There was no specific medical function to the potlatch, but the attack on it by government and missionaries had a diffuse effect on various aspects of Northwest Coast healing. The potlatch came to be viewed by the government as a 'foolish, wasteful and demoralizing custom' as early as the 1870s (R. Fisher 1977:206). To an extent, the objection related to the fact that some Northwest Coast groups had escalated potlatching to the point of destroying, rather than giving away, the various goods in a form of competition. This was the result, in part, of the deadly effects of epidemic diseases that had decimated the villages and blurred lines of ascension. The government was also prodded by the missionaries, who viewed the potlatch as heathen and an obstacle to the Christianization of the Indians. The views of the Rev. Cornelius Brant (Methodist), writing in the 1880s, were likely typical: 'The Church and school cannot flourish where the "Potlatching" holds sway ... Thus all the objects or advantages to be secured by good government are frustrated by this very demoralizing custom; and as the wards of the Government the native tribes should be prevented by judicious counsel and governmental interference, that is by some kind of paternal restraint from indulging in their Potlatching feasts' (cited in LaViolette 1973:42). Brant then added, somewhat prophetically, 'Of course my knowledge of the Indian character suggests the danger of attempting coercive measures.'

In 1883, Prime Minister John A. Macdonald issued a 'proclamation,' stating that the potlatch was 'the parent of numerous vices which eat out the heart of the people. It produces indigence, thriftlessness, and habits of roaming about which prevent home association and is inconsistent with all progress' (cited in LaViolette 1973:38). The proclamation called upon the lieutenant-governor of British Columbia to 'use his best efforts for the suppression' of the potlatch. This was followed in 1884 by an amendment of the Indian Act of 1880, representative of the first attempt to outlaw an Indian ceremonial. As Section 3 of the amendment stated, 'Every Indian or other person who engages in or assists in celebrating the Indian festival known as the "Potlach" [sic] or in the Indian dance known as the "Tamanawas" [sic] is guilty of a misdemeanour and shall be liable to imprisonment for a term of not more than six or not less than two months in any gaol or other place of confinement; and any Indian or other person who encourages, either directly or indirectly, an Indian or Indians to get up such a festival or dance, or to celebrate the same, or who shall assist in the celebration of same is guilty of a like offense, and shall be liable to the same punishment.'[8]

Unlike the potlatch, the 'tamananawas' had more direct relevance to Aboriginal medicine. The term 'tamananawas' referred to shamanistic acts, including healing and ritual cannibalism (Cole and Chaikin 1990:12). It was the ritual cannibalism (involving dogs, corpses, and living individuals), including ritual biting,[9] that was offensive to some non-Aboriginals. Both the Indian agents and the missionaries sought to have this ceremony eliminated.

The 'Potlatch Law' proved to be difficult to enforce, with the federal and British Columbia governments somewhat confused over jurisdiction. Efforts to have the law repealed began as early as 1887, when the Indians of the Cowichin agency sent a petition to the government (LaViolette 1973:57). In 1886, the relevant section was repealed and substituted with a new section making it an indictable offence to participate in or encourage 'any Indian festival, dance or other celebration of which the giving away or paying or giving back of money, goods or articles of any sort forms a part, or is a feature.'[10] This new section broadened the prohibition, however, by outlawing 'any celebration or dance of which the wounding or mutilation of the dead or living body of any human being or animal forms a part or is a feature.' This new clause was directed at both the tamananawas of the Northwest Coast Indians and the Sun Dance of the Plains Indians. The law in some form or another remained on the statutes until the 1951 revision of the Indian Act.

According to Jilek (1982b:14), the potlatch law was used to suppress the Coast Salish healing ceremonial known as 'spirit dancing,' and some older people recalled the prosecutions that ensued. The result was a decline in spirit dancing to the point where dancers from neighbouring groups (especially from the United States) had to be brought in to assist in its revival in the late 1960s.

The Sun Dance of the Plains Indians was also subjected to both legislative action and formal discouragement by government and the churches. This dance (also known as the 'Thirst Dance') was a multi-day ceremony held in the summer to honour the sun and other spirits. Critics were offended by a number of aspects of the dance and related activities. For one thing, the dance took as many as four days to perform, and related activities took many more days before and after. Indeed, the Sun Dance was an important social occasion, and Indians from many different tribes and regions often attended. Furthermore, government agents held the view that dancing was not compatible with a settled, agricultural way of life (E. Titley 1986:165). Second, the dance was viewed repulsively by some non-Aboriginals because of the practice of piercing the flesh on the chest of some dancers as a means of offering more suffering to the Great Spirit. Leather thongs were tied to sticks pushed through the skin and tied at the other end to the central Sun Dance lodge pole. The dancers then attempted to pull the skewers out by straining against the rope.

At first, the government was uncertain as to how to proceed to terminate the Sun Dance. One approach was to implement the 'pass system,' wherein individuals wishing to leave the reserve for any reason were required to obtain the written permission of the Indian agent. This system was conceived in 1885, in part in reaction to the 'rebellion' in the Northwest, but was never formally or legally adopted by the government. As Barron (1988) has noted, it could not be legally enforced, and while the North-West Mounted Police and the Indian agents worked together to enforce the system as a way of reducing the Indians' mobility on the western prairies, they were not very successful. Sun Dances continued to be held, sometimes in open defiance of the pass system, and in other instances more covertly in remote areas.

The 1886 amendment to the Indian Act, described above, was a clear legislative attempt to ban at least some elements of the Sun Dance. And, as with the potlatch, Indian agents were advised to proceed cautiously. Dancing per se was not illegal, but piercing and extensive give-aways were. There were some arrests; the number is unknown, but use of summary conviction facilitated the legal process.[11] Threats of fines and jail sentences were commonplace. Some individuals requested permission to hold the dances, with variable success. For instance, in 1918 the Onion Lake (Saskatchewan) band wrote to Duncan Campbell Scott for such permission, suggesting that the dance was in reaction to the Spanish influenza epidemic, which had been wreaking havoc on the band. They were refused, but attempted to hold the dance anyway, only to be thwarted at the last moment by the police. In contrast, a dance on the Blackfoot reserve in 1921 was allowed to proceed, with a police officer in attendance and without the piercing (Lux 1992, 2001).

A further amendment to the Indian Act, in 1906, made it illegal for Indians to leave the reserve to participate in any 'Indian' dances or to participate in exhibitions without permission.[12] In the years following, a new problem arose for the government: they believed that the large dance camps were also being used for political purposes as Indians began to organize politically (E. Titley 1986:177). Police patrols and police intervention increased at dances after 1921. In effect, the participants were subjected to harassment, as directed in the following circular issued by Duncan Campbell Scott in 1921:

Sir – It is observed with alarm that the holding of dances by the Indians on their reserves is on the increase, and that these practices tend to disorganize the efforts which the Department is putting forth to make them self-supporting. I have, therefore, to direct you to use your utmost endeavours to dissuade the Indians from excessive indulgence in the practice of dancing. You should suppress any dances which cause waste of time, interfere with the occupations of the Indians, unsettle them for serious work, injure their health or encourage them in sloth and idleness. You should also dissuade, and, if possible, prevent them from leaving their reserves for the purpose of attending fairs, exhibitions, etc., when their absence would result in their own farming and other interests being neglected. It is realized that reasonable amusement and recreation should be enjoyed by Indians, but they should not be allowed to dissipate their energies and abandon themselves to demoralizing amusements. By the use of tact and firmness you can obtain control and keep it, and this obstacle to continued progress will then disappear.

To the consternation of the government, Indians began to seek legal advice on the question of holding dances, and they were advised that dances could be held without breaking the law. And they continued to ignore the laws prohibiting the dances and their absences from reserves (E. Titley 1986:178–9). Like the potlatch law, the regulations affecting the Sun Dance and other dancing and religious activities were finally eliminated in the 1951 Indian Act.

The legacy of these repressive measures is still with us today. While there was a time when Aboriginal medicine was open to non-Aboriginals, by the mid-twentieth century Aboriginal peoples had become quite guarded about their knowledge and activities, and the notion that healing and other spiritual activities were 'secret' became pervasive. Clearly, this is a reaction to very real fears in the past that individuals would be prosecuted if they undertook certain ceremonials; it is also likely that the specific laws against the potlatch and the Sun Dance were perceived as laws against many other Aboriginal traditions as well. Indeed, there are many stories in the west of sweat lodges being prevented or disrupted by government agents. Harassment of various kinds continued through the twentieth century; for instance, Kelm (1998:93) described a Kispiox healer who was charged with fraud in the 1920s, after employing the common blowing practice to introduce his power into a patient. In recent years, some healers have begun to discuss their medicine more publicly, the result of the progressive inclusion of Aboriginal healing into clinical settings along with the emergence of a more widespread tolerance and acceptance of a variety of treatment modalities often labelled 'complementary' or 'alternative.' Nevertheless, some individuals who take on more formal roles as traditional practitioners within the contemporary biomedical system may still be chastised by others. These issues will be taken up later in the book.

CONCLUSION

Aboriginal healing traditions, like the cultures themselves, were very complex at the time of first contact with Europeans. It has been possible to examine only a few aspects of these traditions, and we warn against overgeneralization. Furthermore, it is not at all clear precisely which aspects of these healing traditions have survived to the present day, and in what form. However, we do know that Aboriginal medical traditions continued, despite government repression and the introduction of early European medical services in the 'New World,' a topic to which we now turn.

6

Traders, whalers, missionaries, and medical aid

The strong healing traditions of the Aboriginal peoples were not easily pushed aside with the arrival of Europeans and their own medicine in North America. This was due, in part, to the relative lack of sophistication of European medicine (especially in the colonial context), as well as the fact that the delivery of health care services was poorly organized in the first centuries after contact. Indeed, the delivery of health services to Aboriginal people prior to Confederation was primarily on an ad hoc basis by traders and missionaries. As noted in a previous chapter, from the time of contact the Indians and Inuit in what would become Canada suffered somewhat from various epidemic diseases, such as smallpox, influenza, and measles. Much of the rudimentary medical care they received from Europeans had as its intent the rescue of as many disease victims as possible. Although much aid was provided for humanitarian reasons, not all of the motives of missionaries and traders were altruistic. Diseased (and dead) Aboriginal people were a burden on local accounts and were not economically or spiritually productive: they could neither hunt nor trap, and although their souls could be 'saved' on death's doorstep, they certainly could not be truly converted. Furthermore, after the formation of Canada in 1867, the federal government slowly came to see the obvious advantages of allowing the traders and missionaries to continue to deliver medical services.

THE FUR TRADERS

Even though most European expeditions to the northern New World included a physician, it is evident that the skills of these individuals were questionable. While traders and whalers often had possession of basic medical kits or 'chests' from which they could dispense medicines to their employees or charges, very few had any actual medical training. Brett (1969:521) concludes that such individuals likely had little time to treat Aboriginal patients anyway, being overburdened with the demands of treating the ship's crew. Indeed, many crew members suffered extensively from nutritional deficiency diseases such as scurvy, as well as from the effects of cold exposure, including frostbite. As a result, 'instead of the European bringing medical attention to the Eskimo, the latter ministered to the explorer in matters of health by instructing him in the principles of Arctic survival and in preventing scurvy by the simple expedient of eating fresh raw meat or, in the more southerly latitudes, consuming a distillate of the bark of the spruce tree' (Brett 1969:522).

The story of Hudson's Bay Company (HBC) trader and doctor William Todd provides an excellent example of the ad hoc care provided by the company to northern Indians. As Ray (1984) has well documented, Todd's career spanned thirty-five years, from 1816 to 1851, during which time he served as both a trader and a medical doctor, becoming 'the most famous surgeon in the western interior of Canada before 1850' (Ray 1984:13).

In addition to his medical work for company personnel, including HBC Governor George Simpson, Todd played an important role in reducing the effects of disease among the Indian population in western Canada. When, in 1837, it became known that smallpox was afflicting some Indian groups along the Missouri River, Todd commenced a vaccination program using a relatively new cowpox vaccine that had been sent to Canada by the HBC in London; this represents the first use of this type of vaccine in western Canada. Todd even trained an Indian to administer the vaccine to his family and the others in his camp. According to Ray (1984:17), Todd's initiative proved highly successful, and many Indians avoided the dreaded disease. Todd's use of the vaccine was somewhat controversial; not only did he initiate vaccination before confirmation that the disease was, in fact, smallpox, but medical science at the time was not completely convinced of the efficacy of the cowpox vaccine that Todd used. Western medical science in the early 1800s, when Todd entered the service of the HBC, was still rudimentary, with the causes of many diseases and the process of immunization not well understood (Ray 1975:12).[1] Nevertheless, Todd's actions contributed to the development of an 1838 policy directive by HBC Governor George Simpson in London that suggested the basic motives behind treating the Indians: 'We have long endeavoured to impress on the [traders] the importance of introducing vaccination ... both as a measure of humanity ... and with a view to the welfare of the Business ... but we fear that sufficient attention has not been paid ... and that consequences may be very calamitous. We now forward to each of the Factories Packets of vaccine matter, and we desire that it be distributed throughout the Country, and that the Gentlemen in charge of Posts exert their utmost influence ... to induce [the Natives] to submit to inoculation' (cited in T.K. Young 1988b:36).

While his medical endeavours may have been appreciated, Todd was considered by the company to be only an average trader, and hence unworthy of promotion. Indeed, when in 1849 he requested a promotion and remuneration for services rendered as a medical doctor, he was denied on the grounds that 'every medical man in the service is bound to give his professional aid to the Company's Servants and Indians when there is occasion for such aid, although there may be no stipulation to that effect either in his contract when he enters the Service, or in the Deed which he signs on receiving a Commission' (Ray 1984:23). Despite the fact that Todd's medical skills were significant in attracting a loyal Indian following for the company trade, and that only healthy Indians could effectively hunt and trap, his efforts were obviously considered secondary to the ultimate aims of the company as a business.

In general, the medical services that the traders for companies such as the HBC made available to Indians concentrated on groups near the posts themselves, or Indians arriving at the posts from inland. HBC employees were directed to provide aid in times of need and became involved in epidemic control in the late 1700s, not least because 'any death among the hunters or their families, or any disruption in their normal routine, threatened the profits of the Company's stockholders' (F.P. Hackett 2004:579). The desire to protect fur supplies and trade, coupled with humanitarian concerns cloaked in paternalistic attitudes, led early on to practices for preventing the spread of disease, such as quarantine (F.P. Hackett 2004). The 'Homeguard Indians,' in particular, benefited from their proximity to the posts. These northern Indians, usually Cree, Ojibwa, or Chipewyan, congregated around the posts and, over time, became more or less full-time residents. They worked for the traders as hunters and provisioners, as well as labourers. When illness struck them, they were unable to fulfil their roles in the fur trade; furthermore, their suffering was plainly evident to the traders. Indeed, a 1683 directive from the London Committee of the HBC informed Governor Henry Sergeant at the Albany post that the policy of the company was to 'treate the Indians with Justice and humanity ...' (cited in Van Kirk 1980:14). At most coastal posts, listed among the 'officer' class could usually be found a 'surgeon,' whose services were made available to company personnel and Indians alike (Brown 1980:28). As the trade moved inland in subsequent years, only the largest posts were likely to have physicians or apothecaries, although all posts had a dispensary of medicines (T.K. Young 1988b:100).

The availability of medical services (however crude) at the posts, as well as food supplies, was important for the Homeguard Indians, who, according to Van Kirk (1980:16), 'came to look upon the [HBC] Company posts as welfare stations which would provide succour, especially for the crippled, sick or starving' (cf Brown 1980:19; Thistle 1986:65). Food supplies, such as flour and oatmeal, were routinely provided to the local Indians by the traders (Brown 1980:19; Krech 1983b:132). Indeed, trader Andrew Graham described in the late 1700s in self-laudatory terms the provision of such services: 'The hungry are fed, the naked clothed, and the sick furnished with medicines, and attended by the factory surgeon; all this gratis ... I appeal to any gentleman of probity and justice, whether a method so humane, kind, and benevolent, was ever adopted by any people connected with Indians' (Williams 1969:327).

In contrast, Francis and Morantz (1983:93) have suggested that the provision of food supplies to the Indians of eastern James Bay during times of scarcity 'was not an act of charity.' They continue: 'For one thing, it was in the traders' interest to keep the hunters alive and healthy and able to continue gathering furs. But more importantly, it may have been an act of compensation, since starvation among the homeguard was exacerbated by the company itself in its desire to have them present at the spring goose hunt.' Furthermore, these authors present evidence in one instance of an HBC official in 1842 who felt compelled to feed starving Indians because 'I imagine I would be censured did I permit them to Starve under the immediate eye of our Pastor' (1983:163).

As we saw in chapter 5, many of the early traders and explorers had little of a positive nature to say about the medical skills and knowledge of Aboriginal·people. The Earl of Southesk, writing of his travels throughout the west in 1859–60, wrote of the Saulteaux of the Fort Pelly area: 'The Indians are not so healthy a race as is sometimes imagined, stomach and chest complaints frequently occurring, and the women being subject to various female ailments that are common in Europe. As physicians their own "medicine-men" appear to be useless. When an Indian is ill he generally applies at the nearest Fort, where he obtains good medicine, and medical advice if the Company's officer-in-charge has studied the subject, as he often has. Food and shelter too are sometimes given him until health is restored' (Southesk 1875:329). Unclear from this passage, of course, is the extent to which Indians may have been selectively using the traders' medical assistance, perhaps for certain conditions or diseases, or after unsuccessful treatments by their own healers. Alexander Mackenzie, for one, noted that the Cree often sought European medicines as trade items (Williams 1969:327), and these no doubt formed a component of intertribal trading networks.

Fur traders also made efforts to assist the Indians when afflicted by the various epidemic diseases, but their efforts met with mixed, and marginal, success. Thistle (1986:62) has documented the intrusion of smallpox into the Cumberland House area in the early 1780s, noting that many Indians came to the post for medical assistance but that there was little the traders could do. F.P. Hackett (2004) notes that as the epidemic approached Hudson Bay, systematic efforts were made by HBC employees to prevent it from spreading farther. Two subsequent epidemics, in 1824 and 1838, were less virulent as a result of HBC efforts to vaccinate Indians, including the training of Indians and Métis in the methods of vaccination to ensure as wide coverage as possible (Thistle 1986:62). Attempts were also made at isolating non-infected new arrivals to posts. The effects of the epidemics on the company were great, however, and Thistle (ibid.) cites one trader who lamented in 1782 that 'Indeed it is hard labour to keep the House in fuel and bury the dead.' Nevertheless, traders did often collect debts from deceased Indians (through their families), and some even took furs left as sacrifices to 'the good Spirit' by Cree Indians (ibid.:63).

With respect to smallpox, some Indians apparently believed the disease to be so deadly that little hope for recovery was held out for those who contracted it. As William Walker, writing in 1781, stated, 'They think when they are once taken bad they need not look for any recovery. So the person that's bad turns [so] feeble that he cannot walk, they leave them behind when they're pitching away, and so the poor Soul perishes' (Rich 1951: 265). Malnourishment of the sick clearly contributed to their demise, according to Ray (1974:106), as did the practice of jumping into cold lakes and rivers when feverish.

It is clear that the HBC's hiring of Indians led to the development of the Homeguard Indians, with the result that areas around the posts became more heavily populated, at least on a seasonal basis, leading to periodic famine and, of course, the spread of disease. However, company policy must be seen as distinct from the actions of the traders themselves, and it would be wrong to suggest that the company's employees were always focused solely on company business in providing food and medical assistance. As Brown (1980) and Van Kirk (1980) have documented, there were many stable relationships formed between traders and Indians, and hence assistance given to Indians and mixed-bloods often involved assisting kinfolk and loved ones. Indeed, Van Kirk (1980:76–7) has suggested that Indian women were particularly likely to receive assistance from the HBC and North West Company (NWC) traders, and she describes one case of a Carrier woman nursed back to health by NWC traders after being beaten by her husband. When she regained her health, she was allowed to remain at the post, as it became evident that her family no longer wanted her. In another documented case, Van Kirk (1980:17) details the story of an Indian woman left at Albany in 1769 who was 'exceeding ill.' She, too was nursed back to health by the HBC traders, and her children cared for, until the following spring when all four were able to rejoin her husband. While the traders' attitudes towards the women may have been more favourable than towards the men because of their 'bourgeois European notions of how women should be treated' (Van Kirk 1980:17), the fact remains that individual traders' motives extended beyond simply ensuring a profitable business.

Alexander Mackenzie, a Scottish trader who worked for the North West Company, embarked on a journey to the Arctic in 1789. His journals of his explorations in 1789, and again in 1793, demonstrate a willingness to treat sick Indians he encountered. In July of 1793, he described one encounter on the west coast (perhaps a Bella Coola Indian); his description of Indian medicine is ill-informed and unflattering:

At an early hour this morning I was again visited by the chief, in company with his son. The former complained of a pain in his breast; to relieve his suffering, I gave him a few drops of Turlington's Balsam[2] on a piece of sugar; and I was rather surprised to see him take it without the least hesitation. When he had taken my medicine, he requested me to follow him, and conducted me to a shed, where several people were assembled round a sick man, who was another of his sons. They immediately uncovered him, and showed me a violent ulcer in the small of his back, in the foulest state that can be imagined. One of his knees was also afflicted in the same manner. This unhappy man was reduced to a skeleton, and, from his appearance, was drawing near to an end of his pains. They requested that I would touch him, and his father was very urgent with me to administer medicine; but he was in such a dangerous state, that I thought it prudent to yield no further to the importunities than to give the sick person a few drops of Turlington's balsam in some water. (Mackenzie 1971:331–2)

Undaunted, the 'native physicians' took up the challenge of healing the ulcer victim. After 'they blew on him, and then whistled,' 'they also put their fore fingers doubled into his mouth, and spouted water from their own with great violence into his face.' Then, according to Mackenzie, 'they laid him upon a clear spot, and kindled a fire against his back, when the physician began to scarify the ulcer with a very blunt instrument, the cruel pain of which operation the patient bore with incredible resolution' (1971:332–3). This represents an early example of the simultaneous utilization of both European and traditional Indian medicine, a practice that is discussed in greater detail in chapter 9.

The role of traders in the delivery of medical services continued after Confederation, particularly in remote northern areas. There are numerous accounts of HBC employees sending out supplies to families on traplines during the 1918 influenza pandemic, although it has also been argued that inadequate medical care to Aboriginal communities led to a high death rate during the outbreak (Lux 1992). Writing of the early twentieth century, Felton (1959:36) described HBC medical services in glowing, uncritical terms: 'Good medicine chests and surgical implements supplied by the [HBC] Company – and the character of the men they employed – took care of all emergencies and anyone who needed treatment received it.' Noting that nursing stations had begun to supplant the traders' medical role, Felton (ibid.:37) suggested that the latter were relieved to have the 'burden' lifted, having 'shouldered it willingly but often with misgivings.' When influenza broke out at an arctic post in 1928, a company ship organized a 'soup kitchen' and provided blankets to sick Indians; under the supervision of the HBC physician, HBC staff (and some members of the Revillon Frères missionary society) 'tended the sick day and night for two weeks' (ibid.). An outbreak of cerebrospinal meningitis at Cape Dorset in 1943 was met by the delivery of an inadequate supply of sulpha drugs, all that was available at an HBC post some twenty miles away. While awaiting a renewed supply of the drug (which took a month to arrive), the post manager quarantined some Inuit and, travelling by dogsled with an Inuk trapper, did what he could to help. Overall, fifty cases were diagnosed, among which there were twenty deaths. Of course, many of the traders themselves lacked medical training, and if there were no company physicians available, they were forced to resort to what could be referred to as laypersons' knowledge. Hence, Felton (ibid.:38) describes the case of a trader at Bathurst Inlet who, unable to diagnose a problem with an Inuit girl, gave her Oxo (beef bouillon) and rum; she died after two weeks. As Felton notes, these traders often received a 'Post Manager's Medical Guide,' describing common ailments and treatments, and a first aid course (ibid.); otherwise, they received no specialized medical training.

The interest of the HBC in the health of Aboriginal people remained throughout the first half of the twentieth century, despite the fact that the federal government's responsibilities for Indians were clear under the British North America Act. In 1925, the company formed a 'Development Department,' including as one of its responsibilities the welfare of Aboriginal people (Ray 1990:218–19). One project entailed the development of cottage industries. Indeed, Col. E.L. Stone, medical superintendent in the Department of Indian Affairs, 'gave his entire approval to this and stated that his Department was really in need of the Company's help, and in fact had only the Company to turn to' (cited in ibid.:219). With respect to the company's plan to distribute cod liver oil and meal to the Indians, Stone 'stated his desire of joining us in this and obtaining the product from the company for distribution amongst those Indians with whom the Company was not in contact' (cited in ibid.:220).

The head of the HBC's Development Department, Charles Townsend, convened a meeting in 1927 with Dr Frederick Banting (co-discoverer of insulin) to discuss Aboriginal health issues. Banting agreed with Townsend's view that malnutrition was the key reason for high infection rates of Indians with diseases such as tuberculosis and influenza. Banting informed Townsend of a similar program of improving the health of farm labourers in Central America that had had the effect of reducing production costs to the companies involved. Reports authored in 1926 by Drs Stone and Wall of the Department of Indian Affairs strongly advocated for reform to the trapping industry as a measure to improve the health of northern Indians; copies of these reports were submitted to Townsend, for whom they were of obvious interest (Stone 1926; Wall 1926). Ray (1990:220) notes that, by 1928, the HBC was distributing vitamin supplements, powdered milk, and antiseptic to Indians. However, for a variety of economic reasons, by the end of the 1930s the HBC was no longer realizing returns on its labours in the area of medical services to Indians, and the company began to curtail its activities. Nevertheless, as Ray (ibid.:221) suggests, the HBC's role in providing medical services and food to Indians laid 'the groundwork for the modern state welfare system so prevalent in the north today.'

While the HBC had provided medical services and relief to Indians prior to Confederation as a means of retaining a productive and loyal coterie of trappers and hunters, after Confederation the company attempted to convince the federal government to take over these responsibilities; Indian loyalty was no longer assured, and many were trading with rival companies and individuals. However, the government responded by channelling services through other trading companies as well as missionary societies, further undermining the company's tenuous hold on the Indians (Ray 1990:227). As a result, some post managers were reluctant to surrender their relief role. The federal government, in general, was apprehensive about taking on the responsibility of providing relief to the Indians, in part out of fear of costs, but also out of concern that Indians would become dependent wards. Hence, the Indians were continuously bounced between the company and the federal government (a position they would subsequently occupy between the federal and provincial governments). The HBC had little choice but to assist the Indians, through its Development Department, even knowing that such efforts were unlikely to buy Indian loyalty. Ray (ibid.) states unequivocally that 'the northern natives were better off with the company than with government bureaucrats.' But by the end of the Second World War, the federal government's involvement in Indian relief and medical care would begin to dominate.

THE WHALERS

Along the northern coasts, contact between Aboriginal inhabitants and Europeans frequently occurred in conjunction with whaling activities. The effects of the introduction of diseases for these Aboriginal peoples have been described in an earlier chapter. Not surprisingly, the whalers offered periodic medical assistance to those Aboriginals, primarily Inuit, with whom they had sustained contact.

The journal of whaling captain George Comer provides some insight into medical services made available to the Inuit. Comer was the master of an American whaling schooner operating outside the reach of British and Canadian law in the high Arctic between 1903 and 1905. Ship's masters were often called upon to handle a variety of medical problems afflicting crew members, and they were normally equipped with a standard kit of medicines and surgical instruments, though few had any real medical training (Ross 1984: 100, n8). Doctors were also occasionally assigned to whaling expeditions. Although Comer's journal notes occasional diseases affecting the Inuit they encountered, there is little indication of aid provided to any but the crew, with the exception of Inuit working for the whalers. These, it seems, received a great deal of medical attention and were treated as if they were ship's crew. For instance, a 1904 entry describes the return of some Inuit families to the temporary ocean-side camp: 'Two families of our natives came back today. One of the women – Shoofly – has a heavy cold on her lungs with quite a fever, had to be helped off the sled and on board the vessel. The doctor from the steamer *Arctic* has been over twice and is now taking care of her' (Ross 1984:151–2). Over the next two and a half weeks, her progress was periodically charted in Comer's journal. Clearly, she was thought of highly, since she was visited twice daily by the doctor and was given malted milk and scarce oranges until she was able to return to her family's igloo on shore.

Comer's journal also notes that he provided 'sulphur and molasses' to many of the Inuit suffering from 'the itch' (Ross 1984:183) and documents the assistance provided to an Inuk named 'Ben,' who was slowly dying despite medical assistance. The latter situation was, apparently, difficult for Comer, as this man had previously saved Comer's life (ibid.:191).

The journal's introduction also remarks that the Inuit provided some assistance to the whalers. The fresh meat they supplied was seen by whalers such as Comer as essential to preventing scurvy (Ross 1984:18). In this sense, the illness of Inuit working for the whalers threatened not only the whalers' economic fortunes but their physical health as well.

THE MISSIONARIES

Like the traders and whalers, missionaries were among the first Europeans to make sustained contact with Aboriginal people in Canada. Unlike their commercially oriented European colleagues, however, they hoped to convince the Aboriginal people they encountered to undertake radical changes to their cultures and ways of life – or, in a word, to become Christian. Inevitably, missionaries found it necessary to provide medical services to Aboriginal inhabitants, from a humanitarian perspective as well as in the hope of attracting new converts. The historical record suggests that, for a variety of reasons, the missionaries and Indians entered into conflict over the issues of religion, disease, and treatment.

Both Bailey (1969) and Trigger (1985) have documented how Indians in eastern Canada frequently established a connection between the missionaries and their remonstrations on the one hand, and disease and the death of Indians on the other. Baptism, in particular, was seen as both a possible cure for disease and, by some Algonquians and Iroquoians, as the cause of disease. As Bailey (1969:81) writes, 'Of one thing the Indians were certain: the virulent diseases from which they suffered were the direct result of contact with the Europeans. Moreover, it was useless for the priests to say that baptism was not the cause of the abnormally high death rate. They were baptized and they were dying.'

Among the Hurons, the Jesuits came to be seen not only as the source of disease but as great and powerful sorcerers. Trigger (1985:246) notes that the various elements of baptism, such as the baptismal water, were seen by the Indians as charms used against their Indian victims. They were seen to have other powers as well, powers that could cause illness among the people. Fear of the Jesuits increased, and some groups resorted to offering gifts to the 'Black Robes' to convince them to stop killing Indians. On the other hand, one Montagnais shaman, noting that the Jesuits did not suffer from the diseases, believed the source of their power to lie in their black socks, and accordingly he recommended the wearing of such to an Indian patient (Bailey 1969:81).

Aboriginal people were quite clearly able to draw the connection between the arrival of missionaries and the development of deadly diseases, although the missionaries were not the sole sources of disease. Nevertheless, they were often viewed as part of the problem, as well as part of the solution (through their offering of medical assistance and religious rites). As early as 1637, for instance, the Huron council repeatedly discussed administering the death penalty to the Jesuits (Grant 1984:28). Well known to students of Canadian history are the cases of Jesuits Brébeuf and Lalemant, who in 1649 were captured by the Iroquois while ministering to the Huron, and who were subsequently killed by Huron who had themselves earlier been captured and adopted by the Iroquois. These Huron, according to Trigger (1985:268), regarded the Jesuits as sorcerers who had caused the destruction of their people. But the execution of missionaries by Indians was not restricted to the east. According to Southesk, writing in 1859 in the Fort Pelly area of Saskatchewan, among the Saulteaux, 'A few years ago a Roman Catholic priest was killed near this place by the same tribe. Persuaded by his exhortations during a previous visit, the Indians had allowed him to baptize all their children. An epidemic broke out soon afterwards, destroying most of these infants, and the superstitious savages attributed their loss to the mystic rites of the Church. Ignorant of what happened, the priest after a while returned to his flock in the wilderness, but, instead of welcomes, these lost sheep received their shepherd with blows, and added him to the company of martyrs' (Southesk 1875:342).

Certainly, some Indians were perplexed by the Jesuits' 'zeal for saving souls among the dying' and their apparent apathy towards the living, not an attitude conducive to providing medical services. In the words of one Jesuit, quoted in Bailey (1969:80), 'The joy that one feels when he has baptized a Savage who dies soon afterwards, and flies directly to Heaven to become an Angel, certainly is a joy that surpasses anything that can be imagined.' Trigger also notes that, among the Huron, the Jesuits 'were accused of always talking about death rather than hoping for a sick person's recovery, as any decent Huron would do' (1985:246–7). Trigger (ibid.:254) suggests that, after the major smallpox epidemics had waned (around the mid-1600s in Huron country), the Jesuits 'were anxious to avoid a repetition of what they saw as the apostatizing that had occurred during the smallpox epidemic.'

Since the early missionaries were interested in religious conversion, inevitably they encountered some opposition from the Indians' religious practitioners, who, frequently, were also healers. The traditional healers had no experience with the various epidemic diseases, and were at a distinct disadvantage in a struggle with the missionaries. However, the earliest missionaries found curbing epidemics and restoring the health of sick Indians to be a difficult task. Trigger (1985:246) notes that the Jesuits failed conclusively in their attempts to halt the smallpox epidemic of 1636 by conducting rituals in a kind of competition with the Huron shamans. Furthermore, the failure of traditional healing ceremonies had the effect of occasionally spurring the shamans on to more intense efforts to solicit supernatural assistance, thus demonstrating their power; the fact that each round of disease eventually subsided was a positive, supportive sign (ibid.:248–9).

Jesuit efforts to supplant the shamans by undertaking ceremonies and other activities to produce rain or cure sickness were also not particularly successful (Trigger 1985:252). Bailey (1969:80) describes an incident in 1633 in which Jesuits remonstrated with a Mi'kmaq shaman who had treated an ill child in the traditional manner, and who recommended rest, whereupon they were informed by the shaman, 'That is very good for you people; but, for us, it is thus that we cure our sick.'

European medicines, as introduced by the missionaries, seem to have met with mixed responses. French remedies were, in general, opposed by the Montagnais in the early 1600s. On the other hand, a Jesuit hospital in Quebec saw a large Native patient load in 1640, exhausting their supply of medicines and leading the Mother Superior to note that the Indians had 'no difficulty in taking our medicines, nor in having them-

selves bled' (cited in Bailey 1969:76). Grant (1984:39), for one, is not surprised that some French medicines, and elements of Catholicism, were
accepted by the Indians in eastern Canada, arguing that 'There was
nothing in the principles of native religion to limit access to spiritual
power to a single cult, and borrowing from the religious repertoire of
other tribes was a common practice.' Certainly, being able to deal with
the spirit world was an important part of the early missionaries' acceptance by the Indians, and having medical remedies that appeared to
work was important in validating this supernatural power. But supernatural powers, those that in the view of the Indians allowed the missionaries to heal, could also be used to cause harm and disease. This
explains much of the ambivalence that the historical record suggests
existed with respect to Indian acceptance of the medical assistance and
proselytizing of the missionaries.

The evidence that the traditional medical system did not succumb to
the epidemics is not clear for other groups. Among the Montagnais in
the early 1600s, Bailey (1969:81) states that, 'As the sorcerers were ridi-
culed by the priests, and as the imported diseases grew in dimension,
they were discredited, having been thought to have lost power over the
manitou.'

Missionary success varied from region to region and nation to nation.
As European contact increased and Europeans' power over the Aboriginal peoples was consolidated, mission success increased. This is particularly true of the Indians of the east coast and along the St Lawrence River.
In contrast, Indians farther north and west were less affected, perhaps
because 'the system of native medicine was closely woven into the social
fabric' (Grant 1984:53). However, certainly a different lifestyle also
explains, in part, the reluctance of northern groups such as the Ojibwa
and Cree to accept missionaries and their medicines. Involvement in the
fur trade reinforced the high degree of mobility of these Indians, and
except for the 'Homeguard' who began to settle around the posts, most of
the Indians remained mobile and out of effective reach of the missionaries for much of the year. The southern Indians, especially the Huron and
Iroquois, lived in villages and followed a horticultural lifestyle; it was
comparatively easier for the missionaries to develop a congregation. The
Anglicans, in particular, were subsequently accused of creating 'tobacco
Christians' – that is, nominally converting northern Indians with gifts of
tobacco and other provisions, especially in times of need (ibid.:113). Ultimately, however, by the mid-1800s even the northern Indians began to
accept Christianity, in some instances with a fervour that created a great

deal of competition among various Christian denominations; it was believed (with some accuracy) that the first denomination to reach a group would gain a significant foothold (ibid.:114). However, as we have seen in an earlier chapter, while this may have meant some damage to traditional spirituality and medicines, it certainly did not eliminate them completely.

In Labrador, the establishment of missions in the late 1700s and on into the 1800s provided a source of medical care for the Inuit of the region. The Moravians, in particular, found a foothold in Labrador, and although generally lacking in medical training, nevertheless endeavoured to provide what services they could. Nonetheless, from time to time trained medical personnel were available. For instance, in 1897 the Rev. Paul Hettasch, trained in medicine, established a temporary hospital in Hopedale (Ben-Dor 1966:185). In 1903 a hospital with a resident physician was built at Okak. When Dr Wilfred Grenfell was appointed to examine conditions along the coast of Labrador, he was ultimately brought to declare, 'There can be no question the Moravians have so far saved the native population for Labrador' (cited in ibid.). Grenfell would go on to establish the 'International Grenfell Association,' responsible for medical and educational work in southern Labrador, which by the 1950s was officially responsible for services to both Inuit and settlers. By 1959, there was a nurse stationed at Makovik, and the construction of a nursing station followed in 1961 (ibid.:186).

Missionaries continued to be involved in medical care for Indians up to and after Confederation, combining their concern for the health of the indigenous populations with their religious activities. In British Columbia, for instance, William Duncan successfully assisted many Tsimshian people during a smallpox epidemic in 1862, leading to their widespread conversion (Kelm 1998). In British Columbia as in other parts of the country, mission hospitals came to dominate the landscape, providing a unique and fairly successful means of proselytizing. Lux (2001) describes the active medical assistance provided by Methodist John Maclean on the Blood reserve in Alberta, but even here the people's acceptance of his help seemed to ebb and flow. One area in which missionaries maintained some control over Indian health was with respect to schooling. Residential schools, in particular, saw Indian children held under the missionaries' charge for up to ten months each year. It is apparent that many of these schools actually lacked proper medical facilities and that disease, especially tuberculosis, was rampant.

Overall, the conditions in many schools were appalling. Grant

(1984:180) describes attempts by Anglicans to explain a high mortality rate at their schools for Blackfoot Indians by referring to high overall Indian mortality rates. But the schools were 'drafty and crowded, food scanty and often unappetizing' (ibid.). Part of the problem was the low government grants provided to the mission societies to operate the schools, making it difficult to provide adequate nutritional programs and health services. Many schools were sealed shut to conserve energy. And even the propensity for the schoolmasters to promote participation in brass bands may have led to increased rates of diseases of the pulmonary system (Miller 1989:212).

Dr Peter Bryce, appointed in 1904 as Canada's first medical officer for the Department of Indian Affairs, issued a report in 1907 exposing the poor sanitary conditions that led to high mortality rates in these boarding schools and indicating that in their fifteen-year history 24 per cent of all students who had attended were known to be dead (Bryce 1922:4). Tuberculosis was the main disease that affected residential school students. The report resulted in calls to abandon these schools in favour of reserve-based day schools. This course was opposed by many denominations; indeed, in his 1907 report, Bryce commented that 'Everywhere was too apparent the fear that their [tubercular students'] exclusion might lessen the per capita grant' that the schools received (1907:277). So a plan to deal with the poor health conditions was never executed, in part because of the cost and in part 'because it would have undermined the authority of the churches running the schools' (Grant 1984:193). Nevertheless, after 1945 the trend towards day schools developed. These changes came too late for many Indian children, however, as suggested in the words of Duncan Campbell Scott, deputy minister for Indian Affairs in the second decade of the twentieth century: 'It is quite within the mark to say that fifty per cent of the children who passed through these schools did not live to benefit from the education which they had received therein' (cited in Miller 1989:213). Further, as became publicly evident only in the latter part of the twentieth century, the long-term consequences of the schools included the development of a variety of mental health and social problems, and the emergence of a 'residential school syndrome.'

Under the control of the missionaries, many schools fulfilled multiple purposes, and the children were not the only ones 'educated.' For instance, 'industrial homes' developed in conjunction with many mission hospitals in the Arctic. The first such home was established at Chesterfield Inlet in 1938 by the Roman Catholics, followed within a few years by Anglican hospitals in Pangnirtung and elsewhere. These homes provided care for the elderly and infirm, and taught them handicrafts. Medical care was a part of the services offered, and although the number of patients in any given home rarely exceeded twenty at any one time, the role of such homes was seen as important (Jenness 1972:69).

The missionaries were also responsible for developing the first hospitals throughout much of Canada. Heagerty (1928:143), in his highly romanticized history of medicine in Canada, identified the logical connection between missionization and medical care: 'The hospital is an expression of Christianity. With the dawning of the era of Christianity there arose the desire for the accomplishment of good works, and this found ready expression in the care of the sick and needy, who abounded in every locality ... Little wonder then that, with such a background, the French should have been burning with zeal to establish in Canada a hospital for the care of the sick Indians who were reported to be dying by thousands from diseases.' The first such hospital was established in Quebec in 1639, to be followed in 1644 by a hospital in Montreal. Both were operated by the 'Hospital Nuns,' the Ursulines.

It is difficult to document all of the hospitals that the various missionary societies and church groups developed. Some were simple tent structures, or were combined with other facilities, and lasted for very short periods. But others were of a more permanent nature, and no doubt made a valuable contribution to the delivery of medical services to Aboriginal peoples. Some of these are discussed in the following chapter.

RECIPROCITY IN THE DELIVERY OF MEDICAL SERVICES

The provision of medical services was not entirely unidirectional. In a variety of ways, Indians assisted the traders, whalers, missionaries, and settlers in medical matters. In the early years of contact, scurvy was a particularly pervasive problem. One of the earliest known examples occurred during the winter of 1535 when Jacques Cartier's men experienced a severe bout of scurvy, ameliorated when Iroquoians taught them to concoct a vitamin C-rich drink from white cedar (cited in Trigger 1985:131–2). James Isham, an HBC employee at York Factory in the 1740s, referred to the use of a plant by Indians and traders alike to treat scurvy and a variety of other disorders (Rich 1949:216–17). Decker (1989:45) cites an 1843 case at York Factory in which the Indian women and children gathered cranberries, gooseberries, and currants to help the HBC traders stave off scurvy. Indeed, many deaths from smallpox during the 1780s reduced the number of hunters for the HBC to such an extent that scurvy outbreaks occurred. Other services were provided as well. For instance, Zimmerly (1975:77) notes that in Labrador in the late 1800s, the death of an Inuit woman was particularly mourned by many of the Euro-Canadians because of her active role as a midwife to them. Additional aids, especially various herbal preparations and the treatment of wounds and injuries, were provided as well. Missionaries and settlers also benefited from the Indians' extensive knowledge of herbal remedies, which they used alongside, and in some cases as substitutes for, various European aids (Lux 2001).

THE INTRODUCTION OF ALCOHOL

The introduction of alcohol to Aboriginal people is often associated with the practices of the fur trade, and our discussion of the traders and missionaries would be incomplete if we were not to examine this controversial issue. Aboriginal people in Canada at the time of contact lacked a brewing tradition and had no experience with alcohol. With the introduction of the fur trade, alcohol came to be used as a gift item as well as an item of trade. Its use among the Indians created a variety of health and public safety problems, and put the traders into conflict with the missionaries, who opposed the use of alcohol.

The French fur trade in eastern Canada introduced alcohol as early as the 1670s, and as competition between the English, Dutch, and French traders heated up, alcohol became more prominent. The HBC and other fur trading companies used alcohol in a variety of ways. As Hamer and Steinbring (1980:7) have noted, 'Alcohol was used as an inducement to participate, as a medium of exchange, and as a standard of competitive access.' Presents of alcohol were made to Indians when they arrived at trading posts, and Indians often demanded such, threatening to take their furs to other posts where the alcohol policy was more liberal. According to Ray (1974: 85, 142), lavish gift giving involving alcohol and tobacco intensified at the height of competition in the mid-eighteenth century; at York Factory, for instance, 864 gallons of rum and brandy were traded in 1753. Traders realized that there was a need to stock alcohol to deliver to the Indians, and shortages hampered trading activities. However, it would be erroneous to suggest that ample supply of alcohol alone was required to prosecute a successful trade; indeed, the Indians also demanded a large stock of high-quality trade goods (Ray 1974:143).

Not surprisingly, traders would use alcohol, especially rum and brandy (invariably cut with water) to entice trappers away from rival company posts. North West Company trader Alexander Henry wrote in 1805 that, 'if they misbehaved at our houses and were checked for it, our neighbours [HBC] were ready to approve their scoundrelly behavior and encourage them to mischief' (cited in Hamer and Steinbring 1980:9). Alcohol was also used as a trade item itself, along with other items of European manufacture. For instance, in 1744 the HBC had a standard of one gallon of brandy for four beaver pelts, and Norwester Alexander Henry set a standard price on alcohol in 1800 of two gallons for every ten animals killed by Indian hunters and delivered to the post for food; he refers to one case in which a trapper traded 120 beaver pelts for two blankets, a small mirror, and eight quarts of rum (Hamer and Steinbring 1980:8).

The trade in alcohol had many disruptive effects, according to European commentators. The Jesuits, who were strongly opposed to the use of alcohol, wrote extensively of the problems it caused among the Indians. They wrote, for instance, that 'Every night is filled with clamours, brawls, and fatal accidents, which the intoxicated cause in their cabins,' and 'It [drunkenness] is so common here, and causes such disorders, that it sometimes seems as if all the people of the village had become insane, so great is the license they allow themselves when they are under the influence of liquor' (cited in Dailey 1968:47). Alexander Mackenzie (Garvin 1927:101) in the late 1700s contrasted the behaviour of Cree Indians under the influence of alcohol with that when sober, noting that 'They are also generous and hospitable, and good natured in the extreme, except when their nature is perverted by the inflammatory influence of spirituous liquors.' Similarly, Andrew Graham (Williams 1969:152) wrote in the late 1700s that, 'They are much given to fighting and quarrelling when drunk; but at other times are seldom seen passionate or guilty of maiming the person of another.' Daniel Harmon, writing in 1802, lamented his considerable loss of sleep due to constant, all-night drinking parties by the Cree (1911:11). And for some Indians, the quest for alcohol became serious; George Simpson wrote in 1820 of the Indians 'tormenting us for liquor' (Rich 1938:120).

Assault and murder were just two of a variety of social problems that were caused by alcohol, according to the Jesuits and traders who commented. To the list can be added rape, marriage breakdown, and food deprivation. Indeed, for the periods in which alcohol was consumed, there was a general breakdown in the social norms characteristic of such consumption. Consumption tended to occur over a day or more, until the supply was gone. As David Thompson wrote in 1785 of the Cree along Hudson Bay, 'No matter what service the Indian performs, or does he come to trade his furs, strong grog is given to him and sometimes for two or three days, men and women are all drunk and become the most degraded of human beings' (Hopwood 1971:80). Many observers agreed with John Franklin's (1969:56–7) assessment of the Cree, that 'They were formerly a powerful and numerous nation ... but they have long ceased to be held in any fear ... This change is entirely attributed to their intercourse with Europeans; and the vast reduction in their numbers occasioned, I fear, in a considerable degree, by the injudicious introduction amongst them of ardent spirits.'

Alcohol consumption was not a uniquely male activity. Women also engaged in consumption to the point of intoxication. According to Van Kirk (1980:27), many traders noted in their journals that the Homeguard women in particular seemed to become more rapidly addicted to alcohol than the men, and that 'not only did it make them prone to jealous acts of violence and the neglect of their children, but it debauched their morals.' Prostitution of Indian women was one product of this alcohol problem.

It is also important to stress that many Indians abstained from alcohol consumption altogether and many recognized the social problems it caused. Indeed, some western band chiefs welcomed the formation of the North-West Mounted Police in 1873 as a means of stemming the American whisky trade. Some trading captains requested that the traders not make alcohol available to band members. Measures were sometimes taken to reduce the carnage wrought by drunkenness, such as restraining individuals by tying them up, or hiding their weapons when they were drinking (Dailey 1968:51). There were also instances where some chose to stay sober, in effect to watch over those that were drinking. And the consumption pattern of most Indians often involved binge drinking at the posts followed by long – even year-long – periods of total abstinence. The consumption of alcohol was primarily a trading post activity; as such, true alcohol addiction was likely rare.

As the competition between the HBC and the North West Company in western Canada heated up, the availability of liquor increased, and this proved to be a heavy drain on the accounts of both companies. In 1821, when the two amalgamated, the newly reorganized HBC no longer needed alcohol to propagate the trade. Consequently, in 1825, it passed a new regulation 'that the use of Spiritous Liquor be gradually discontinued' (R. Fleming 1940:126). The policy, however, did not mean that the trade in alcohol stopped immediately, for the Indians were able to keep the liquor flowing to some extent. Indeed, in 1840 the HBC at Cumberland House was informed by one Indian 'that the effects of this new law would be perceivable in the amount of our Return's by next June' (Thistle 1986:91–2). And HBC Governor George Simpson clearly exempted the Indians of the plains from the new policy, for a time, because these Indians continued to provide important provisions to the company (Rich 1938:303n)

Over the latter part of the nineteenth century, supplies of alcohol to Indians dried up throughout much of the north, aided in part by an Indian Act prohibition for registered Indians. Access to alcohol was not completely severed, especially in southern areas, but certainly it became more difficult in other areas. By the 1960s, many northern Aboriginal communities were resorting to periodic consumption of home brew, referred to cryptically in some areas as 'white lightning' or 'moose milk.' Home brew supplies were readily available from local traders, though not all promoted brewing. Home brew represents an interlude linking the historic introduction of alcohol in the fur trade to the reintroduction of alcohol in the post-1960 years of increasing access to Euro-Canadian society.

CONCLUSION

Medical services for Aboriginal people in the pre-Confederation era were largely in the hands of the fur traders, whalers, and missionaries. They all had some interest in assisting the Aboriginal inhabitants, but despite their efforts, the toll that the epidemic diseases took was significant. Lack of organization, lack of formal medical training, and limited access to medical supplies meant that their victories in treating Aboriginal patients were often overshadowed by their defeats. When Canada was formed in 1867, the new country demonstrated little concern for the health of Aboriginal people and did not immediately develop strategies for combating disease. As we shall see in the next chapter, the government remained content with the level of service provided by the traders, whalers, and missionaries, supplemented by new government agents in the form of the police and the military.

7

The emergence of government health services

As we noted in the opening chapter of this book, the formation of Canada in 1867 with the British North America Act effectively transferred the responsibility for 'Indians and the lands reserved for Indians' to the new federal government. This did not immediately translate into the development of medical services for Indians by the federal government, however; Brett's (1969:521) assertion that 'until the commencement of the twentieth century, the development of medical services in the north was conspicuous by its absence' pertains to most Aboriginal areas of Canada. The Inuit, who were eventually recognized as a federal responsibility, and the Métis, who never were, received organized government medical services even later than the Indians. Missionaries, traders, and government agents continued for many years to provide medical care on an ad hoc basis throughout most of the new country and territories.

THE 'MEDICINE CHEST' CLAUSE AND TREATY PROVISIONS

One of the most controversial areas of discussion in the field of Aboriginal health care concerns the treaty *right* to free, comprehensive medical services for Indians. Although the issue has essentially been settled in the courts, supporting the federal government's view that no such right exists, many Indian organizations maintain that the treaties, in general, must be interpreted liberally, with an eye towards the 'spirit and the intent' of the agreements. From their view, this means that the right to medical care is a treaty right, notwithstanding any previous legal decisions.

In order to properly understand the issue of treaty rights to medical care, it is essential first to understand the historic context of the treaties.

The first 'numbered' treaty was signed in 1871 in southern Manitoba; and between 1871 and 1877 a total of seven such treaties were executed. In general, the Indians in the 'northwest angle' in northwestern Ontario, and especially across the southern prairies, were somewhat anxious to sign the treaties. By 1870, eastern settlers had begun to encroach into the west, and the formation of Canada three years earlier had foreshadowed a likely westward expansion. Furthermore, many Aboriginal groups in the west were beginning to experience the negative effects of the decline in the bison herds. Starvation and deprivation were becoming more common, and many Indian leaders began to see the treaties, and their provisions for federal agricultural assistance and education, as a means to ensure a future for their people. That these leaders were thinking of the future is clear when one reads Alexander Morris's *The Treaties of Canada with the Indians*, first published in 1880. As Morris was the chief treaty commissioner for many of these first treaties, his observations are pertinent to this discussion.

Unfortunately, when examining the issue of treaty promises, we must appreciate that the Indian side of the story is less precisely documented than the Euro-Canadian side. The best source of information from an Indian perspective comes from the oral tradition and, in rare instances, from research undertaken with, or in accounts dictated by, Indians present at the negotiations. Recent research and court cases have affirmed the importance of the oral tradition as a source of information on Aboriginal-European relations, and so we can put to rest the idea that this form of knowledge acquisition and transmission is less valid than a written record (see, for example, Ray, Miller, and Tough 2000). As we shall see, the Indian perspective tends to vary somewhat from the official treaty text and versions offered by Morris and other Euro-Canadian officials witnessing the events.

The only treaty that specifically mentions medical care is Treaty Six, which contains two relevant clauses: 'That in the event hereafter of the Indians comprised within this treaty being overtaken by any pestilence, or by a general famine, the Queen, on being satisfied and certified thereof by her Indian Agent or Agents, will grant to the Indians assistance of such character and to such extent as her Chief Superintendent of Indian Affairs shall deem necessary and sufficient to relieve the Indians from the calamity that shall have befallen them.' And, 'That a medicine chest shall be kept at the house of each Indian Agent for the use and benefit of the Indians, at the discretion of such Agent.' It is very apparent from Morris's (1880) description of the Treaty Six negotiations that these two clauses were added into the official text of terms to be offered to the Indians; this represents one of the few instances in which this was the case. These Indians, primarily Plains Cree and Saulteaux, were clearly concerned about the recent turn of events in their region. Morris (1880:177) wrote that 'The Indians were apprehensive of their future. They saw the food supply, the buffalo, passing away, and they were anxious and distressed ... They desired to be fed. Small-pox had destroyed them by hundreds a few years before, and they dreaded pestilence and famine.' In his dispatch of 4 December 1876, Morris recounted the discussions he had had with the Indians that led to the inclusion of these two clauses in the treaty. As he wrote at the time, 'At length the Indians informed me that they did not wish to be fed every day, but to be helped when they commenced to settle, because of their ignorance how to commence, and also in case of general famine ... They were anxious to learn to support themselves by agriculture, but felt too ignorant to do so, and they dreaded that during the transition period they would be swept off by disease or famine – already they have suffered terribly from the ravages of measles, scarlet fever and small-pox' (ibid.:185).

The demands of the Indians were clearly articulated to Morris, and these included 'provisions for the poor, unfortunate, blind and lame,' 'the exclusion of fire water in the whole Saskatchewan [district],' and 'a free supply of medicines' (Morris 1880:185). Morris records his response to these demands as follows: 'I replied ... as to our inability to grant food, and again explaining that only in a national famine did the Crown ever intervene ... We told them that they must help their own poor and that if they prospered they could do so' (ibid.:186). Morris records no response with respect to the provision of medicines.

Less than a week later, Morris met with another group of Indians in the region to sign the treaty. In response to Cree chief Beardy's comments that, 'when I am utterly unable to help myself I want to receive assistance,' Morris once again replied that 'we could not support or feed the Indians ... If a general famine came upon the Indians the charity of the Government would come into exercise' (Morris 1880:188).

A scribe by the name of A.G. Jackes accompanied Morris and the treaty party and made a record of the events and dialogue leading up to the signing of the treaty with various bands. Here we see some additional insights into the question of medical services. For instance, Jackes quotes Morris as telling one band that 'the fire-water which does so much harm will not be allowed to be sold or used in the reserve' (Morris 1880: 206). Furthermore, Morris stated that 'I cannot promise, however, that the Government will feed and support all the Indians; you are many, and if we were to try to do it, it would take a great deal of money, and some of you would never do anything for yourselves... [but] that the sympathy of the Queen, and her assistance, would be given you in any unforeseen circumstance' (ibid.:210–211). Morris (ibid.:212) advised that 'some great sickness or famine stands as a special case.' Jackes also records the Indians' request that 'we be supplied with medicines free of cost' (ibid.:215). In response, Morris apparently stated quite clearly that 'A medicine chest will be kept at the house of each Indian agent, in case of sickness amongst you' (ibid.:218).

There is some evidence that health matters may have been discussed at other treaty signings as well, despite the fact that no references to such appear in the treaty documents. For instance, concerns for the health of Indians in northern Saskatchewan and other areas of the north led to requests that treaties be signed with them. Thomas White, superintendent general of Indian Affairs in 1887, described 'repeated applications ... made by Indians inhabiting the regions north of the boundary of Treaty No. 6,' adding that 'quite recently the Hudson's Bay Company has renewed its solicitations in the same behalf, alleging that serious sickness is now prevalent among the Indians of the Peace River District, and that there is an apprehension of there being an insufficiency of food during the Winter ... The diseases from which they are stated to be suffering are stated to be measles and croup.' Indeed, according to White's report, the Hudson's Bay Company took the position that 'the expense of providing and caring for sick and destitute Indians should devolve upon the Government as their natural protectors, and that the Hudson's Bay Company should not charge itself with the same' (cited in Fumoleau 1973:36). Fumoleau (ibid.:37) also described an 1887 *Calgary Tribune* article entitled 'Starving Indians' in which it was suggested that destitute northern Indians needed a treaty in order to alleviate their suffering.

At the negotiations for Treaty Eight, Fumoleau (1973:113) argues that the treaty commissioners indeed promised medicines and medical care, citing a 1919 report by D. McLean, assistant deputy and secretary of Indian Affairs, who wrote that the Indians were 'assured ... that the Government would always be ready to avail itself of any opportunity of affording medical service' (cited in Fumoleau 1973:113). The report of the treaty commissioners apparently suggests that the Indians requested 'assistance in seasons of distress' and that 'the old and indigent who were no longer able to hunt and trap and were consequently often in distress should be cared for by the government' (R. Daniel 1987:98). The treaty commissioners 'promised that supplies of medicine would be put in charge of persons selected by the Government at different points, and would be distributed free to those of the Indians who might require them.' Furthermore, 'We explained that it would be practically impossible for the Government to arrange for regular medical attendance upon Indians so widely scattered over such an extensive territory. We assured them, however, that the Government would always be ready to avail itself of any opportunity of affording medical service just as it provided that the physician attached to the Commission should give free attendance to all Indians who he might find in need of treatment as he passed through the country' (cited in ibid.).

Fumoleau (1973:114) also notes that medical doctors often accompanied treaty parties after the signings, dispensing medicines and treating Indians. Although inadequate from the perspective of alleviating the widespread ill-health of these peoples, the apparent promises and provisioning of medical services were, arguably, linked to the treaties themselves.

Fumoleau (1973) documents a similar story for the signing of Treaty Eleven. The need for a treaty in the far north was explained in part by the poor health conditions of the Dene Indians who lived in that region. Starvation, combined with diseases such as tuberculosis ('consumption'), dysentery, whooping cough, measles, and Spanish influenza, were taking a serious toll, and the Indians in many cases appealed to be taken into treaty as a way of ameliorating their suffering.

It is clear, then, that the provision of medical services was either a partial justification for, or entered the discussions of, at least three treaties. Quite likely, similar concerns were expressed at other treaty negotiations as well. The degree to which there is disagreement over the terms of these treaties is profound and continues to plague government-Indian relations to this day. Indeed, it did not take long for some detractors to begin to argue that, whatever the Treaty Six promise was, it was too much. For instance, in 1880 Manitoba's Dr John Shultz suggested in Parliament that the need to provide food to Indians was 'one of the vicious conditions of Treaty # 6,' and Donald Smith, also of Manitoba, referred to the clause as 'a most unfortunate one and never ought to have been agreed to by the Indian Commissioners' (cited in Ray 1990:41). Prime Minister John A. Macdonald's response to the Treaty Six provisions is enlightening of his Indian policy: 'Of course the system is tentative and it is expensive, especially in feeding destitute Indians, *but it is cheaper to feed them than to fight them, and humanity will not allow us to let them starve for the sake of economy'* (ibid.; italics ours). Needless to say, the lack of adequate government food supplies was one of the reasons for the Indian 'uprising' during the 1885 'rebellion' in Saskatchewan.

With respect to medical care, the promises can easily be interpreted in many ways. On one hand, the treaty commissioners indicated that medicines would be available, and the provision of free medical services at the annual treaty ceremonies would further cement in the Indians' minds the link between the treaty and medical care. But the treaties also indicate that the provision of such services would be at the discretion of the government, in the person of its agents, and that there were limitations on the extent to which services could or would be delivered. Cost factors clearly limited the government's commitment. W. Morrison (1985:149) describes the anger of Indians at York Factory in 1915 when a physician failed to pay an annual visit, as they believed they had been promised by Treaty Five. And there is evidence that the treaty promise as understood today is far from agreed upon even among Indians. So, while authors such as Fumoleau (1973) and R. Daniel (1987) would suggest that the treaty promises regarding medical care have not been fulfilled, at least one Treaty Seven (Peigan) elder interviewed by Daniel (1987:142) stated very clearly that 'the only two promises they kept were with regard to medicine and education.'

As the question of treaty rights to medical care attracted attention, especially after 1945, the views of the federal government and Indian political organizations diverged. The federal position was self-serving; for instance, Dr P.E. Moore, superintendent of Indian Health Services, wrote in 1946 that, 'Although neither law nor treaty imposes such a duty, the Federal Government has, for humanitarian reasons, for self-protection, and to prevent spread of disease to the white population, accepted responsibility for health services to the native population ...' (P.E. Moore 1946:140). The federal government noted in 1957 that medical care was a treaty obligation only under Treaty Six, but that medical services for all Indians were provided on 'humanitarian rather than on legal grounds' (cited in Barkwell 1981:9). In 1964, they reiterated that 'the Federal Government has never accepted the position that Indians are entitled to free medical services by Treaty rights' (ibid.), and again, in 1970, that 'despite popular misconceptions of the situation and vigorous assertions to the contrary, neither the federal nor any other government has any formal obligation to provide Indians, or anyone else, with free medical services' (ibid.). In contrast, Indian organizations have taken the view that medical services are, indeed, a treaty right. For instance, the Indian Association of Alberta wrote in 1970 that 'the intent was that Indians should receive from the Federal Government whatever medical care could be made available,' which they interpret to mean the latest technology, medicines, and services (Indian Association of Alberta 1970:33). The Assembly of First Nations has taken a similar position, arguing that 'the Indian treaty negotiators sought, and the Crown negotiators guaranteed, establishment of a free, guaranteed health care package as a perpetual right, to be available to all Indian people, regardless of income or place of residence,' which in effect means *all* registered Indians, whether or not they have treaty status (Assembly of First Nations 1979:3).

The Canadian courts have been asked to rule on the extent of the treaty promise to medical care for treaty Indians, and their interpretations have guided government policy in this area. The first case occurred in 1935, known legally as *Dreaver v. The King* (unreported case; Barkwell 1981:14). Dreaver was a chief of the Mistawasis Band in Saskatchewan, and under his name the band launched a suit against the federal government to recover monies it had spent on medical supplies between 1919 and 1935. Dreaver had actually been present as a young man at the signing of Treaty Six, and in his testimony argued that all medicines were guaranteed free to Indians under that treaty. Furthermore, evidence indicated that medicines had, in fact, been supplied free from the time of the treaty in 1876 until 1919. The trial judge agreed with Dreaver's interpretation of the treaty.

In 1965, another Treaty Six Indian, Walter Johnston, was charged with failure to pay a 1963 tax under the Saskatchewan Hospitalization Act, and he used as his defence the provisions of Treaty Six, which gave him tax-exempt status (Barkwell 1981:15). Johnston was found not guilty because the act exempted those who were entitled to receive hospital services from the federal government. The judge noted that, 'I can only conclude that the "medicine chest" clause in Treaty No. 6 should be properly interpreted to mean that the Indians are entitled to receive all medical services, including medicines, drugs, medical supplies and hospital care free of charge' (cited in ibid.). However, upon appeal to the Saskatchewan Court of Appeal, the court ruled that a more literal interpretation of the treaty promise was appropriate, and that 'the [medicine chest] clause itself does not give to the Indians an unrestricted right to the use and benefit of the "medicine chest" but such rights as are given are subject to the direction of the Indian agent' (ibid.:16). Hence, according to this appeal judgment, only a 'first-aid'-type kit was required to be provided, and the court agreed with the federal government that it was not the latter's intent to provide comprehensive and free medical services to Indians. Furthermore, even the provision of medicines from the 'medicine

chest' was at the discretion of an Indian agent, or other federal representative. The judgment in this case even questioned the validity of the judgment in *Dreaver*.

In 1969 in Manitoba, a member of the Peguis Band claimed the right
to free medical care on the grounds that she was a treaty Indian. After
an accident, she had obtained money from the government to cover
medical expenses, as she was uninsured and lacked the means to pay. In
response, the Manitoba Hospital Commission attempted to recover
from her their expenses in treating her. In *Manitoba Hospital Commission
v. Klein and Spence* (1969), Judge Wilson noted that there were no provisions for medical care in treaties One or Two, and that the Treaty Six
provision was offered to those Indians by Alexander Morris as lieutenant-governor of the Northwest Territories, and not Manitoba, and therefore the medicine chest provision could not be extended to Manitoba.
Furthermore, Wilson supported the ruling in *Johnston* that a literal reading of the treaties was the most appropriate (Barkwell 1981:17).

The final case to be noted is *R. v. Swimmer*, in which in 1969 Andrew
Swimmer was charged with not paying a tax under the Saskatchewan
Hospitalization Act, and the Saskatchewan Medical Care Insurance Act.
The judge accepted that Treaty Six entitled Indians to free medical care,
and that Swimmer was therefore exempt from the tax. But on appeal the
decision was overturned in a judgment written by the same judge as in
the *Johnston* appeal, and for essentially the same reasons (Barkwell
1981:18).

In essence, the judgment in *Johnston* has become the leading one for
purposes of interpreting the medicine chest clause and the question of
Indian treaty rights to free medical services. There clearly exist irrecon-
cilable differences between the viewpoint of Indian organizations and
the federal government on this issue.

A number of points emerge from this discussion. First, at the time of
the signings of at least some of the treaties, the Indians were concerned
about their future and expressed a desire for assistance in some form if
famine or disease were to afflict them. The fact that by the early 1870s
Aboriginal people in western and northern Canada were already suffering extensively from disease and starvation suggests not only that relief
from these conditions was on their minds but that the treaties were seen
as a way of improving their lot. Second, the federal government, through
its agents, clearly made offers in some instances to provide medical care;
the question remains as to the extent of this care. Third, both a literal reading of the treaty and the discussion of the negotiations as described in
Morris (1880) suggests that the government intended limits to be placed

on medical care and that it would retain control over such care. Fourth, other evidence suggests that the Indians heard somewhat different promises, perhaps understanding that a 'medicine chest' represented state-of-the-art medical care that would evolve over the years. Fifth, subsequent visits by government officials to pay treaty annuities and other benefits under treaty often included a physician who examined and treated patients at no cost to them, supporting in the Indians' eyes the link between the treaty and medical services.

As a result of these legal cases, the federal government has been supported in its position to provide medical services to Indians as a matter of *policy*, rather than legal obligation. This effectively allows the government to alter services as it wishes, which it does periodically. Indian organizations, in contrast, remain firmly committed to the view that the 'spirit and intent' of the treaties be honoured, and that the Indian view, as currently evident in the oral tradition, should be accepted as the true version of the promises. Even some scholars accept the premise that Treaty Six 'became the basis for free health care for all Amerindians' (Dickason 1992:282; see also Favel-King 1993), the legal judgments notwithstanding. More recent court cases on other treaty matters have suggested that the courts today are more accepting of the oral tradition and use the idea of the 'spirit and intent' of the treaties in their deliberations; it is possible, therefore, that a new legal case based on the treaties would be better received than these earlier ones. Yet, even if the federal government or the courts were to acknowledge that a treaty right to health care exists, such a right would still have to be translated into policy to be implemented (for example, the contents of the 'medicine chest' would have to be defined in a mutually agreeable manner). This would no doubt entail serious negotiations and likely opposition from some sectors of Canadian society, since Canadians in general do not really have a 'right' to specific health care services. At any rate, the whole treaty issue with respect to health care was overtaken by the introduction of more-or-less-universal health insurance in Canada in the 1960s and 1970s; today, most of the debate centres on selected health services not provided by government plans and on issues relating to the process of health transfer (Jacklin and Warry 2004).

THE POLICE AND THE MILITARY

The North-West Mounted Police (NWMP), formed in 1873, provided some medical services to Aboriginal people, often acting as agents for the Department of Indian Affairs (DIA). Established in part as a

response to Indian requests to end the American whisky trade, which
was wreaking havoc upon the southern Plains Indians (as well as to
demonstrate Canadian sovereignty in the sparsely settled west), the
force's role in controlling the Indians' access to alcohol remained a central activity throughout its early history. Even today, in remote areas,
the Royal Canadian Mounted Police (RCMP), the successor to the
NWMP, continues to deal with alcohol-related problems. But the police
provided other services as well. In the Yukon, for instance, Coates
(1991:174) suggests that NWMP surgeons routinely provided services to
Indians in the early part of the twentieth century. In 1905, the Department of Indian Affairs had four such doctors on retainer, treating Indians at no cost but charging the federal government two dollars per visit.
Medicines and hospitalizations were also made available free of charge
to Indian people. However, by 1914 'those [Indians] of means were
expected to pay their own bills. When Indian prospector Skookum Jim
Mason, co-discoverer of the Klondike strike, fell ill in 1916, the DIA
refused to pay the $100 hospital charge' (Coates 1991:174).

The NWMP also played a role in effecting quarantines when diseases
struck particular Indian groups. When smallpox struck the Poundmaker
and Little Pine reserves in 1912, and the Red Pheasant and Stoney
reserves in 1913, the NWMP was called in to enforce quarantines. These
initiatives sometimes had far-reaching effects on local economies. A prolonged smallpox quarantine at John Smith reserve in 1913 was supported by an NWMP constable whose duties included forestalling
attempts to hunt, freight, work in logging camps, or sell wood and fur.
These actions further debilitated the community (Lux 2001:182–3).

Fetherstonhaugh (1940), in his tribute to the force, described a number
of 'humanitarian' efforts engaged in on behalf of Indians on the prairies.
In 1881, in the Fort Qu'Appelle district of Saskatchewan, a constable
named Holmes endeavoured to assist Indians affected by smallpox. Having studied medicine and acquired some nursing experience, Holmes
undertook to vaccinate as many Indians and settlers as possible, and otherwise care for the sick, as there was no doctor available. Fetherstonhaugh (1940:123) describes Constable Holmes in rather heroic terms:

This meant travelling many miles on snowshoes, camping in the open with no
protection from blizzards and cold other than a hole in some deep drift of snow.
It meant days spent in the lodges of the stricken Indians, where sanitation was
unknown and the air was foetid with the odour of the disease. It meant all these
things and more, but it wrought the district's salvation. Finally, after many

deaths, the vaccine took effect. New cases ceased to appear. Immunization triumphed. And Holmes, rewarded only by his pay of seventy-five cents a day, returned to routine duties in the Force as an acting hospital steward.

Fetherstonhaugh (1940:123–4) also described the efforts of another constable at Norway House who, when scarlet fever and diphtheria broke out in 1881, 'quietly tackled the grim problem which the epidemics provided,' including caring for the sick and the dying, burying the dead, and disinfecting the tents. When influenza attacked the Inuit and Indians in the Coronation Gulf and Mackenzie River areas between 1926 and 1928, the police offered assistance despite falling ill themselves. The same is true for the 1918–19 influenza pandemic, when the force was sent to enforce quarantines at Alberta and Saskatchewan, assisting in relief work in the process (Lux 2001:186). The enforcement and assistance roles of the NWMP often clashed. In the wake of the devastating effects of the First World War and the 1918 influenza pandemic, and to celebrate their end, chief and counsellors at the Onion Lake reserve in northern Saskatchewan twice petitioned D.C. Scott to hold a two-day Sun Dance in the summer of 1919. The request was refused both times, but preparations proceeded anyway, only to be stopped when the NWMP were sent to suppress the event. Similar circumstances occurred at the Piapot and Big River reserves (Lux 2001:187).

In contrast to Fetherstonhaugh's praise for the force, W. Morrison (1985:143) argues that, at least in the north, the police viewed Aboriginal people 'with a mixture of paternalism and contempt,' perhaps a view conditioned by the 'noble redskin' image many police had of Plains Indians (ibid.:59). References to 'lazy' Indians, for instance, occur repeatedly throughout police reports in the early 1900s, though as Morrison notes, this apparent laziness could have been caused by disease or other factors (if, indeed, the Indians were actually 'lazy'). In the Yukon, Morrison notes that 'The attitude of the police towards the Indians they encountered ... was generally that they were a lazy, dirty nuisance, to be given meagre aid if they were actually starving, but to be ignored as much as possible' (ibid.:145). The attitude of the police in the Mackenzie Delta and Hudson Bay 'was much the same.' However, some police realized that the Indians were victims of circumstances over which they had no control, and the HBC was often criticized by the police for their actions (ibid.:146).

For much of the north, in both treaty and non-treaty areas, the police acted as agents of the government; this included making treaty payments, undertaking the census, and delivering medical services. Police doctors often provided medical services to Aboriginal people, including vaccinations against smallpox (Lux 2001:140), but, as Morrison (1985:148) explains, the police were sometimes angered over what they perceived to be refusals to follow their medical instructions. Morrison (ibid.:148) quotes one police doctor in Churchill in 1915, who stated, 'I have repeatedly explained to them the infectious nature of the disease [tuberculosis], how it spreads, and how it could be lessened. My advices seem to have been of very little use, and results have been very discouraging.' The fact that the Indians probably did not comprehend the doctor is suggested by Morrison. Nevertheless, the poverty and poor health that characterized many Aboriginal people living around the fur trade posts and police stations desensitized the officers and led them to become callous about their plight. In contrast, the force developed more positive views of the Inuit, 'who had all the qualities the Indians lacked,' including thriftiness, cleanliness, and morality (ibid.:152). Nevertheless, by 1910, and especially after 1920, the police found themselves dispensing relief to starving Inuit as well as Indians (ibid.:158). Change, and colonization, had reached into the high Arctic.

The NWMP, then, like the missionaries and traders, provided medical services and relief to varying degrees to Indians and Inuit, in some instances for humanitarian reasons and in others, grudgingly, because it was part of their job. Their services also included enforcing quarantines and in this area, at least, encountered some opposition.

The military also played a role in the delivery of medical services to Aboriginal people. In many instances, they simply supported the efforts of others, such as the missionaries in the Arctic; this included providing transportation and delivering medicines. However, military doctors were also called upon to provide medical services.

The years following the Second World War saw the military become involved in a variety of medical areas, concomitant with military expansion in the north as a means of securing Canadian sovereignty during the Cold War. In the high Arctic, radar bases were established as a means of warning against a polar attack by the Soviet Union. These bases collectively were known as the Distant Early Warning Line, or 'DEW Line,' and the military personnel employed Inuit to construct the bases and provide other services. Medical assistance was provided to these Inuit and their families, but the experiences were not always good. Schaefer (1959:81) describes how the construction of the DEW Line base near Davis Inlet on the Labrador coast in the mid-1950s seriously affected the Inuit, many of whom found employment in construction.

The resultant noise severely reduced the availability of game in the area, and these Inuit workers became dependent on a carbohydrate-based diet. But when the construction ended in 1957 and the Inuit were laid off, the military decided not to further their dependence by administering rations. A series of infections struck their camp, including tuberculosis and measles. By late 1957, almost half of the forty Inuit who had been living in a nearby camp were either dead or had been evacuated south for medical treatment.

Foulkes (1962a) has provided a view of military medical services, based largely on his own experiences as a physician with the Royal Canadian Air Force (RCAF) at Fort Nelson, British Columbia, from 1955 to 1957. The first medical services in this region were supplied on an ad hoc basis, often by United States military personnel (attached to the Alaska Highway construction project), or by private physicians under contract to the Department of National Defence. By the mid-1950s, RCAF medical officers had taken the place of these private practitioners. Part of Foulkes's job involved providing medical services to the 'Slave' Indians (a Dene- or Athapaskan-speaking people, also known as the Slavey). The living conditions for these people were atrocious, according to Foulkes, particularly for those who lived in the village by the air base. Other Aboriginal people lived throughout the region, and Foulkes was required to provide services to them as well. Emergency medical advice was often provided by telegraph. He writes of the Canadian National Telegraph, 'I can recall talking with anxious parents about a sick child, with interpreters who had received a message from an Indian runner about some calamity in the bush, with the consultants in Edmonton and Vancouver regarding an extraordinary case, and with the various individuals within the chain of command for the calling of an aircraft for an urgent air evacuation' (Foulkes 1962a:535). Private citizens were required to pay for medical services, although the Department of Indian Affairs picked up the costs for registered Indians. Indian and Northern Health Services of National Health and Welfare also employed a nurse in the region, whose work focused more on preventive medicine.

There were many problems encountered in the treatment of Aboriginal patients. Foulkes (1962a:548) suggested that 'Treatment, recommended without due consideration of all of the difficulties inherent in the home environment, especially in the Indian settlement, could lead at times either to near-tragedy or to a display of ingenuity.' He describes ways in which Indian patients afflicted with scabies managed to bathe and wash clothes frequently despite a lack of running water, including one who created a bathtub by lining a trench with canvas and heating water on an open fire next to it. Foulkes also notes the continued existence of traditional medicine 'in the hinterland,' mentioned by some of his patients. For instance, he describes seeing patients 'with wounds dressed in obnoxious concoctions of bear grease and assorted unidentifiable ingredients' that he then treated 'in a more orthodox manner.' He also describes an incident in which parents' fear of hospitals led one couple to hide their child in the bush for many months; when he was finally found, he was on the verge of dying from what Foulkes describes as 'a once operable tuberculosis in the brain' (ibid.:549).

Aboriginal and other patients were required to share the military hospitals' wards, and Foulkes (1962a:550) notes that, 'even though the North country is far from free of discrimination and prejudice, there was no loudly expressed objection.' Despite his rather narrow view of traditional medicine, Foulkes presents some enlightened viewpoints on the state of health in the region, including the effects of poverty and other social conditions on it. For instance, with respect to sexually transmitted diseases, he notes that the major source of the problem lies with the civilian workers and 'their lack of respect for the dignity of Indian girls' (Foulkes 1962b: 676).

When the RCAF's Tactical Air Command was dissolved in 1959, the small hospital was transferred to the Fort Nelson community as a civilian hospital. The role of the military in providing medical service in this region was formally relinquished at this time (Foulkes 1962c:750–1).

Grygier (1994) has documented the role that the military played in the detection and treatment of tuberculosis among the Inuit. Their participation included X-raying and transporting patients, and providing other services and facilities. For instance, the Department of National Defence hospital in Edmonton was transferred to Indian and Northern Health Services and opened in 1946 as the Charles Camsell Indian Hospital. The notorious Coastguard ship *C.D. Howe*, about which more will be said later in this chapter, became the cornerstone of much Arctic screening for Inuit tuberculosis, and some of the medical staff were officers in the RCAF. Given the militarization of the Canadian north after 1945, the role of the military in health as well as other administrative areas is not surprising.

INDIAN AGENTS AND RELIEF MEASURES

The first Department of Indian Affairs was established in 1880, with Prime Minister Sir John A. Macdonald as its superintendent general.

This department was not originally concerned with Indian health problems and initially made no provision for medical services and personnel (Graham-Cumming 1967:123). Some Indian bands voluntarily paid for medical services, and Indians were directed to use local physicians and hospitals on a fee-for-service basis.

The Indian agent system was a quasi-military approach to handling the administration of Indian affairs. Although 'agents' were used by the colonial government prior to Confederation, the era of the 'Indian agent' really commenced after the treaties were signed in western Canada, beginning in 1871. The Indian agents, responsible for virtually all aspects of the administration of Indian affairs and the implementation of elements of the treaties in large 'agencies,' were all-powerful. Often working in conjunction with the police and the missionaries, the Indian agents executed federal policies, designed to facilitate the 'protection, civilization and assimilation' of their charges (Tobias 1976). Medical assistance and food rations or 'relief' in times of 'famine or pestilence' were a part of these policies.

While some Indian agents actually had medical training, for the most part they had little more than lay knowledge of medical matters; indeed, many agency postings were simply political patronage appointments. In the early years, the 'medicine chest' represented the embodiment of medical services available through the agent, but by the early twentieth century government-employed medical officers became more readily available. The government always retained a strong element of control in the hiring of such physicians, and many were placed on salaries rather than being paid on a fee-for-service basis.[1] Private physicians were also utilized, particularly in emergencies or where a government physician was not at hand. A choice of physicians was not readily available to Indians, although Col. E.L. Stone, medical superintendent in the Department of Indian Affairs, was confident that 'The Department does not contemplate that a sick Indian who is genuinely dissatisfied with the regular physician should be denied the services of another' (1935:84).

One of the problems that faced the new government was the impoverished circumstances of Aboriginal people on the western prairies. Disease was rampant on many reserves, and with the collapse of the bison herds many were attempting to make the transition to an agricultural life (the provisions of which were included in the treaties).[2]

The federal government, working through the Indian agents, provided rations to Indian bands, but often under tight restrictions. In some instances, rations were withheld entirely. In 1882, Chief Moosomin of the North Battleford agency in Saskatchewan was brought to write that 'There is to-day great distress in my band. The rations are suspended now for 41 days ... It is impossible to work on an empty stomach' (Department of Indian Affairs 1882:195). In other instances, 'able-bodied' Indians were refused rations on the assumption that they could work instead. Indian agents exercised a great deal of autonomy to limit rations and thereby effect savings for the government; conversely, they were often rebuked when their designations of destitute Indians were challenged by superiors. Rations were clearly used as a mechanism of social control: Indians who left their reserves without permission or refused to take up agricultural work could be cut off. Even hungry children, or those suffering from illness, could be refused.

There is also little question that, in general, inadequate rations were provided, and that the Department of Indian Affairs and the Indian agents were aware of this fact. Flour and bacon were the staples of the rations diet, and only occasionally was fresh meat allowed (the government retained tight control over the cattle herds on Indian reserves). Well into the twentieth century, the government went to great lengths to avoid defining any Indian as 'destitute.' Quantities were limited, and the food was of inferior nutritional value. The nutritional health implications of the rations program are clear when one keeps in mind that Aboriginal people were undergoing a transition away from a high-protein diet of fresh meat; indeed, some local government administrators often encouraged Indians to keep hunting, despite a formal agricultural policy. By the end of the nineteenth century, some western bands had begun to develop small cattle industries and to grow vegetables, but these endeavours came somewhat late for many who succumbed to diseases while dependent on a rations diet (see Lux 2001:33–6).

FEDERAL INDIAN HEALTH SERVICES

In 1904, Dr Peter H. Bryce was appointed as the first federal official responsible directly for Indian health. As 'General Medical Superintendent,' he proved to be an active and persistent advocate for improving health conditions on reserves.

Bryce had been the secretary of the Ontario Provincial Board of Health prior to his appointment and had been a leader in the public health movement in Canada (T.K. Young 1984:258). The health of Indian people was clearly a priority for him. In 1903, he began to argue that the province's Indian Department required better organized medical services to offset the effects of the many contagious diseases on reserves. But these measures would be costly in the eyes of the Government of Ontario, an increase in expenditures of between $10,000 and $15,000 each year. His suggestion was turned down (E. Titley 1986:83).

After his appointment to the federal government in 1904, Bryce came into direct conflict with Duncan Campbell Scott of the Department of Indian Affairs, whose own personal mission seemed to focus on reducing government expenditures. For his part, Bryce became particularly concerned with the tuberculosis problem, one that necessitated increasing expenditures. His repeated requests for a special grant for $20,000, to be used for preventive programs among the Indians, were rejected by Parliament in 1907. The seeds for Bryce's downfall were sown, but not before he was able to bring the severity of Aboriginal health conditions to national attention.

In 1907, Bryce launched an investigation into the conditions at industrial and residential schools on the prairies. The results of his investigations were made available to politicians and the press, and ultimately published in part in 1922 as *The Story of a National Crime: An Appeal for Justice to the Indians of Canada*. He found the schools to be rife with disease and lacking proper medical facilities. According to his fifteen years of survey data, from 25 per cent to 35 per cent of all children who had been pupils had died, primarily from tuberculosis but also from other diseases, such as measles (Bryce 1914:137).[3] Bryce even suggested that the Indian schools be transformed into sanatoria, so bad was the health situation! As we saw in the previous chapter, the church officials who operated the schools reacted defensively, but the Indian agents tended to corroborate Bryce's report. Nevertheless, one high-ranking government official accused Bryce of exaggerating the magnitude of the problem (E. Titley 1986:84).

Bryce's plan to improve the health conditions in these schools was reasonable. Each school could employ a health nurse to improve sanitation and environmental conditions, and a program of better exercise and fresh air for the students could be implemented. The churches, Bryce suggested, should not be involved. Realizing that the government was likely to baulk at the increase in expenditures that such a program would entail, Bryce suggested it be tested on an experimental basis in one province. But he failed to get Duncan Campbell Scott's approval for the plan. The churches were very upset with Bryce's report and would not likely cooperate, according to Scott. Scott's response was to propose improvements in ventilation, exercise, and diet, presumably at a lower cost to the government. Bryce's publication of 1922 contained a critical comment on the way the tuberculosis problem had been handled by Scott and the minister of health, Dr W.A. Roche. With respect to Roche, Bryce scorned his 'transparent hypocrisy' and suggested 'how little the Minister cared for the solution of the tuberculosis problem' (Bryce 1922:8). Invoking the treaties as a last resort, Bryce stated that 'The degree and extent of this criminal disregard for the treaty pledges to guard the welfare of the Indian wards of the nation may be gauged from the facts' of the widespread devastation caused by tuberculosis.

By 1913, Bryce's railing against the government appeared to render him persona non grata among his superiors. His efforts in 1920 to have Indian health removed from the Department of Indian Affairs to a new Department of Health were thwarted. According to Arthur Meighen, then superintendent of Indian Affairs, such a transfer was not possible, in part because it would create a duplication of services, 'and there would be a sort of divided control and authority over the Indians which would produce confusion and insubordination and other ill effects among the Indians themselves' (cited in T.K. Young 1984:259). This meant that the responsibility for health would remain with Indian Affairs for another twenty-five years. However, Bryce was ultimately successful in seeing another of his projects adopted: in 1922, a mobile nurse-visitor program was implemented that would see the medical officer's work being complemented by the work of nurses at the community level. The first nursing station was opened in 1930 on the Fisher River reserve in Manitoba. Bryce also introduced some degree of health education, having circulars on tuberculosis translated into Cree, for instance, as well as issuing a 'Book of Regulations' on medical services to Indian agents. Finally, it was Bryce's idea to fill the obvious vacuum of physician services by contracting local physicians (Hader 1990:107).

Maundrell (1942; cited in Graham-Cumming 1967:125) suggests that Bryce 'ignored all consideration of money' in his work, a fact that clearly clashed with Scott's acute sense of fiscal responsibility, as well as with other government priorities. Bryce remained in the position of chief medical officer until he retired in 1921, bitter and disillusioned over the failure of many of his proposals and at being denied the position of deputy minister in the newly formed Department of Health in 1919. His strident, perhaps abrasive, approach left a legacy, however; his position was not refilled until 1927. In the meantime, according to Maundrell (ibid.), 'A study of the reports and correspondence impresses one with the disorganization of the services. The natives received medical treatment but there was little effort to overcome the worst epidemics. The appointment of a Medical Superintendent might have been postponed indefinitely but for the increasing friction between field doctors and the departmental accountant who taxed their fees. Something had to be done to prevent these quarrels ...' Financial concerns, once again, proved to be paramount in these early years of government services to Indians.

In 1927, a medical doctor named Col. E.L. Stone was appointed medical superintendent in the Department of Indian Affairs. Stone had been a physician in the department, travelling throughout Indian agencies undertaking health surveys and treating patients. In 1926 he was a physician at Norway House, Manitoba, and in charge of the hospital there. The hospital served a number of more remote communities, where missionaries acted as dispensers of medicines. But the hospital itself was small, only sixteen beds, and inadequate to meet the needs of long-term patients.

Stone's 1926 report, 'Health and Disease at the Norway House Indian Agency,' provides some indication of his approach to health matters. The Norway House Cree were impoverished, though not necessarily starving, and the rampant tuberculosis they experienced was the result. According to Stone (1926; rpt 1989:246), 'Disease here means one malady, and one only, for all practical purposes. That is tuberculosis. Practically nobody dies of anything else.' But while poverty was a contributing factor to this disease profile, Stone placed greater emphasis on sanitation and personal sanitary habits. He wrote, 'There is no need to go into details about the sanitary habits of these people in their houses. It is enough to say that they are not likely to help limit the spread of infection from the sick to the well.' [4] In an effort to appear as unbiased as possible, he then added, 'And they are not much, if any, worse than those of many white people' (ibid.:249). In an oblique reference to the apparent laziness often reported by police, traders, and others, Stone wrote insightfully, 'One is often led to wonder what these Indians might be able to accomplish if they were freed, by some miracle, from consumption. There is no doubt that their energy would increase enormously.' But then lapsing into a racial argument common at the time, he adds, 'It must be remembered that they have much white blood, and many of the instincts peculiar to the white race' (ibid.:242). The ultimate answer to the tuberculosis problem lay with improving the economic fortunes of the people, particularly their ability to earn a living in the trapping industry through better conservation and restrictions on outside trappers. He argued that an increase in rations would not help the population, and that 'the present

Medical Services [were] not meeting the needs in that it is dealing with effect rather than cause' (ibid.:256). Nevertheless, Stone had collaborated with Bryce and others in the establishment of a committee in 1924 to investigate the tuberculosis problem among Indian people, and he ultimately presided over antituberculosis surveys and projects in British Columbia and Saskatchewan (Hader 1990:111, 113).

Stone's critical comments pale in comparison to those of Bryce, with whom he had some contact. Stone was clearly more popular with his superiors. Nevertheless, with his appointment in 1927, Stone was still somewhat of a pioneer. His Norway House reports were taken seriously, and led to the establishment of the Qu'Appelle Medical Health Unit in Saskatchewan to treat tuberculosis patients (Graham-Cumming 1967:125). He also continued Bryce's work in providing circulars on health matters. But, as Bryce had found previously, the lack of funds provided for Aboriginal health care prevented much progress from being made.

At the time of Stone's appointment, a formal Medical Branch was established within Indian Affairs. Writing in 1935, Stone described the workings of this branch in the *Canadian Medical Association Journal*. The Indian agent retained a great deal of power within the new framework, for as Stone noted, 'The Indian agent ... is responsible for every matter affecting the interests of the Indians under his charge, including ... the administration of the medical and health services' (Stone 1935:82). While some agents were also physicians, most had to rely on branch medical officers to provide services. Nevertheless, the agent's concern was more one of cost, and the medical officers were relatively free to treat patients of their own accord. The Indian agent's permission was required to have a patient hospitalized, and the head office in Ottawa had to consent to a transfer to a sanatorium. The system had holes, but Stone firmly believed 'that no Indian need lack the services of a physician or the advantages of a hospital when he is sick or injured, if by any means of transportation the doctor can be conveyed to him, or he be brought to the doctor or hospital' (Stone 1935:83).

Stone was not alone in his fight against tuberculosis. In 1928, Dr Robert Ferguson, a pioneer in the treatment of the disease and superintendent of the Fort Qu'Appelle sanatorium from 1917 to 1948, reported the results of a survey on Indian tuberculosis at an international conference; but despite the alarming incidence of the disease that he identified, federal resources remained relatively slim. Indeed, in its 1933 budget, the Medical Branch suffered a 20 per cent cutback. As a result, the Department of

Indian Affairs was forced to state in 1934 that 'it is impossible to admit to sanatorium more than a very small proportion of Indians who are recommended for such care.' Sanatorium care was to be reserved for the homeless. And in 1935, when a Battleford (Saskatchewan) agency physician requested a sanatorium admission for a child, he was told that 'The Department is in the unfortunate position of not having sufficient funds to maintain in hospital an increased number of *ordinary* cases of tuberculosis' (cited in Hader 1990:114; italics ours). The government's response in this case was to supply a tent for the child! The problem of shortage of funds was put into perspective in 1937, when an editorial appeared in the *Canadian Tuberculosis Association Bulletin* arguing that 'the facilities for early diagnosis, treatment and prevention that have been used to such good advantage in the White population have never been made available for the attack on the Indian problem' (cited in Hader 1990:117).

In 1935, there were eleven medical officers in the Medical Branch who were employed full-time, and eight Indian agents with medical training. Another 250 physicians were employed part time, or as needed, including urban-based specialists and still others who saw Indian patients privately. There was little in the way of dental services, outside of basic services such as extractions. A total of eleven field nurses was employed by the branch, supplemented by others employed by missionary or provincial organizations. The first nursing station, opened at Fisher River, Manitoba, in 1930, would be followed by the construction of many more. A network of some 200 hospitals was available, including tuberculosis sanatoria, most of which were quite small and not definable as 'hospitals' per se. Stone (1935) states that only seven could be so classed, with the smallest having eight beds and the largest forty. Many of these facilities were operated by provincial governments as public facilities, or by missionary organizations. The revenue accruing to many hospitals as a result of treating Indians was extremely important to their viability.

The costs of medical services remained an issue throughout Stone's tenure. His efforts to deal with the tuberculosis problem and other communicable diseases and to expand the scope and magnitude of medical services were hampered by a lack of funds. According to Maundrell (1942; cited in Graham-Cumming 1967:126), 'The medical services provided are the more impressive when it is remembered that the Branch has never had at its disposal any more than about one-half the amount per capita expended by the Canadian population at large, and that the Indians are relatively a sickly people. In 1934 the per capita cost was $9.60, approximately the same as in 1930, whereas the per capita cost for the white population was $31.00.' It is hard to imagine that medical coverage could have been as good as Stone suggests, given the relatively low expenditures and the fact that the branch was responsible for at least 112,500 people spread over 800 communities.

In 1936, the Department of Indian Affairs was absorbed by the Department of Mines and Natural Resources, including the Medical Branch of Indian Affairs and the 'Eskimo' Health Service of the Northwest Territories Branch. Stone remained as the medical superintendent, and Dr P.E. Moore became his assistant. When war broke out in 1939, Stone returned to military service and Moore took his place. Moore was ultimately appointed director of the Indian health service in 1945, and when Stone returned after the war the latter concentrated on having a hospital for Indians and Inuit built in Edmonton (Graham-Cumming 1967:126).

Moore, like Stone and Bryce before him, wrote numerous articles on the Indian health service. Writing in 1946, Moore described a health service that had grown somewhat since 1935. Twenty-seven full-time physicians were now employed in Indian and Northern Health Services, seven of whom were assigned to the Northwest Territories and the eastern Arctic. Some 700 physicians were employed part-time, providing services on demand to Indians in their regions. The service was now operating sixteen hospitals in addition to provincial facilities available to Indians across the country, including tuberculosis sanatoria. Twenty-four field nurses were employed, plus many more part-time 'field matrons' and 'field dispensers,' who administered medicines, often under the direction of a physician at the other end of a two-way radio. The persistence of traditional Indian medicine, based on 'ignorance and superstition' according to Moore, was still seen as a roadblock in the delivery of medical services, especially in remote areas (P.E. Moore 1946:141).

Physicians were required to travel extensively in this period, and visits to smaller Indian communities were often timed to coordinate with the payment of treaty money. Cameron Corrigan (1946), the physician based at Norway House, described accompanying the Indian agent on annual treaty parties, sojourns that took a month. The doctor undertook medical examinations and vaccinations, as well as pulling teeth, while the agent paid out the annual five dollars per capita stipulated by the treaty. In all, some 4,000 people were given this whirlwind treatment, and since they were not required to pay for the medical services, it is easy to see how such joint treaty-medical expeditions appeared, to the Indians, to be simply an exercise in fulfilling the treaty right to free medical care.

How did the early physicians view their Indian patients? While most never recorded their thoughts in a manner that would be available to researchers, a significant number could not resist writing of what to them were adventures in the wilds of the country. Their ill-informed (even racist) attitudes, for the most part, can be seen as typical of general Canadian attitudes regarding Indians, as well as formal government policy. William Shaw, a physician among the Kwakiutl in British Columbia, for instance, supported the banishment of the potlatch, arguing that 'A new Indian is rising on the ashes of the old, many now have modern houses and motor cars, and are rapidly taking a useful place in the White Man's civilization' (1923:659). Wall's report on the Indians along the Quebec-Ontario border noted for one band that 'The Chief here is a careless and indolent man of low mentality, and the mentality of the Band as a whole appears to be lower than the average' (1926; rpt 1989:269). Corrigan, the resident physician at Norway House in the mid-1940s, described the Indians there as being 'promiscuous, and amoral,' adding, 'I do not believe an Indian can be treated for any sickness unless he is hospitalized, as he cannot be trusted to take medicine intelligently' (1946:221). The general disdain that most physicians held for traditional medical approaches has been discussed in a previous chapter. In the end, it becomes clear that the physicians believed, as did many in government, that Indian people were clearly threatened with extinction from disease and that their only hope was assimilation (including intermarriage with non-Aboriginal people to 'strengthen' their gene pool).

The construction of Aboriginal health in medical writing from the first half of the twentieth century reveals how the 'Indian problem' and Indian bodies themselves became pathologized and infused with concerns about contagion, gender, and race (Kelm 1998, 2005). The period is marked by worries about disease spreading *from* First Nations *to* settler communities, signalling a shift in blame back onto Aboriginal communities themselves. With the emergence of epidemic tuberculosis in western Canada and the decline in the health of Aboriginal people in general, reserves began to be feared as reservoirs of infection (Hackett 2002:244). It appeared to many that 'conditions peculiar to the Indians ... are responsible for the excessive death rate' (Department of Indian Affairs 1908:xxiii) and that they were an inevitable part of the Aboriginal condition. Also evident in medical and government reports of the time are beliefs about 'the failings of [Aboriginal] men and women to live up to their "natural roles" either as providers or caretakers' (Kelm 2005:384). There was a tendency, for instance, to blame Aboriginal mothers for their children's deaths (Moffat and Herring 1992). 'Probably much of this infantile mortality may be traced to premature marriage, which result in weakly offspring, and to ignorance of inexperienced mothers as to what constitutes suitable nourishment for their children, and as to their care when sick' reads a Department of Indian Affairs sessional report (Department of Indian Affairs 1911:xxii). This was part of a wider discourse on 'mother's ignorance' and the inherent deficiency of Aboriginal mothers. Aboriginal men, by the same token, were depicted as having declined from hunters in the bush to idlers on reserve. 'Physicians agreed that tuberculosis was the physical manifestation of the transition from nomadism to the confinement on reserve' and that 'Indian men were "degenerating" and had ceased to be good providers for their families' (Kelm 2005:387).

Racism to some degree was evident with respect to certain aspects of tuberculosis treatment. Many Indians experienced more or less forced evacuations to northern and southern hospitals for treatment. In the Yukon, for instance, tubercular Indians were sent to the general hospital in Whitehorse and, in some instances, south to the Camsell Hospital in Edmonton in the late 1940s and 1950s (Coates 1991:105, 215). While efforts to treat and prevent tuberculosis among the Indians were, in part, the result of humanitarian motives, and while quarantining tuberculosis patients was the accepted practice for all, it is also true that 'the regular appearance of disease among the Natives and the perception of non-Natives that such illnesses threatened their communities added support to government and public efforts to segregate the Natives' (ibid.:107). Indeed, as Coates (ibid.:95) documents for the Yukon, racial segregation in the area of medical care was the norm in the 1940s: 'In most centres, the people consistently demanded the segregation of hospitals and refused to share wards with Native patients. The Mayo Hospital, funded by the Treadgold Mining Company, refused to admit Natives to its general wards. Instead, Indians received treatment in a tent to the rear of the main structure ...' In Whitehorse, similarly, there was a general hospital and, for a time, a small building 'fitted for the infirm and tubercular Indian patients.'

Some physicians shared the views of the non-Aboriginal public; in 1939 several doctors refused to treat Indians at the same fee rates as for non-Indians, despite the lament of the Department of Indian Affairs that it was 'not prepared to admit that sick Indians are less desirable patients than white people' (Coates 1991:96). Views of Indians as 'dirty' and 'diseased' were pervasive, and while the existence of widespread disease among these peoples is not contestable, the underlying attitude at the time that the Indians were inferior certainly is. The link between poverty and disease was clear, and even reports that implied inferiority of moral or physical standards among Indians betrayed the real causes. Coates (ibid.:104) quotes a North-West Mounted Police surgeon, writing in 1903: 'They [Yukon Indians] are a squalid, pitiable looking lot of people. Those who do not exhibit advanced symptoms of disease show signs of the existence of germs. They are particularly unclean in their habits and almost entirely destitute. I declare I have not seen in the different tents I have had occasion to enter, a decent pair of blankets; they have but small flimsy things, and in most cases a mere heap of rags. It is a fact as incontrovertible, as it is deplorable, that disease, actual want and destitution prevail among the majority of them.' The postwar years saw an increase in the medical services available to Indians. A new federal department, National Health and Welfare, had been formed in 1944, and in 1945 Indian and Northern Health Services, including services to Inuit, was transferred over. All other aspects of Indian administration remained with the Indian Affairs Branch, however, and these ultimately were transferred to a new Department of Indian Affairs and Northern Development in 1966, an arrangement that would come to create much frustration among those attempting more holistic health programs. Even at the outset, the Indian agents, renamed 'Superintendents,' retained control over health matters by virtue of their designation as 'Health Officers,' despite the fact that the services themselves were to be delivered by a separate department. As the years passed, however, it became increasingly evident that the poor socio-economic conditions of the Indians, leading to poor sanitation and education, among other problems, were to a large extent responsible for their relatively poor health. Indeed, according to Graham-Cumming (1967:128), officials with the Department of Mines and Natural Resources were upset with the transfer of Indian health matters to the new department, viewing it as a critical comment on their abilities, and hence interdepartmental cooperation was difficult to achieve.

By 1956, National Health and Welfare was operating eighteen hospitals (growing to twenty-two by 1960), thirty-three nursing stations (thirty-seven in 1960), fifty-two health centres containing dispensaries, and thirteen other health centres employing full-time physicians or nurses (eighty-three health centres in 1960) (P.E. Moore 1956:229; T.K. Young 1984:260). Employment had grown considerably, and there were now 39 field medical officers, 43 hospital medical officers, 11 dental surgeons, 106 field nurses, and 232 hospital nurses. Additional services were provided by 63 part-time physicians and more than 1,200 private physicians and 125 dentists. More than $17 million was appropriated for these medical services in 1956.

In 1962, another government reorganization saw the elimination of Indian and Northern Health Services and the creation of a new branch, Medical Services, which amalgamated the services of seven programs: Civil Aviation Medicine, Public Service Health, Indian Health, Northern Health, Quarantine, Immigration, and Sick Mariners' Services. In effect, any Canadian whose medical services fell outside the domain of provincial programs became the responsibility of this new branch. Aboriginal health services were facilitated by the existence of a region and zone structure across the country (T.K. Young 1984).

The 1960s saw the closure of some Indian hospitals and sanatoria as the need for them decreased; there were only nine hospitals left by the mid-1970s. In contrast, the number of nursing stations and health centres increased to more than 100. Indeed, nursing station services developed as the backbone of the Medical Services Branch. Overall expenditures on Indian health continued to increase, and by the end of the 1960s the budget was more than $28 million (compared to only $4 million in the 1950s). Hospital insurance was also introduced, and by 1971 all provinces were covered by universal medical care insurance. Questions of medical indigence – or treaty rights to medical care for that matter – became increasingly irrelevant in a country where everyone had access to medical services. In some provinces, where insurance premiums were implemented, the federal government assisted in their payment by Indian bands. Medical services offered directly to Indians by the federal government were concentrated in the more remote and northern areas; in other instances, Indians sought services from provincial facilities and private physicians, who then billed back to the federal government.

THE DEVELOPMENT OF MEDICAL SERVICES FOR THE INUIT

The Inuit were among the last to experience organized medical services delivered by the federal government. The missionaries, traders, military, and police continued to have a prominent role until after the Second World War in some areas.

The first hospitals constructed in the Arctic were operated under the auspices of the churches. For instance, the Anglicans erected a small hospital on Blacklead Island, in Cumberland Sound, in 1902 and in Pangnirtung in 1929; the Roman Catholics did likewise at Aklavik in 1926 and Chesterfield Inlet in 1929. The Anglicans and Roman Catholics collaborated with the federal government to construct a six-bed facility at Coppermine in 1929 (Jenness 1972:8). These were not always permanent facilities, however, and hospitals often closed only a few years after their construction.

That missionary medical services in these early hospitals were a part of an overall attempt to Christianize the Inuit is clear. One report on the development of the hospitals at Blacklead Island and Pangnirtung noted that the hospitals represented great medical advances, 'since at that time the Eskimo were pagan, and often made it very difficult for the Mission-aries to treat the patients properly in their tents and snow huts' (A. Fleming nd:1). This report, issued by the Arctic Mission, concluded by saying: 'The Hospital has been established following the example of the Master Who went about healing the sick and afflicted. Pray that through its means the Saviour may be made known to many – both Eskimo and white' (A. Fleming nd:7). As we shall see shortly with respect to tuber-culosis treatment, medical care and culture change were often viewed by the Euro-Canadian caregivers to be interrelated.

The medical officers at these church-run hospitals were usually federal employees. The Department of the Interior, followed by Indian Affairs and, after 1935, the Department of Mines and Natural Resources were responsible for recruiting and employing the medical staff (P.E. Moore 1974:132). However, since there were relatively few hospitals in the early years of the twentieth century, much medical care still remained in the hands of the missionaries and traders in the more remote areas, and the federal government supplied northern missions with medicines during the early part of the twentieth century (Jenness 1972:44). Between 1918 and 1923, the government spent some $30,800 on relief for the Inuit, most of which was paid to the police and trading companies who provided the aid (Jenness 1972:32). During the years of the Second World War, when relatively few medical personnel were available for Arctic service, the Canada Medical Procurement and Assignment Board posted some med-ical officers of the Department of National Defence to staff some of the northern hospitals (P.E. Moore 1974:133).

In 1921, the federal government created the Northwest Territories Branch, in the Department of the Interior, to administer the north. It had become apparent that relief measures were required in some Inuit settle-ments and that health care required some attention. As Jenness (1972:32) notes, the federal government at that time assumed that it had a legal responsibility to the Inuit, though in 1932 this responsibility was clari-fied to mean 'they have not the status of Indians, and the provisions of the Indian Act do not apply to them.' Yet, since 1880, in matters of health and education, the federal Department of Indian Affairs had made no distinction between the Inuit and Indians in the north. In 1924, Indian Affairs officially took responsibility for the Inuit (through an amendment to the Indian Act), extending medical services into the eastern Arctic. In 1928, the responsibility for Inuit was transferred to the commissioner of the Northwest Territories, and in 1932 the Indian Act was amended to delete the Inuit provision (Jenness 1972:33). In 1945, the care of both Indians and Inuit was transferred to the Department of National Health and Welfare, and the Inuit began to receive family allowance benefits for the first time (Jenness 1972:77).

In 1955, the Northern Health Service was established by the federal government, and the responsibility for medical services to the Northwest Territories was placed with the Department of National Health and Welfare. One of the pioneers in the delivery of medical services in the Arctic in this era was Otto Schaefer. The conditions in which he operated were crude, to say the least, and frequently called for innovation and, in the eyes of the doctors themselves, a certain amount of heroism. For instance, here is how Schaefer described one incident that occurred in 1956:

In March 1956, a dog-team came racing into Pangnirtung from a camp 60 miles distant where a woman had suffered a severe haemorrhage associated with an incomplete abortion. The patient had become unconscious and had been regarded as unfit for dog-sled transportation. I rapidly collected blood-grouping sera, transfusion bottles and gynaecological instruments and, with our own dog-team, raced to that camp. There, I grouped and cross-matched a number of Eskimos, transfused 1000 c.c. of blood into the unconscious patient and, after overcoming the shock, proceeded to evacuate the uterus. All these procedures took place in a small, crowded sealskin winter tent, where the low ceiling kept my back bent all the time and the only sources of light were a dim seal-oil lamp and my flashlight. (Schaefer 1959:81)

Schaefer cites other similar incidents, including one in which a missionary, an HBC manager, and a 'wise old Eskimo woman' removed the retained placenta from a bleeding woman, under the direction of a physician 500 miles away communicating by means of a two-way radio (Schaefer 1959:81).

The consequences of the Inuit's anomalous position vis-à-vis Canada are perhaps best demonstrated with respect to the Ungava region of Quebec. As Vanast (1991) has documented, when Quebec gained the northern territory in 1912, it became the only province with an indigenous Inuit populaton. Quebec's response was to assume that the Inuit were 'Indians' under the British North America Act, and hence a federal responsibility. Canada, on the other hand, believed the Inuit to be Quebec citizens. A battle raged on this issue until 1939, when Quebec achieved a Supreme Court ruling that the Inuit were 'Indians' in law, and hence a federal responsibility. Nevertheless, Canada was slow to act upon its responsibilities until the 1950s, leading Vanast (1991:74) to conclude that, while 'There was no conspiracy to keep Ungava's Inuit unfed and unhealthy ... the outcome was not much different than if there had been one.'

One of the easiest ways to reach Inuit settlements throughout the first half of this century was by boat or ship. In some cases, travel facilities were on a modest scale. For instance, in 1930 the physician at Aklavik was provided with a small boat so that he could travel throughout Coronation Gulf. But medical services were also provided by ships that plied the coastal waters. In the 1920s, with the advent of the Eastern Arctic Patrol, the vessel *Arctic* travelled the eastern coast with a medical doctor as it replenished supplies at coastal trading posts (later, the *Beothuk* took over this role). When a medical station was established at Pangnirtung in 1924, the patrol doctor managed to examine more than 500 Inuit in the region over two winters (Jenness 1972:44). The Eastern Arctic Patrol ship *C.G.S. Nascopie* regularly supplied coastal missions with medicines between 1918 and 1947 and was eventually provided with a medical staff and X-ray equipment as part of the fight against tuberculosis. When it ran aground in 1947, the government was forced to build a new ship, the *C.D. Howe*, which was commissioned in 1950. The *C.D. Howe* was designed with medical work in mind (Graburn 1969:143). However, before the *Nascopie*'s demise, that ship managed to X-ray more than 1,500 Aboriginal people in 1946 alone. The years from 1947 until the the *C.D. Howe* came into use saw the Royal Canadian Air Force and even the United States Air Force involved in removing tubercular Inuit to Quebec City or the Charles Camsell Hospital in Edmonton for treatment (Jenness 1972:85).

The medical ships in the eastern Arctic had a relatively short season, leaving Montreal at the end of June and returning in late October because of ice threats. For the rest of the year, medical evacuations were undertaken by the RCAF. In some instances where landings were impossible, medical supplies with instructions, and occasionally even physicians, were parachuted into camps (P.E. Moore 1956:232).

The manner in which the federal government attempted to control and eradicate tuberculosis in the north was controversial and has left a legacy of bitterness among many Inuit to this day.[5] According to Jenness (1972:88),

Very few tubercular Eskimos at that period left their homes willingly; the great majority went in silence, offering no resistance, and their relatives stood silently by and watched them depart without tears. But there were occasions when the Royal Canadian Mounted Police officer had to use his authority, and a number of families deliberately kept away from any settlement when the hospital ship was due to make its annual call. In the south the evacuee, strictly confined to hospital, unable to speak more than a few words of English, could hardly fail to be lonely and depressed, although both the doctors and the nursing staff lavished on him more than usual sympathy and care. His low morale imperilled his recovery and restitution to his home, while his kinsmen in the north, lacking news of him, despaired of ever seeing him again.

The situation as described by Jenness is only partly compatible with that offered by others. For instance, where Jenness describes how government officials provided reading materials in syllabics and facilitated the exchange of letters with relatives back home, it has also been suggested that these officials were so inefficient in their paperwork that sometimes relatives and even spouses were kept in separate wings of the same hospital without anyone's apparent knowledge. There simply was no formal program to keep families together, or keep them informed, until the mid-1950s, ten years after tuberculosis evacuations had begun (LaPointe 1986). Government attempts to implement a 'disk list' system, a means of keeping track of Inuit whose Inuktitut names were incomprehensible to them, were largely a failure (D.G. Smith 1993). In some cases, families were not informed of the deaths of members until many years later.

The handling of Inuit patients throughout this period was scandalous. It was not uncommon for individuals to board the medical or patrol ships for X-rays and then be refused permission to return to shore when the results positively indicated tuberculosis. They were simply taken away (Grygier 1994:96). And once in the southern hospitals, according to a federal official whose job it was to reunite families, 'The Inuit people were treated like cattle ... To the bulk of the federal staff in Ottawa, they were just numbers' (LaPointe 1986). But these numbers kept getting mixed up. Another official with the Department of Northern Affairs and Natural Resources in the north in the 1950s recalled a young boy of perhaps six, speaking only French, who was dropped off by plane in a small northeastern Quebec Inuit village. He was wearing only shorts, sandals, and a shirt, despite the wintry conditions. Having been in the south so long, he was unable to adjust to living in an igloo and eating traditional foods (LaPointe 1986). Other patients were not even lucky enough to be returned to their families; in some cases they were dropped off at settlements hundreds of kilometres from home, often with little recollection of their families. Some children never returned to the north at all; they were adopted by southern families, or else perished in the hospitals. Not surprisingly, the Inuit came to regard the arrival of the medical ships and their X-ray equipment with apprehension, leading Schaefer (1959:249) to comment in1959 that, 'many old Indians and Eskimos are still more afraid of evacuation to the white man's land than of death ...'

The potential that hospital treatment had for culture change among the Inuit was clearly recognized at the time; indeed, this was seen as a positive by-product by government. According to Jenness (1972:89), the 'protracted stay in southern Canada has made it more difficult for many Eskimos to return to the primitive conditions of their earlier life.' Some, Jenness argued, were no longer physically capable of enduring the Arctic rigours, as a result of their poor health, while others 'will resent its hardships and privations ... and ... will prefer to remain in the south and enjoy the flesh-pots of our civilization.' Jenness's support for assimilation is clear:

And why, indeed, should they not remain [in the south]? Why should we force them to return, for the rest of their days, to an environment which very few white men are willing to endure for a single winter – an environment in which not many Eskimos can maintain themselves and their families today without continuous help from our government ... Why then should we subsidize our Eskimos to keep them in barren Arctic regions where without our subsidies many of them would die of starvation? Should those to whom we have carried our deadliest diseases, and then brought south to cure them of those diseases – should they not be allowed, even encouraged, to stay among us if they wish, and helped to earn in the south the livelihood that the underdevelopment of the north, and nature herself, deny them today in their homeland? (ibid.:89)

The Eurocentric biases inherent in Jenness's observations are painful to read today, and they must be seen in the context of his view that all Aboriginal people were destined to be assimilated sooner or later. Nevertheless, it is quite clear that cultural change was an important by-product of tuberculosis treatment and that, combined with the separation of families and kin, it served to undermine Inuit society to some extent. Medicine and social change do go hand in hand. Indeed, as early as the 1920s the director of the Northwest Territories Branch, O.S. Finnie, assumed that 'it was the duty of the federal government to civilize the Eskimos and to safeguard their health and welfare' (Jenness 1972:30). Jenness himself argued in his policy paper on 'Eskimo Administration' that 'Integration with other citizens of the Dominion is the only goal possible for Canada's Eskimos' (ibid.:30).

A large number of Inuit were taken south for tuberculosis treatment from the 1940s through the 1960s. At the height of treatment, one-sixth of the 9,500 Inuit were being treated for the disease (LaPointe 1986), with an average hospital stay of twenty-eight months (Grygier 1994:83). Although the tuberculosis epidemic that swept the country through these years required serious measures, there can be little question that the Inuit were not treated on a par with the Euro-Canadian victims of the disease.

Many government administrators and doctors were unable to pronounce and spell Inuit names. The Inuit themselves had a low literacy rate, and some had only one name, while others had European surnames and still others had common or first names that could change over time. In the 1920s, one doctor suggested that a universal system of identifying Inuit would greatly facilitate medical record keeping and vital statistics. Apparently, other northern government personnel, such as the police, had also thought that a system was needed, and some recommended fingerprinting. As Derek Smith (1993:50) notes, 'A simple and necessary system of medical patient identification had grown into something different and much more comprehensive, if not also much more insidious.' But fingerprinting was quite logically associated by the Inuit with criminal activity, and they were not anxious to participate. It was an unidentified doctor who suggested in 1935 'that at each registration [of vital statistics by the RCMP] the child be given an identity disk on the same lines as the army identy [sic] disk and the same insistance [sic] that it be worne [sic] at all times.' Thus, the 'Eskimo Disk List' system was born.

There was some government opposition to the disk list system, in which each Inuk would be expected to wear a tag around his or her neck or wrist with a unique identification number. In part, this opposition was due to the fact that neither Indians, who had registration numbers, nor any other 'wards' of other dominions wore them. Proponents of the system saw it not only as an efficient way to record vital statistics and medical records but also as a way of facilitating overall administration of the Inuit, including a general hunting and fishing licensing system. But some Inuit refused to wear their disks, some simply threw them away, and even government administrators were sloppy in their use of the numbers. An administrator at Aklavik was brought to lament that, 'In trying to sort out hospital accounts and other matters concerning Eskimo [sic – the usual plural at this time] I am encountering more confusion than should be necessary. There seems to be no clear lines exactly as to who is counted as a native Eskimo and thus a charge on the Department and who is of white status and not. I find children of white men with disc numbers and children of Eskimo without. I find at least two cases where Indians also have Eskimo discs' (D.G. Smith 1993:58). Not surprisingly, it was evident by the 1960s that the disk list system was not working, and it was abandoned officially in the early 1970s with the adoption of 'Project Surname,' an effort to have all Inuit select surnames and standardize the spelling of names.

By 1943, the Northwest Territories had eleven hospitals in operation, nine owned and operated by missionaries and the other two by mining companies; however, the eastern Arctic was considerably less well served, with only 48 hospital beds for 3,762 people, compared to 213 beds for 8,000 people in the west (Duffy 1988:52–3). By 1946, only nine physicians served in the Northwest Territories. The hospitals at Aklavik, Chesterfield Inlet, and Pangnirtung continued to operate throughout the 1940s, although at least one government official referred to the latter as 'disease traps ... unfit for human habitation' (ibid.:57). The federal government began to shift its medical services in a new direction by establishing nursing stations. The first was opened in 1947 at Port Harrison in the eastern Arctic, and the next at Coppermine in the western Arctic. The advent of the DEW Line radar network improved access to medical facilities for some Inuit, particularly employees of the military bases, although the corporation operating the bases was often in conflict with the federal government regarding precisely who was eligible for medical services (ibid.:60–1).

By the early 1960s, twelve major Inuit settlements had nursing stations, the staff of which could service another fourteen smaller outposts, and dependency on the mission hospitals and the ship patrols began to be phased out. The nurses were in contact with physicians via radio (although radio signals were often unclear due to atmospheric conditions). Medical evacuations by plane became more common, with patients often transported to the southern urban hospitals for more comprehensive treatment (Jenness 1972:86–7). The government continued to expand the nursing stations, and by the mid-1960s there were twenty-five in all, supported by federal hospitals in Inuvik and Frobisher Bay (now Iqaluit) and by the Charles Camsell and Moose Factory hospitals, as well as seven smaller mission hospitals (P.E. Moore 1974:134). As for the Indians, the nursing station model was well on its way to being entrenched as the core of the medical services to be delivered to northern Inuit.

There does not appear to have been any great effort to recruit Inuit nurses for these stations at this time; this was a trend that would come later. But one telling incident occurred at Sugluk, where an Inuk nurse was the first hired when the nursing station opened there in 1960. She was not well accepted by the community, who preferred the services of the missionary who had been treating them for more than a decade, and who was 'White'; despite the nurse's training, it was difficult for them to accept the nurse as being qualified because she obviously did not look 'White' like the other medical practitioners they had experienced (Graburn 1969:149). The change in attitudes required for self-determination was obviously a few years away yet in this community.

THE DEVELOPMENT OF MEDICAL SERVICES FOR THE MÉTIS

Government services for the Métis in western Canada developed very slowly and in an ad hoc fashion. This was no doubt due to the anomalous position of the Métis vis-à-vis the Indians: the federal government undertook no official responsibility for the Métis, and it was largely left up to the provinces to render medical aid. The provinces, it seems, were reluctant to do so until the Métis population in the west began to experience widespread ill health and were therefore perceived as somewhat of a threat to the Euro-Canadian population. This seems to have come to a head in the 1930s in Saskatchewan and Alberta. Because of the inadequacy of data on the Métis, we will examine only some important aspects of the development of medical services for those in Alberta.

By the end of the nineteenth century, many western Métis could be found living on the margins of both Indian and Euro-Canadian societies. Many lived on lands adjacent to Indian reserves; but despite often strong kinship connections to the reserve, they were denied treaty and other benefits and services because of their legal status. Many others lived along road allowances, squatting on provincial lands on the outskirts of Euro-Canadian communities. Even the northern Métis settlements were impoverished, and diseases such as tuberculosis and syphilis quickly became rampant.

In 1932, the Métis Association of Alberta was founded by Malcolm Norris, Jim Brady, and Joseph Dion. Events leading up to its formation included petitions demanding that the Métis obtain rights for, among other things, land, education, and health care. They lobbied for a commission of inquiry into the state of the Métis in Alberta, and were ultimately successful. A royal commission was established in 1934 to examine 'the problems of health, education and general welfare of the half-breed population of the province' (cited in Pocklington 1991:12).

This commission, which became known as the Ewing Commission, after the chair, included a medical doctor, Dr E.A. Braithwaite, who had played an important role in organizing public health services in Alberta. Evidence presented by the Métis Association at the commission hearings indicated that the Métis were experiencing extremely high rates of infant mortality, tuberculosis, and venereal diseases (Pocklington 1991:14). In the process of gathering their data, the association had obtained testimonials from six doctors and Indian agents in the Grouard area, where many believed the worst health conditions existed. One doctor reported that 50 per cent of the Métis in this area were afflicted with venereal diseases, but were destitute and unable to pay for treatment (Dobbin 1981:77). According to Jim Brady, in his testimony at the Ewing hearings, 'At a distance of 300 miles from this very spot there are settlements who I don't think ever saw a doctor in their lives' (cited in Dobbin 1981:101).

The reliability of the Métis Association's data was challenged by the government in the form of Dr Harold Orr of the Alberta Department of Health. Orr had previously alerted his minister to the political implications of increased health expenditures on the Métis, and had advised his minister against sending a doctor to the Grouard area because 'the cost would be prohibitive unless the Venereal Disease Vote was very greatly increased' (cited in Dobbin 1981:101). At the hearings, Orr suggested that the prevalence of tuberculosis and venereal diseases was only slightly higher among the Métis in comparison to the 'Whites.'

When the Ewing Commission report was issued, it ran to only fifteen pages, and it is unclear which way the commission truly leaned on the questions of disease and treatment for the Métis. Nevertheless, the report did agree that the Métis were experiencing serious health problems and identified a number of possible reasons. They noted that many Métis lived far from doctors and nurses and lacked the money both to cover travel costs to consult them and to pay them. Travelling doctors and nurses, who commonly visited Indian reserves, rarely came to these Métis communities. The report also noted the poor sanitary conditions that characterized Métis homes and the lack of proper food (the report implied that some Métis were, in effect, periodically starving). However, in the end the commissioners wrote, 'On the whole, the Commission is of the opinion that while the health situation is serious, it is not, except as to the particular diseases mentioned [presumably tuberculosis and venereal diseases], more serious than among the white settlers' (cited in Pocklington 1991:16).

Clearly, the Alberta Métis were once again victimized by their anomalous legal status. The Ewing Commission made it clear that any assistance was to be provided to them out of 'considerations of humanity and justice,' but not because the Métis held any special rights as Aboriginal people (cited in Pocklington 1991:17). The Ewing Commission did not want the Métis to become wards of the state, as the Indians were. However, they did recommend that land be set aside for the Métis, parcels that were referred to then as the Métis Colonies and today as the Métis Settlements, where small hospitals could be constructed (these colonies were established under the authority of the Métis Population Betterment Act of 1938). The Métis living in these colonies would be periodically provided with the services of a travelling physician, with the anticipation that ultimately a resident physician would be hired. It is not clear to what extent the Métis were to be required to pay for these services.

The report of the Ewing Commission was tendered in February of 1936. Subsequently, some efforts were made to deal with the health status of the Métis, especially to provide tuberculosis treatment. While the systematic tuberculosis treatment of reserve Indians had begun in southern Alberta in 1935, the Métis did not receive similar attention until later, primarily in the 1940s, and with the establishment of the colonies. Card and colleagues (1963:25–6) present data showing that, between 1934 and 1939, Métis constituted only 6.9 per cent of the patients discharged from treatment facilities, but that this figure began to rise thereafter, until by 1960–1 the Métis constituted 23 per cent of the patients, disproportionately high relative to their overall population in the province. Most Métis patients tended to be treated at the Aberhart Memorial Sanatorium, constructed in 1952 to service the northern half of the province. According to Card and colleagues (ibid.:27), the number of 'walk-outs,' or patients leaving hospital prior to completion of treatment, began to increase in the 1950s, as Métis patients became more numerous (the implication that these walk-outs were Métis is clear, if not stated directly). This led to a provincial law in 1958 designed to enforce the confinement of 'recalcitrant infectious tuberculosis sufferers.'

The prevalence of disease remained high among the Métis for many years, despite these health programs. Again unlike the Indians, who received regular programs of diagnosis and treatment, the Métis were subjected to only 'irregular' screening. The report by Card and colleagues (1963), *The Métis in Alberta Society*, provides an interesting snapshot of perceptions of the Métis at the time. Subtitled 'with special reference to social, economic, and cultural factors associated with persistently high tuberculosis incidence,' the report documented that the Métis tuberculosis rate was, by the early 1960s, about half that of the treaty Indians. These authors appeared to be moving away from simple biological explanations of disease prevalence (that is, that the Métis have high tuberculosis rates because of the ancestral Indian heritage, and therefore a genetic susceptibility). They argued that, 'the major determinants of Métis status, and hence contributing factors to tuberculosis incidence, are economic poverty and what, by all criteria, amounts to a lower-class way of life, not an aboriginal way of life' (Card et al. 1963:398). The Métis, they suggested, occupied a class position within the context of the larger Euro-Canadian class structure, and this position was inherently one of poverty. This apparently radical (for the time) observation must be tempered, however, with the remnants of attitudes from an earlier era that still influenced the authors, for they suggest that the solution to the disease problem lies in 'extending civilization northward and increasing Métis participation in it,' hence promoting Métis 'individual and group upward mobility' (ibid.).

CONCLUSION

It is clear from this chapter that there was no grand strategy for the development of government services for Aboriginal people. Such development occurred on an ad hoc basis depending on the region, the legal status of the Aboriginal group in question, and even the personalities of the various caregivers and administrators who, in one way or another, were charged with the responsibility for Aboriginal health. Aboriginal perspectives on the development of medical services are largely absent in the literature for this period. As we shall see in the next chapter, the development of medical services in the contemporary era has not been without its problems, too.

8

The organization and utilization of contemporary health services

The previous chapter discussed the constitutional and legislative basis for Aboriginal health services and traced the involvement of the federal government since Confederation. This chapter describes and analyses the way the contemporary health care system 'works' – how services are organized and delivered, how much they cost, and how they are used. Attention is paid to both the bureaucratic machinery and health professionals within the system on the one hand and to the users of services – Aboriginal people themselves – on the other. The broader political aspects of health care delivery, particularly how health care as an agent of Aboriginal self-determination is regarded and applied, forms the subject of chapter 10.

HEALTH SERVICES DELIVERY BY THE FEDERAL GOVERNMENT

The major government agency in Canada responsible for health services to the majority of registered Indians has been the Medical Services Branch (MSB) of the federal health department, which changed its name to First Nations and Inuit Health Branch (FNIHB) in 2000. Until the late 1980s, when health services in the Northwest Territories were devolved from the federal to the territorial government, it was also the agency responsible for the Inuit, the Dene, and all other residents in the Northwest Territories. Originally organized in 1962 (then only a 'directorate' rather than a 'branch'), it was formed by amalgamating seven independent services that had come into existence with the department in 1944: Indian Health, Northern Health, Civil Aviation Medicine, Civil Service Health, Immigration, Quarantine, and Sick Mariners' Services. Although no longer administratively distinct, these original divisions remained identifiable as spheres of activity within the branch. Over the years, new activities were added and others dropped (such as Sick Mariners' Services). Like many other federal government agencies, MSB/FNIHB has been afflicted by a penchant for periodic administrative reorganizations – each time associated with an inflation in job classification and titles of the key management staff! This chapter is not intended to be an administrative history of MSB/FNIHB; rather, it describes in some detail the system as it had evolved up to 2005.

It is important to understand the role of the federal health department in Canada, where, constitutionally, health care is the primary responsibility of the provinces. A federal health department has existed since 1919. In 1928 it became the Department of Pensions and National Health, taking on responsibility for the welfare of First World War veterans. This latter function was given over to the new Department of Veterans Affairs when the Department of National Health and Welfare (DNHW) came into being in 1944, under the Department of National Health and Welfare Act. Health care is no different from many other aspects of Canadian politics, where there have been frequent federal-provincial squabbles concerning overlapping responsibilities and charges of intrusion into each other's jurisdiction. There have been provincial politicians who regarded the existence of a federal health department as unnecessary. The federal role in health care has primarily been regulatory, particularly in such areas as safety of food and drugs, protection from health hazards, and disease control and surveillance. With the introduction of universal hospital and, later, medical care insurance, DNHW became responsible for administering transfer payments to the provinces for such programs. Because of such statutory expenditures (health insurance, family allowance, old age security, and other forms of social assistance and welfare), to which all Canadians are entitled, DNHW was a behemoth among federal departments. In 1993 the 'Welfare' arm of DNHW was separated from the 'Health' arm. DNHW then became simply Health Canada. (The department also sets broad national standards in a variety of public health fields and funds public health research.) There remained a mixed group of clients, to whom some direct health services were provided, who were the main responsibility of MSB/FNIHB. Among these special client groups, registered Indians across Canada as well as all residents (including non-Aboriginal Canadians) in the northern territories prior to the transfer to the territorial government received a range of preventive and curative health services. The other groups, such as federal public servants, immigrants, refugees, international travellers, and civil aviation personnel, were provided only a limited range of services, consisting mostly of health advice, screening examinations, and emergency assistance. With the transformation of MSB to FNIHB in 2000, these groups are no longer the responsibility of the branch, which now serves only Aboriginal clients. In 2004, the Public Health Agency of Canada was created as a separate entity from Health Canada, responsible for national coordination of disease surveillance, control, and prevention as well as emergency preparedness and response. Although some aspects of Aboriginal health were included in this agency's functions, its precise role vis-à-vis FNIHB of Health Canada has not been clearly defined.

Since its inception MSB/FNIHB has been administered in a regionalized structure, with regions and zones. Over the years the boundaries have also changed. Initially the Northwest Territories was divided into zones administered along a north-south axis – thus, the Keewatin Zone was part of Central Region, which encompassed also Manitoba and northwestern Ontario. Later, there was one Northern Region, which included both the Northwest Territories and the Yukon. The Northern Region eventually split into two regions. By the late 1980s, all MSB regions corresponded to a province or territory, with the exception of the multiprovince Atlantic Region. The assistant deputy minister for MSB has overall responsibility for all of the branch's programs. While there have been various intervening layers at one time or another, the line authority runs through the regional directors and zone directors. At all levels, various health professionals act in an advisory/consultant capacity to the line managers.

Until the 1970s, there were usually a base hospital and more peripheral units such as health centres, nursing stations, and clinics within each zone. The typical system in more remote zones has been described: for example, the Keewatin Zone in the Northwest Territories (L. Black 1969) and the Sioux Lookout Zone in northwestern Ontario (T.K. Young 1981). A 1970 paper in the *Canadian Journal of Public Health* by the then director general of MSB listed a variety of operational problems faced by MSB staff in the north (Wiebe 1970). The sheer geographical expanse of each zone posed immense difficulties in supply and logistics, affecting the cost and timeliness of facility construction, transportation of patients and staff, and intra-agency communication. On the human scale, there were problems with insufficient quantity and poor quality of the staff employed. The conditions of employment, whether in terms of remuneration, fringe benefits, or general ambience, often made MSB uncompetitive with other health agencies. Furthermore, employees had to recognize and be prepared for the cultural differences and need for mutual understanding between non-Aboriginal staff and Aboriginal users. Adding to these problems were the legion of 'do-gooders' who volunteered their services to MSB, but often with conditions attached, and assorted short-term researchers and adventurers whose uncoordinated visits and demands were more trouble than they were worth (Wiebe 1970).

The performance of MSB has been evaluated periodically by the Auditor General (AG) of Canada. Federal auditing has gone beyond simply checking ledgers and uncovering 'waste' to determining 'value for money' and scrutinizing the internal workings of government departments. In 1987, the AG pointed out that 'existing planning, evaluation and management information systems are so deficient that the Department cannot be sure that it is providing an adequate level of health care ... with due regard to economy, efficiency and effectiveness' (Auditor General 1987: Section 12.43). Where data were collected, they were often not analysed or used. Much of what MSB did was not, or could not be, evaluated. The AG mentioned that an evaluation of the National Native Alcohol and Drug Abuse Program (NNADAP) had gone on for ten years and finally was abandoned for lack of data. On the positive side, the AG commended the more than 3,000 community health representatives, health liaison workers, and lay dispensers for serving their population well (ibid.: Section 12.48–12.50).

In the late 1980s MSB operated some 500 health facilities, including eight hospitals, across the country. The AG reported that four of the hospitals were in an advanced state of deterioration and seven of the eight had such low occupancy rates that they were half-empty most of the time (Auditor General 1978: Section 12.79). While MSB has been keen on 'getting out of the hospital business' since the early 1970s, and has successfully extricated itself in places such as North Battleford, Saskatchewan, many small hospitals were difficult to close because of community pressures, mostly related to fears of erosion of the federal commitment to Aboriginal health care, economic consequences, and reduced access to facilities where Aboriginal patients were in the majority. In the case of Sioux Lookout, Ontario, where a small town of 3,000 residents (though serving a catchment population of an additional 15,000) has had two hospitals, one federal and one provincial/municipal, a merger has long been debated. However, little action was taken until the early 1990s, when a multiparty (Aboriginal, federal, provincial, and municipal) negotiation process was initiated. Amalgamation of the two hospitals was finally accomplished in 2004, with a single governing board. Plans were also developed to build a completely new facility. In the Northwest Territories, MSB contributed substantially to the construction of the new hospital in Yellowknife in the mid-1980s. The successful transfer of the Frobisher Bay (now Iqaluit) hospital to the territorial government heralded the later complete transfer of all MSB activities. This model was followed in the Yukon, with the transfer of the Whitehorse hospital in the early 1990s.

Throughout much of its existence, the declared mission of MSB has been to assist Aboriginal people to attain a level of health comparable to that of other Canadians living in similar locations through direct services or other means. With the reorganization in 2000, the newly established FNIHB articulated its mandate as follows:

- to ensure the availability of, and access to, health services for First Nations and Inuit communities;
- to assist First Nations and Inuit communities to address health barriers and disease threats, and attain health levels comparable to other Canadians living in similar locations; and
- to build strong partnerships with First Nations and Inuit to improve the health system.

FINANCING ABORIGINAL HEALTH SERVICES

The actual cost of health services to all Aboriginal people in Canada has never been comprehensively determined. Even in the case of on-reserve Indians, where the federal government has been the main source of services, accurate attribution of costs has proven difficult. A true, comprehensive picture must also include costs related to services provided by provincial and territorial governments and out-of-pocket costs incurred by patients themselves. The provincial governments, for example, have shared-cost arrangements with the federal government for patient care in MSB-operated hospitals in their territory. On the other hand, the federal government also tries to recover from the provincial governments the costs of services provided to non-status Indians and non-Aboriginal residents who live in communities where MSB/FNIHB operates the only health facility – such as a nursing station. Even more elusive are indirect costs and how far one should go in labelling something as health-related. A detailed economic analysis is beyond the scope of this chapter. One can only look at how much MSB/FNIHB spends on Aboriginal health services within the context of overall federal government expenditures.

Figure 22. Growth in First Nations and Inuit health annual expenditures

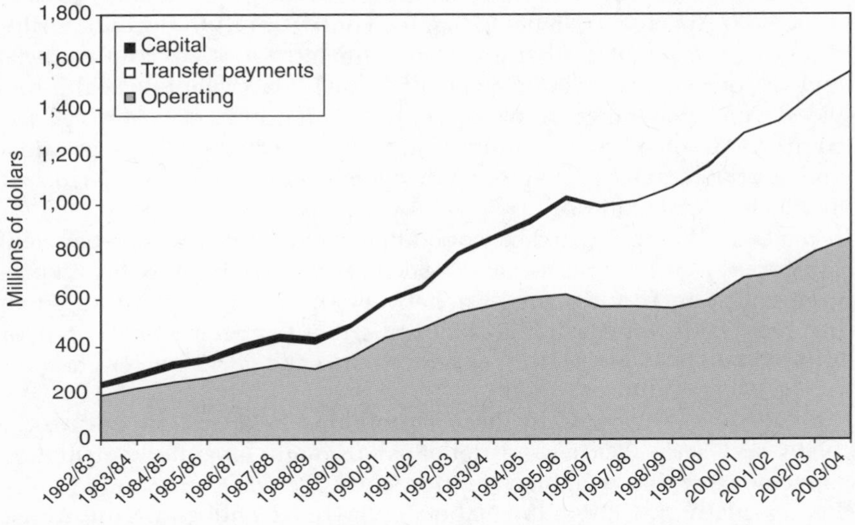

Source: *Public Accounts of Canada* (Receiver General for Canada, relevant years)
Note: This is a stacked area graph. The top curve indicates the combined expenditures of all three categories.

The trend in the three categories of expenditures attributed to the First Nations and Inuit Health activity or business line by Health Canada is shown in figure 22, based on data published in the *Public Accounts of Canada* (which reports on how much was actually spent, rather than what the government intended to spend). In 2002–3, the total expenditures amounted to $1.5 billion. It can be seen that capital expenditures (for example, for construction and renovation of facilities) have declined since their peak in the mid-1980s, when there was a burst of new construction of nursing stations and health centres, whereas transfer payments and operating expenditures have increased substantially. The growth of transfer payments is particularly rapid. In the 1980s, they accounted for less than 15 per cent of expenditures, but by 2005 they constituted 45 per cent of expenditures. Note that all expenditures are expressed in 'current' rather than 'constant' dollars; in other words, they represent dollars at face value in the year they were spent and are not adjusted for inflation.

The increasing importance of transfer payments in the operation of MSB/FNIHB's programs reflects the shift from providing services directly to Aboriginal clients to making contributions to the two territorial governments and Aboriginal governments (such as band councils and regional treaty/tribal councils) to provide a variety of health services, which may range from total control of all health services to specific components such as community health representatives, transportation, and support services. Chapter 10 discusses in detail the transfer policy and its implementation.

Instead of being divided into operating, capital, and transfer-payment categories, expenditures can also be classified as community health programs, hospital services, program delivery and administration, and non-insured health benefits. In the early 2000s, these categories accounted for approximately 48 per cent, 2 per cent, 7 per cent, and 43 per cent, respectively, of expenditures.

Many of the community health programs in operation during the 1990s and early 2000s were delivered through separate contribution agreements with Aboriginal agencies. These include Community Health Representatives (CHRs); the National Native Alcohol and Drug Abuse Program (NNADAP), Brighter Futures, and Building Healthy Communities; the Canada Prenatal Nutrition Program; and the First Nations and Inuit Home and Community Care Program. The Auditor General observed that balancing the need for flexibility with fulfilment of obligations posed a challenge. Some programs had overlapping objectives – for example, Brighter Futures, Building Healthy Communities, and NNADAP all dealt with some aspects of mental health. Specific expectations and activities under agreements were often not clearly stated, and activity reports were not provided consistently (Auditor General 1997: Chapter 13). With regard to clear objectives and activity reporting, the 2000 follow-up audit found that they were present in only 42 per cent and 51 per cent of agreements respectively (Auditor General 2000: Chapter 15).

Non-insured health benefits (NIHB) expenditures have assumed increasing importance in the First Nations and Inuit health 'envelope.' The term refers to health insurance premiums (in provinces where they are levied), patient transportation, prescription drugs, various prosthetic devices and medical appliances, dental care, eyeglasses, and some health services such as mental health crisis interventions. NIHBs generally fall outside of coverage by provincial health insurance plans, and for non-Aboriginal Canadians these have to be paid for either out of pocket or by third-party insurers. Prior to 1978 MSB provided such benefits to status Indians on reserves and to Inuit on the basis of need. An attempt to tighten fiscal control in 1978, with the release of a 'Policy Directive for the Provision of Uninsured Medical and Dental Benefits,' led to widespread protest from Aboriginal groups. The dispute was superseded, first by a change in government as a result of the general election and later by the announcement of the 'Indian Health Policy' in 1979. The policy was widely interpreted in practice to mean the extension of NIHBs to status Indians and Inuit, as an entitlement regardless of ability to pay and often also regardless of place of residence (Auditor General 1982).

In the early 2000s, FNIHB operated on a 'sliding scale' of services based on residence: (1) all eligible First Nations and Inuit receive supplementary health benefits including drugs, dental care, vision care, medical equipment, and mental health counselling (under NIHB expenditures); (2) First Nations living on a reserve receive public health services, alcohol and drug addiction services, and medical transportation; and (3) residents of isolated and remote communities receive primary health care services delivered by nurses and/or physicians, emergency treatment, and referral to other health care facilities.

The total amount of NIHB expenditures escalated from $36 million in 1979–80 to $80 million in 1982–3 (Auditor General 1982), and $166 million in 1986–7, accounting for 40 per cent of all spending by Indian and Northern Health Services (Auditor General 1987). Since that time, the actual amount has continued to skyrocket, although its share of total spending remains at about 40 per cent. By 1992–3, this sum had grown to $442 million. When adjusted for inflation, and including the growth of the eligible population both naturally and as a result of Bill C-31 (which reinstated the status of many Indians, particularly women), the per capita increase averaged 7 per cent annually in constant dollars (Auditor General 1993). In 2002–3, NIHB expenditures reached $688 million (figure 23). Of these, pharmaceuticals accounted for the largest proportion (42 per cent), followed by transportation (30 per cent) and dental care (19 per cent). Pharmaceuticals also showed the greatest increase, having more than doubled in dollar figures in the decade since 1993–4 (Health Canada 2003d).

When the Indian Health Policy was approved in 1979, the federal Cabinet imposed a spending ceiling beyond which MSB had to seek supplemental appropriations. Such annual requests became a regular feature and increased year after year. In fact, non-insured benefits have become an almost open-ended expenditure and a bureaucrat's nightmare – they

Figure 23. Growth in non-insured health benefits annual expenditures

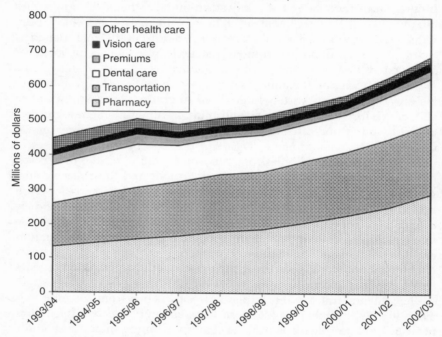

Source: Health Canada 2003b

are deemed uncontrollable because they are authorized by health professionals in the private sector and can be directly accessed by the clients.
This fact did not escape the notice of the Auditor General. The Auditor
General's report for 1982 indicated that high staff turnover, the absence of
nationally established standards, and insufficient procedural and administrative guidance from branch headquarters to regions and zones
resulted in inconsistent availability of such services across the country.
Non-insured benefits also proved a bonanza to health professionals providing services to Aboriginal people. The Auditor General's office
reported cases of excessive charges that were duly paid by MSB, often
without assurance that the services had even been rendered (Auditor
General 1982:372). Several biennial audits later, in 1993, the report still
found MSB 'administering the program without agreement on its exact
nature, without complete information on its costs, and without an effec-

tive management control framework.' While MSB established national program directives in 1989, the auditors found that, had these guidelines been followed, the total 1992–3 NIHB expenditures would have been reduced by 20 per cent (Auditor General 1993:500). NIHB continued to be a target for criticism by the Auditor General in subsequent reports in 1997 and 2000.

As already mentioned above, drug costs are the most important, and fastest-growing, component of NIHB expenditures. In its 2004 audit of all federal drug benefit programs administered by several departments (which also serve, in addition to Aboriginal people, military personnel, the RCMP, veterans, inmates of federal prisons, and certain classes of immigrants), the Auditor General chastised Health Canada for its inability to resolve serious and persistent management problems. The number of clients receiving fifty or more prescriptions in a three-month period had tripled since 1999. This clearly did not reflect changing medical needs. The audit also uncovered hundreds of clients who were receiving two or more narcotics from multiple doctors and multiple pharmacists (Auditor General 2004: Chapter 4:9–11).

From the Aboriginal perspective, there is solid reason on constitutional and political grounds for NIHBs to be an integral part of the federal government's responsibilities towards Aboriginal people. Yet, given that NIHBs have at best only a marginal impact on the health status of Aboriginal people, the fact that they constitute such a substantial proportion of total health expenditures by MSB/FINHB, in a climate of fiscal restraint, can only skew and distort overall health priorities. The vast amounts paid to diverse private dentists, optometrists, pharmacists, and taxi companies can surely be better spent on the development of preventive dental programs, vision screening, a formulary of essential and efficacious drugs, and a triage/referral/evacuation policy.

HEALTH PROFESSIONALS IN THE SYSTEM

In the early 2000s, there were some 1,400 full-time-equivalent public servants under the First Nations and Inuit Health 'business line' of Health Canada (Health Canada 2003d), down from some 2,500 in the late 1980s. The decline reflects the 'outsourcing' of services to Aboriginal communities under transfer and other contractual arrangements. The largest of the occupational groups employed by MSB/FNIHB, in terms of both numbers and breadth of geographical distribution, is nurses. There are hospital-based and community health nurses – the HOS and the CHNs, in public service parlance. Few in and out of MSB/FNIHB would dispute the fact that nurses constitute the backbone of service delivery programs. With justification, they are the unsung heroes, often under stress and not very often appreciated. Particularly in the northern zones, the conditions of work are such that Canadian graduates, in times of high demand, often shun the government's enticements.

Nurses have been the subject of much inquiry over the years. In the 1970s an Interdepartmental Committee on the Nursing Group, composed of representatives of all federal departments that hired nurses (Veterans Affairs, National Defence, Penitentiary Service, and National Health and Welfare), perceived a high degree of dissatisfaction over issues of salary, effective utilization, career progression, professional development, management relations, quality of supervision, and the work environment (Department of National Health and Welfare 1974). While none of these were unique to nurses working in Aboriginal communities, the cross-cultural setting and the geographical isolation seemed to accentuate these difficulties.

Canitz (1989a) examined the factors associated with the high stress levels and high turnover of MSB nurses, particularly in the isolated north. Life in the nursing station setting, where the boundary between the personal and professional was blurred, demanded substantial lifestyle adjustments. The expanded occupational responsibilities but decreased professional support, inadequate preparation and orientation prior to employment, and lack of direction and support while in their postings all contributed to dissatisfaction and burnout. A nurse working in Aboriginal communities as an MSB employee was faced with additional challenges. Cultural awareness and tolerance are not qualities that can be taught overnight. Gender and age issues were often magnified when predominantly young, female nurses were perceived to be in authority positions. Issues of power and control vis-à-vis the government bureaucracy, medical dominance, and community pressures all came to the fore in the nurses' exercise of their professional duties. The actual voices of nurses retelling how these issues affect their daily lives are captured in *GOSSIP: A Spoken History of Women in the North* (Canitz 1989b).

Canitz (1989a:178) provided a vivid description of the enormous scope of the northern nurses' daily activities:

Providing medical care, they deal with colds, pregnancy, chest pain, marital problems, depression, employee physicals, and more. They are public health nurses providing pre- and post-natal clinics, immunizations, and home visits to the elderly. They are the resident dentist applying temporary fillings or pulling teeth that can't wait for the next dental visit. At night, they mysteriously turn into an entire emergency room rolled into one person. They are alone to suture, bandage, resuscitate, and console. Northern nurses are x-ray technicians and radiologists through the lens of the primitive x-ray machines they have to use. They are laboratory technicians and pathologists as they draw blood, collect urine, and utilize swabs as a means of pinpointing and identifying the etiology of a disease. They are public health inspectors responsible for the hygiene of all public services.

The idea of nurses working in isolation, diagnosing and treating diseases – thought to be the preserve of physicians – often frightened physicians, administrators, and not a few nurses themselves. Yet, a Committee on Clinical Training of Nurses in 1970 suggested that 50 per cent of cases seen in a nursing station were totally manageable by a nurse without additional training, while less than 1 per cent were completely beyond the scope of a nurse even with additional training and available consultation. The remaining 49 per cent could be managed with training and consultation. While improved skills in physical assessment and case management would better prepare nurses for work in isolated settings, this would be perceived as encroaching upon the realm of practice claimed by physicians. No Canadian medical or nursing licensing bodies have tackled such legalistic issues head-on. Such grey areas in the remote margins of the country appeared to be best left undisturbed. Provincial nursing licensing bodies tend to recognize only what are traditionally considered 'nursing' duties. The issue of liability is further complicated by the transfer of control of some nursing stations to First Nations and tribal councils, which often cannot afford to offer the same amount of insurance coverage formerly provided by MSB. Despite experimental projects in the 1970s, the concept of the nurse-practitioner never did take root in southern Canada. In this respect, MSB can take some credit for having the longest tradition of employing nurses in an expanded role in large swathes of the Canadian hinterland.

In the 1980s, nursing leaders in MSB embraced the health promotion rhetoric (as did much of the public health profession). Emphasis on clinical training for nurses gave way to talk of the nurses' changing role from one of service provider to 'facilitator, supporter, and resource worker' and a shift from treatment to health promotion (Doucette 1989). However, in the communities, nurses continue to be overloaded with acute health problems requiring immediate attention, and the shift from a curative to a preventive orientation remains very much an unrealized goal.

With the increasing number of First Nations communities controlling their own health care, many nurses, formerly federal public servants, found themselves working in entirely new, and often unfamiliar, occupational environments. A few case studies have investigated nurses' views of Aboriginal-controlled health services. Hiebert and colleagues (2001) conducted focus groups with nurses working in three northwestern Ontario First Nations communities under a regional Aboriginal health authority. The informants indicated that collaboration between nurses and community members had improved after transfer, and nurses felt that they were now more than just service providers, having a stronger role in program planning with the community. Morale had improved, which resulted in a higher retention rate of staff. With community empowerment, acts of vandalism directed at the nursing station and harassment of the nurses, which had been endemic, declined.

While their number has greatly dwindled, physicians – referred to as medical officers or MOFs – once exercised great authority within MSB. Until the late 1970s, most senior line manager positions – from the deputy minister, assistant deputy minister, director general, and regional directors down to the zone directors – were occupied by MOFs. In some zones, the zone director dashed from the operating room to the office and alternated ward rounds with bursts of bureaucratic chores. As health care became increasingly complex, a managerial revolution swept through all echelons of government. MOFs were considered amateur administrators, and increasingly they have been replaced by 'pure' administrators, many of whom have risen through the clerical ranks. From health practitioners with little or no administrative training, the system was soon taken over by administrators with little or no health background.

Physicians who work on salary in the government have traditionally been held in low regard by the rest of the medical profession. The loss of 'clout' within the MSB organization would further deter prospective fresh recruits from entering the service. In the early 1980s, the remaining senior MOFs in MSB perceived a crisis with regard to the number, quality, and role of MOFs. A Task Force on Medical Officers was convened in 1983 to make recommendations to reverse the fortunes of the MOFs within MSB. Little came of the task force, however. The position of MOFs within MSB continued to be eroded. By the end of the 1980s few management positions were held by MOFs. The 1980s and 1990s witnessed the burgeoning of the rejuvenated medical specialty of 'community medicine.' Compared to provincial and municipal health departments, MSB has not been successful in tapping into this pool of physicians more sympathetic to, and better skilled in, health care management, planning, and evaluation (Department of National Health and Welfare 1983).

The crisis in physician recruitment towards the end of the 1960s led MSB to seek assistance from medical schools, teaching hospitals, and professional associations. The poor quality of the clinical staff and their generally short duration of stay throughout most of the 1950s and 1960s was a common complaint of the employer (T.K. Young 1988b:104).

The medical schools came to the rescue and relieved MSB of the headaches of physician recruitment and retention. This new arrangement was a symbiotic one. The prestige of affiliation with a medical school, generous salaries and benefits and continuing education leave, housing subsidies, and the availability of clinical back-up by specialist consultants were seen to be attractions to potential recruits, who generally tend to be young, recent graduates. The universities benefited by gaining access to new community sites where teaching and research could take place in conjunction with the delivery of services. The image of universities' developing a social conscience and stepping out of the ivory tower to help the impoverished and underserved was also one that universities were keen to project.

Physician services in various northern zones were contracted out by MSB to the universities: Queen's in the Moose Factory Zone, McGill in the Baffin Zone, the University of Toronto in the Sioux Lookout Zone, and the University of Manitoba in the Keewatin Zone. The lifespan of these programs varied, and by the beginning of the 2000s only the University of Manitoba Northern Medical Unit remained.[1] The largest of these in terms of staff size, geographical coverage, and budget, it has actually expanded to cover more than thirty communities in Manitoba and Nunavut, and its contractual relationship is no longer solely with MSB but is also with the provincial and territorial governments and other funding sources.

An important consequence of the involvement of universities in service delivery is the establishment of special programs to promote the entry of Aboriginal students into health professional faculties. The University of Manitoba took the lead, initiating a Special Premedical Studies Program in 1979 to prepare students for admission into medicine, dentistry, pharmacy, and medical rehabilitation. This program has since been extended to include also a Professional Health Program as the original students gained entry into, progressed through, and graduated from these faculties (Stephens 1991; Stephens et al. 1998). Other universities have since established similar programs.

Accurate statistics of Aboriginal health professionals are difficult to obtain. One source estimated 800 Aboriginal nurses and 67 physicians in the whole of Canada in 1998 (Commission on the Future of Health Care 2002:220). Aboriginal communities have also begun to take steps to address the issue of health human resources. For example, in 2004 the Six Nations Council and the Chiefs of Ontario developed '2020 Vision: Strategy for Training Aboriginal Physicians in Ontario,' which called for major government investments in and partnerships with the province's four medical schools to improve recruitment, training, and support of Aboriginal students.

In addition to universities, a few professional associations have also taken a keen and sustained interest in the health of Aboriginal people, notably the Canadian Pediatric Society (CPS), which has since the late 1960s set up an Indian and Eskimo Child Health Committee. The Canadian Psychiatric Association also established a Native Mental Health section, which in 1989 formed its own association, the Native Mental Health Association of Canada.

Over the years, individual medical schools also offered short elective periods that enabled undergraduate and postgraduate students to work in Aboriginal communities. An early example is Queen's University's program on the Tyendinaga Mohawk reserve (Read and Strick 1969). Many students, thus exposed, later returned for full-time practice as general practitioners, and a few even devoted a considerable portion of their later professional career to the field of northern and Aboriginal health care.

Canadian faculties of dentistry, notably those at Toronto and Manitoba, also became actively involved in providing services to Aboriginal communities through university-MSB contracts. The University of Toronto's dental involvement in the Sioux Lookout Zone dates back to 1970 (K.C. Titley 1973). An evaluation of changes in dental health status after ten years of service showed little change. While dental manpower woes have largely been overcome, the program's coordinator was honest in admitting that 'until solidly based preventive programs incorporating fluorides, fissure sealants and education become a major component part of the service, the dentist's role in controlling dental disease will be mainly palliative' (K.C. Titley and Bedard 1986).

A unique contribution to dental manpower development – beyond merely supplying southern, non-Aboriginal dentists – is MSB's School of

Dental Therapy (Davey 1974). The first (and so far only) of its kind in North America, the school was started in 1972 in Fort Smith, Northwest Territories, but moved to Prince Albert, Saskatchewan, in 1982. Dental therapists can be considered dental auxiliaries with an expanded role in both prevention and treatment. Its curriculum and training methods have been emulated overseas in some developing countries. Indeed, several African and Carribean countries began sending students to the school, accounting for as much as one-third of the student body (Torbert 1990). In Canada, however, attempts to expand into the provinces were thwarted by provincial dental associations over the issue of licensing and the threat of competition posed by a low-cost, but effective, alternative.

The need for on-site psychiatric consultations to reduce institutionalization at distant mental hospitals has long been recognized. A multi-university team of psychiatrists, for example, assessed mental health needs in the Northwest Territories on behalf of MSB in the late 1960s (Atcheson et al. 1969), and most university northern programs introduced a psychiatry component in the early 1970s (Levine et al. 1974; Pelz et al. 1981; Hood et al. 1993). These programs send psychiatrists and trainees to provide individual therapy to patients referred by local nurses, physicians, and CHRs, conduct interagency conferences and community meetings, and provide continuing education for local staff. The Sioux Lookout program won a merit award in community psychiatry from the American Psychiatric Association in 1978. In the early 1980s, it was one of the first programs to begin the training of Aboriginal counsellors (Timpson 1984).

UTILIZATION OF HEALTH SERVICES BY ABORIGINAL PEOPLES

There is a widespread perception among health professionals and administrators in Canada that Aboriginal people use health care services differently than non-Aboriginal people do. Many factors are believed to play a role in accounting for such differences. The health planning literature conceives of *use* as dependent on *supply* (the availability of services) and *need* (the burden of ill-health), which is expressed as *demand* by those willing to seek or pay for health services to satisfy the need. Thus the type of services that are made available (or not made available) to Aboriginal people, particularly those living in remote areas, would affect utilization. The higher (or lower) prevalence of many health conditions would also affect utilization related to the relief of those conditions. Cultural and socio-economic barriers, even in situations where the need is great, may result in reduced demand and reduced use. On the other hand, the same cultural and socio-economic factors can result in the opposite – apparent overuse.

Many commentators on Aboriginal health have simplistically re-garded health service utilization as merely an issue of 'cultural differ-ences' (usually expressed in stereotypes, as in 'Indian time'). Waldram (1990c) referred to a body of 'medical folklore' held by health care prac-titioners that Aboriginal people underuse or even avoid medical care. On the other hand, there is an equally strongly held belief that Aborigi-nal people overuse or abuse the health care system – for example, by 'pestering' nurses in off-hours for minor illnesses.

The stereotypes about Aboriginal health care utilization are perva-sive. For instance, the 1969 Booz-Allen report, a major review of Indian health services conducted by an international health service consultancy firm for MSB, stated that,

Many Indians have little understanding of the meaning of good health because of cultural differences and education deficiencies. Indians exhibit little aware-ness of what is meant by good health and because of this lack of awareness there is a tendency to both over and under-utilize health services ... Indians frequently fail to recognize significant symptoms and delay seeking treatment until they are acutely ill. (Booz-Allen 1969:13)

In order to establish that differential utilization exists, one can look at a variety of data sources at the national and regional levels: hospital admissions, visits to ambulatory care offices, and survey-based self-reports of health service use. An important point that should be recog-nized is that differential use relative to Canadians in general does not mean that Aboriginal people receive 'better' or 'worse' health services, or receive such services more or less efficiently. Using Canadian health ser-vices utilization rates as the yardstick for comparison should not imply that the national level is necessarily the appropriate one.

As all Canadians are covered by universal hospital and medical care insurance, and all hospitals and physicians bill their provincial health insurance agencies for reimbursement, the enormous databases main-tained by these agencies can serve as important sources of data on health service utilization. Unfortunately, it is possible to examine utili-zation by Aboriginal people only in some provinces, namely those in western Canada (British Columbia, Alberta, Saskatchewan, and Mani-toba). Furthermore, it is only status Indians who are separately identifi-able through special coding of their health insurance plan number.

Figure 24. Age-sex-specific hospitalization rate, late 1990s

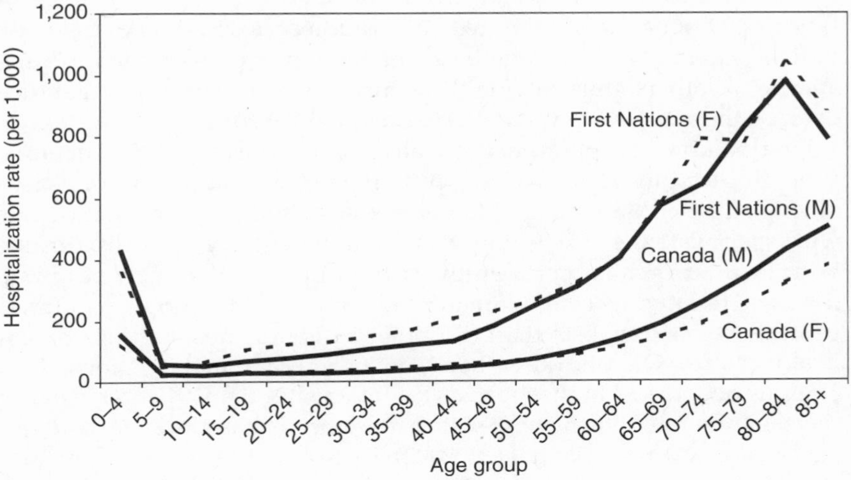

Source: FNIHB, Health Information and Analysis Division 2004
Note: First Nations data cover only British Columbia, Manitoba, and Saskatchewan.
Pregnancies are excluded.

Data from three western provinces in the late 1990s illustrate that in all age groups the hospitalization rate of status Indians exceeded that of the total population (figure 24).

Manitoba First Nations had higher rates of hospitalization than the non-Aboriginal population in the province in the late 1990s: 2.2 times the hospital discharge rate and 1.7 times the total days of hospital care. About 16 per cent of First Nations people (compared to 11 per cent of all other Manitobans) were admitted to hospital at least once in a year. The pattern of higher hospitalization among First Nations occurred in all tribal council areas and health regions. Moreover, hospitalization rates were lowest in the major urban centres of Winnipeg and Brandon, where hospital services are most readily available (Martens, Bond, et al. 2002).

In a study to determine if acute-care hospitals were used appropriately, the Manitoba Centre for Health Policy and Evaluation reviewed a sample of hospital charts from each of twenty-six Manitoba hospitals during 1993–4, using a set of well-validated, objective, clinical indicators of the severity of illness and intensity of service. They found that a high proportion of medical admissions in the province were inappropriate, with about half of all admissions being for non-acute conditions or conditions that could have received care through alternative methods or facilities. Despite their high rate of utilization of hospital services, treaty Indian patients had the same levels of appropriateness (or inappropriateness) as others, thus belying the commonly held perception that they overuse the acute-care system (DeCoster et al. 1999).

First Nations people also used physician services more frequently, averaging 6.1 physician visits per person per year, compared to 4.9 visits among all other Manitobans. However, the ambulatory consultation rate with specialists (i.e., excluding visits to inpatients by specialists inside hospitals) was similar between the two groups. In Winnipeg and Brandon, where most specialists are located, First Nations people had fewer contacts with specialists than did other residents, despite their poorer health status. On the other hand, in northern remote regions, First Nations people had higher specialist contact rates than other residents in the same region, which suggested a more needs-based delivery of specialist care (Martens, Bond, et al. 2002). It also suggests that, despite geographic remoteness, equity in some services can be achieved through outreach programs (such as those operated by the Northern Medical Unit) and subsidized medical transportation for appointments (under NIHB).

Given the poorer health status of First Nations people, their higher health care use (of both hospital and physician services) would indicate that the health care system appeared to be responsive to the needs of those in poorer health. However, in terms of preventive health care, First Nations people did not fare as well. First Nations children had far lower complete immunization rates than other Manitoban children at ages one (62 per cent vs 89 per cent) and two (45 per cent vs 77 per cent). At the time of discharge from hospitals, only 54 per cent of First Nations newborns were started on breastfeeding, compared to 80 per cent among non-Aboriginal newborns. Among women aged fifty to sixty-nine, the rate of mammography (an effective breast cancer screening procedure for this age group) was 26 per cent among First Nations women, compared to 56 per cent among other women (Martens, Bond, et al. 2002).

Information on the use of health services can also be obtained in the course of a survey. The Canadian Community Health Survey (CCHS) of 2000–1 was a national survey of Canadians that sampled more than 3,500 Aboriginal respondents living off reserve, including those in the northern territories. Overall, there was no difference in the proportion of respondents who had had a contact with a general practitioner in the past year between Aboriginal and non-Aboriginal people nationally, whether in urban or rural areas. However, the rate for Aboriginal people in the northern territories was much lower (59 per cent vs 76 per cent). In addition, Aboriginal people were less likely to have a regular doctor than other Canadians (76 per cent vs 84 per cent). The disparity was particularly severe in the territories (31 per cent vs 67 per cent), and detectable in the rural areas of the provinces (79 per cent vs 84 per cent), but disappeared in the urban areas. The proportion with contacts with a dentist was lower among Aboriginal than non-Aboriginal people nationally, in both urban and rural areas, and also in the territories. About 20 per cent of Aboriginal people reported that in the past year there was a time when they needed health care but did not receive it, a measure of unmet health needs that was higher than the 13 per cent among non-Aboriginal Canadians. The reasons for this unmet need were classified as unavailability (48 per cent – service not available where or when required or waiting time too long), inaccessibility (51 per cent – due to cost or lack of transportation), and unacceptability (17 per cent – concerned attitudes and competing responsibilities) (Tjepkema 2002).

The 1991 Aboriginal Peoples Survey (APS) indicated that within the Aboriginal population, health care utilization varied according to such demographic and socio-economic factors as age, sex, income, and education. The pattern was similar to those observed in other populations. Thus women used health services more frequently than men, and the elderly more than the young. Those with more education, higher income, and living in urban areas were more likely to have a physician contact. An attempt to identify the role of cultural factors in health care use yielded mixed results. Those who were fluent in an Aboriginal language were less likely to have consulted a physician, whereas those who participated in traditional activities were more likely to have consulted one (Newbold 1997).

It is important to balance such national/provincial perspectives on use of health services with more in-depth inquiries at the local/regional level. Thouez, Foggin, and Rannou (1990) surveyed the Cree and Inuit in northern Quebec and found that, as expected, functional incapacity and perceived morbidity variables were linked to the degree that primary health care and hospital services were used. However, they also found that negative perceptions about the services provided and doubts about the physician were also significant determinants of health service use.

Waldram (1990c) surveyed inner-city residents in Saskatoon and compared the pattern and determinants of visits to physicians by Aboriginal and non-Aboriginal patients. To his surprise, he found little difference between the two groups. Just under 80 per cent of Aboriginal people indicated that they had a regular physician, and were able to provide that person's name. A similar proportion reported having consulted their regular physician at least once in the previous three months, while 57 per cent had undergone a physical examination within the last year. These differences were not statistically significant from the proportions reported by non-Aboriginal patients, thus discounting conventional wisdom that Aboriginal people in the city had a tendency to avoid physicians.

The study further demonstrated that persons who had lived in the city the longest, those with children, females, and those who were married were most likely to have a regular physician and to have had a recent contact with that practitioner. While Waldram did show that only 33 per cent of the Aboriginal patients had arrived with an appointment on the day of their interview, compared to 59 per cent of the non-Aboriginal patients, he also found that only 29 per cent of the Aboriginal patients had telephones, compared to 82 per cent of non-Aboriginal patients, and that most patients with telephones had made appointments. The most problematic group in Waldram's research, in terms of underuse or avoidance of the urban health care system, were single White males, yet no medical folklore seemed to exist among medical practitioners with respect to their problematic use.

The use of health care services should also be viewed in the political context, particularly the power relationship between Aboriginal 'users' and predominantly non-Aboriginal 'providers'. (The conventional use of such terms is in itself problematic.) The pattern of health service use can be profoundly altered in communities that have assumed control of their health care delivery. The William Charles First Nation, located at Montreal Lake in Saskatchewan, was the first band in Canada to obtain control over health care delivery under the Health Transfer Agreement of MSB (see chapter 10). Prior to transfer, amid a high level of physical and social health problems, the community practised little self-care and home management of minor childhood illnesses. Immunization rates were low. Some residents, particularly seniors, avoided contact with the nursing station, while others made constant demands on the nurses after hours. After the transfer of control in 1988, this pattern of behaviour was changed dramatically (M. Moore et al. 1990).

O'Neil (1986, 1990) studied the provider-client relationship in the Arctic and how it could be affected by personalities. Nurses and physicians who are sensitive and open to cross-cultural differences and who have a high degree of commitment to community issues generally find it easier to develop satisfactory relationships than those with rigid ideas about their professional role and who have little interest in community life. O'Neil believed that the existing structure of federal health care tended to frustrate the efforts of sensitive and committed practitioners but reward those with an aloof, detached, and 'colonial' approach.

Health care encounters involving Aboriginal people and non-Aboriginal medical practitioners are often affected by ingrained racial stereotyping. Sherley-Spiers (1989) documented the perceptions of Dakota patients in southwestern Manitoba. In their view, seriously ill patients were often assumed to be intoxicated by the attending physicians. Physicians often scolded mothers for not taking proper care of their children and for bringing them to the clinic either too early and when they were not sick enough or too late when the illness was too far advanced.

Many Aboriginal people have made known their views of the health care system in numerous community meetings across the country conducted as part of public inquiries. Common concerns range from systemic ones – such as the infrequency of doctors' visits, inaccessibility of nursing stations after hours, lack of Aboriginal health personnel, inflexible referral and evacuation policies, and inadequate boarding arrangements – to highly personal accounts of insensitive treatment, misdiagnosis, and delayed evacuation. The Scott-McKay-Bain Health Panel was convened by MSB and the Nishnawbe-Aski Nation of northern Ontario in response to a hunger strike by Aboriginal leaders in the Sioux Lookout Zone Hospital in 1988. On the national scene, the Royal Commission on Aboriginal Peoples during 1991–4 also invited Aboriginal communities to voice their health care concerns, among other issues.

In summarizing the personal accounts of the health care system by 'users' who made presentations in community hearings to the Scott-McKay-Bain Health Panel, Madeline Beardy wrote:

The Native women of the Sioux Lookout Zone had a lot to say about the present health care system. They expressed views about the nursing stations, hospital experiences, nurses, doctors, transportation and communications. Often when people are asked what their views are on medical matters they associate the question with pain, discomfort, frustration and some anger. Also the family and friends of people involved in health problems face fear, anxiety, confusion and shock. (Scott-McKay-Bain Health Panel 1989a:4–5)

There was a widespread perception among Aboriginal people that they did not receive health care of comparable quality to that experienced by non-Aboriginal people. In the First Nations and Inuit Regional Health Survey of 1997, only a third of the respondents thought their care equivalent. Groups that were particularly dissatisfied were those with chronic conditions, the disabled, and those living in small and isolated communities. The Manitoba component of the survey were also asked about discrimination from health care workers: 16 per cent reported having experienced discrimination inside their community and 30 per cent outside their community (First Nations Information Governance Committee 2004:50–1).

In 2002, the National Aboriginal Health Organization (NAHO) commissioned a commercial polling firm to conduct a telephone survey of on-reserve First Nations people on a variety of health issues. Regarding satisfaction and experience with the health care system, 67 per cent rated the quality of health care they received in the past month as 'excellent' or 'good.' There was regional variation, with the highest proportion of satisfaction (>80 per cent) reported by those residing in the Atlantic provinces and Quebec, and the lowest in British Columbia, Yukon, and Manitoba (60 per cent or less). Those residing in isolated and remote communities were least likely to have a favourable impression of their health care (National Aboriginal Health Organization 2004:75–7). We hasten to add here that perceptions, while important in so far as they affect health care utilization, are only partial indicators of the adequacy or appropriateness of health services. Such perceptions can be influencd by other factors, some not directly related to health care. It is important to note that non-Aboriginal people also often express dissatisfaction with the health care system.

THE FUTURE ROLE OF GOVERNMENTS

What role will the federal government play under the era of 'new relationships' with Aboriginal people? Since the 1990s the federal role in services to Aboriginal people, whether provided by Indian Affairs or by FNIHB, is increasingly viewed as one of 'funder' rather than 'provider.' As is already evident from figure 23, the role of 'transfer payments' has assumed a predominant position within FNIHB. The federal agency perceives itself as having a residual role in strategic policy development, information management, and financial accountability. Already, FNHIB in 2005 is unrecognizable compared to the Indian and Northern Health Services at the time of the creation of DNHW in 1945 and MSB at the time of the 1962 major reorganizations.

The provincial and territorial governments have become major players in health care delivery to Aboriginal people, altering the long-standing 'special relationship' between the federal government and Aboriginal people. Provincial governments have traditionally shied away from involvement in direct provision of health services to Aboriginal people on reserves, preferring to let the federal government worry about them (and pay the lion's share). Aboriginal organizations traditionally have also insisted on dealing only with the federal government, in accordance with a 'nation-to-nation' mode of discourse, except when it comes to eligibility for provincial services. The truth of the matter is, however, that universal health insurance plans administered by the provinces and territories cover Aboriginal people within their respective jurisdictions. (In the few provinces that have at one time or another levied health insurance premiums, FNIHB pays for them on behalf of Indians and Inuit, under the NIHB provisions).

In recognition of the multijurisdictional nature of Aboriginal health care, a Tripartite Working Group on Aboriginal Health was struck in 1991 as a result of a meeting between the federal, provincial, and territorial health ministers and the leaders of the four national political Indian, Inuit, and Métis organizations. This working group reported to the Conference of Health Ministers in 1993, bringing to the national level the recognition, if not the solution, of structural barriers to the delivery of Aboriginal health services.

Within several provincial health ministries (in Ontario and British Columbia, for example), small, tentative steps have been taken to include Aboriginal health in the organizational structure. After extensive province-wide consultations in 1992, the Ontario government launched the Aboriginal Healing and Wellness Strategy in 1994, with the signing of implementation agreements with major provincial Aboriginal organizations representing First Nations, Métis, friendship centres, and Aboriginal women. These agreements were renewed in 1999 for another five years. Funding was contributed by the provincial health and community services ministries as well as the Native Affairs and Women's Directorates. The strategy has two components, one of which specifically targets family violence while the other is concerned more broadly with health and wellness. It aims to promote integration of traditional and culturally appropriate approaches to healing and wellness in Aboriginal communities with mainstream services. It has supported a network of Aboriginal Health Access Centres across the province, providing holistic, comprehensive, primary care services, including healing lodges and treatment centres for addictions and family violence; women's shelters; a maternal centre employing Aboriginal midwives; the Healthy Babies, Healthy Children Program to promote healthy child development and support families; and a variety of training projects (Aboriginal Healing and Wellness Strategy 2003).

After the final report of the Royal Commission on Aboriginal Peoples was released in 1996, the federal government announced 'Gathering Strength: Canada's Aboriginal Action Plan.' The plan was government-wide, although the majority of the actions fell under the responsibility of the Department of Indian Affairs and Northern Development. Health Canada's role was limited to initiatives directed at diabetes and tuberculosis control and developing the Aboriginal Healing Foundation and a healing strategy addressing the legacy of Indian residential schools.

In 2002, Roy Romanow, a former premier of Saskatchewan who was appointed commissioner to examine the future of health care in Canada by Prime Minister Jean Chrétien in response to a widespread perception of a health care crisis in the country, submitted his final report. 'Aboriginal Health' constituted one chapter (Commission on the Future of Health Care in Canada 2002:211–31). In it, Romanow identified a 'disconnect' between Aboriginal peoples and the rest of Canadian society when it comes to sharing the benefits of the highly touted Canadian health care system. This disconnect was attributed to five factors:

- competing constitutional assumptions;
- fragmented funding for health services;
- inadequate access to health care services;
- poorer health outcomes; and
- different cultural and political influences.

These issues have been thoroughly examined in this book, in both this and preceding chapters. As a solution, Romanow recommended consolidating Aboriginal health funding from all sources and creating Aboriginal health partnerships with a clear structure and mandate to manage Aboriginal health services. Such bold, cross-jurisdictional remedies are particularly difficult to implement in the Canadian context, and it remains to be seen if health care arrangements for Aboriginal people will change fundamentally in the future.

CONCLUSIONS

This chapter began with a description of the Aboriginal health care system, primarily from a 'technocratic' viewpoint. It ends with an examination of the changing role of the various levels of government. A health care system has many components, but the most important of these are the 'providers' and the 'users.' Yet 'users' as a term is inadequate to depict the central role played by Aboriginal people in such a system. No longer satisfied as passive consumers of services, albeit services generally competently delivered and at great expense, Aboriginal groups have entered a new era of self-determination in health care since the 1980s and 1990s. This will be the subject of chapter 10. An Aboriginal health care system has Aboriginal people not only as 'users' but also as 'providers,' and everything in between as well. Not surprisingly, then, parallel to the continued development of medical services and related initiatives, discussed in this and previous chapters, there has been a re-emergence of 'traditional' health care, the subject of the next chapter.

9

Aboriginal healing in the contemporary context

As we suggested in chapter 5, Aboriginal medicine and healing approaches began to re-emerge (from the perspective of non-Aboriginal observers) in the 1980s. By this time, many Aboriginal communities had experienced significant losses of traditional healing knowledge, and there were relatively fewer healers than in the past. These losses are part of the legacy of colonialism, epidemic diseases, missionization, residential schools, and government policies of assimilation (including the outlawing of some healing-related ceremonies, as we saw in chapter 5). But not all was lost. It might be just as accurate to say that many aspects of Aboriginal healing and spirituality were shielded from the scrutiny of non-Aboriginal people, including but not exclusively law enforcement officials. For instance, predictions of the demise of the Midewiwin and shaking tent were simply wrong, and these activities have continued to this day. The sweat lodge has experienced a resurgence, and it is being introduced back into communities where it has been absent for generations, and into new communities where it likely never existed. The Sun Dance and the potlatch remain very much a part of Aboriginal traditions among the Plains and Northwest Coast peoples, respectively. In recent years, these and other healing and spiritual ceremonies have been opened up more to non-Aboriginal people, to the extent where we are now hearing calls to incorporate elements of Aboriginal healing into biomedicine, even to the point of formal collaboration between the practitioners in the two systems. Further, some Aboriginal people have begun to allow the limited scientific study of some of their practices, especially their use of plant medicines. The issues surrounding these developments are complex, and are linked to a reversal of the processes of deculturalization and despiritualization and the continued expansion of self-determination. In this chapter, we will examine some important issues with respect to this resurgence.

UNPACKING 'TRADITIONAL ABORIGINAL HEALING'

'Traditional healing' has become a ubiquitous term these days, yet no succinct and agreed-upon definition exists. The term simultaneously speaks to both psychological and physiological processes but adds an element of metaphysics and spirituality as well. It also denotes the significance of past acquired knowledge handed down successively from generation to generation. The problem of definition is evident in the following explanation offered by the Royal Commission on Aboriginal Peoples (RCAP):

Traditional healing has been defined as practices designed to promote mental, physical and spiritual well-being that are based on beliefs which go back to the time before the spread of western 'scientific' bio-medicine. When Aboriginal Peoples in Canada talk about traditional healing, they include a wide range of activities, from physical cures using herbal medicines and other remedies, to the promotion of psychological and spiritual well-being using ceremony, counselling and the accumulated wisdom of elders. (RCAP 1996, Vol. 3:348)

Unfortunately, the adjective 'traditional' implies a static, past-oriented approach to well-being that is of little utility in a contemporary context, a seriously flawed notion. While traditionality speaks to the past, to the accumulated knowledge of generations of healers and patients, it cannot be seen as separate from the very contemporary context in which it exists and is offered. Not surprisingly, there are many relatively new ideas, some emanating from biomedicine and from popular culture, which have been incorporated into so-called traditional healing practices. Similarly, it is common to find elements of Christian symbolism and doctrine entrenched within 'traditional' healing practices. In this sense, traditional Aboriginal healing must be seen as ever-evolving systems of knowledge and practices that synthesize borrowed and newly developed ideas, whatever the source, with existing ideas to maintain a more or less coherent healing approach. Unlike biomedicine, 'traditional healing' is anchored in a cultural context that is celebrated as the source of its knowledge. Traditional healing is as much cultural as it is medical. And we must also be vigilant about how we use the term 'healing.' As Manson and colleagues (1996:275) have suggested, the term 'healing' may simply represent 'the best available metaphor by which non-Natives could describe and understand ... what was happening' in the various activities they witnessed. Despite common usage of the term among Aboriginal people today, one must be alert to the many and varied ways it is used. The same holds true for the term 'medicine,' which exhibits a wide variation in meaning, from deeply held beliefs in spiritual power, to Aboriginal healers, to biomedical practice.

It is our view that the term 'traditional' is no longer useful as an adjective, and therefore we will refrain from its use from this point onward, except in specific contexts. Further, while the term 'Aboriginal medicine' remains popular (including 'medicine man'), 'medicine' is so clearly linked with the scientific paradigm, which largely precludes the central role of spirituality, that it is best to avoid this term. In this chapter, for the most part, we employ 'Aboriginal healing,' a term that encompasses a wide variety of practices and associated knowledge, from the use of herbal medicines to spiritual ceremonies, from the utilization of active pharmacological compounds to what the mainstream would see as psychotherapeutic practice. As important, this term more readily allows for an understanding of the innovation and change that exists in the efforts of Aboriginal people to restore health and prevent illness. Again, however, there will be contexts in which the term 'medicine' remains the most suitable – for instance, when referring to plant-based or herbal treatment compounds.

THE RE-EMERGENCE OF ABORIGINAL HEALING

It has become fairly common in hospitals, clinics, and other institutions in many parts of Canada to see an Aboriginal healer undertaking a ceremony for a patient. This development really accelerated in the early 1980s, as hospital administrators grappled with the complexities of having so many culturally different patients who were going to consult healers with or without hospital involvement. Accommodating healers certainly required some flexibility. For instance, the simple act of a sweetgrass ceremony tended to violate hospital regulations against 'smoking,' and the subsequent solution of disconnecting smoke detectors was not well received, for obvious reasons. Tension often occurred around the issue of drugs and medical devices, such as intravenous tubes; many healers demanded that patients be free of all biomedical accoutrements. Nevertheless, through compromise and dialogue, accommodations have been made.

An early and prominent example of the complexities of involving an Aboriginal healer within a hospital is that of the Lake of the Woods Hospital in Kenora, Ontario. Indeed, a plaque in the lobby of the hospital states that 'We believe traditional Native healing and culture have a place in our provision of health care services to the Native people' (cited in Gagnon 1989:176). In 1980, the Ontario Ministry of Health provided funding to hire a healer to work within the hospital. The move was a controversial one, with some Aboriginal people arguing against it. According to a report on this program (Seaby 1983:2), several complaints were made that, in essence, are often still uttered when institutions and healers come together. These included the following:

- The hiring of a single healer did not recognize that healers, like physicians, have areas of specialization.
- It was breaking traditional practice for the government to pay for the services of the healer, as it is the responsibility of the person who is consulting the healer to provide payment.
- The flurry of media attention at the outset of the program detracted from the healer's credibility within the Native community.
- The location of the healer in the hospital did not meet the approval of the elders.

When the healer died suddenly, within a year of his appointment, some observers were led to believe that this was a sign of the inappropriateness of the arrangement. Nevertheless, soon thereafter a program coordinator was hired to arrange healer services for patients according to family preferences and the specialization of the healer. Efforts were made to have more Aboriginal input into the program as well, to prevent the type of conflict that had arisen under the first program. By the mid-1980s, more than half of the hospital physicians were referring patients to healers for a variety of treatments (D.E. Young and Smith 1992:45). Subsequently, a healer was hired within the hospital's Department of Psychiatry.

In Winnipeg, an initiative to develop a medical interpreters' program at two hospitals led to the introduction of Aboriginal healing into the hospitals themselves (Kaufert and Koolage 1985; O'Neil 1988). These Aboriginal interpreters found that, among their many duties, there was a need to facilitate Aboriginal healing for some patients. Since many of these patients were hospitalized far away from their communities, they lacked a connection to the urban Aboriginal healing network. The interpreters facilitated the process by helping to identify healers and by working with the hospital physicians and administrators to make the necessary arrangements so that such healing could occur in as culturally appropriate a manner as possible.

More recent developments have seen the establishment of entrenched programs and facilities in hospitals and clinics. Throughout the country, especially in areas with high concentrations of Aboriginal people, healing rooms and related programs have been developed that target the Aboriginal population and facilitate complementary and alternative approaches to treatment. In doing so, these hospitals and clinics are following the lead of groundbreaking alcohol and drug abuse treatment programs, such as Poundmaker's Lodge, where Aboriginal treatment rooms are mainstays.

Insofar as the biomedical system has accepted Aboriginal healing, there has been a tendency to marginalize it somewhat within the realm of 'mental health.' One of the pioneers in this area is B.C. psychiatrist Wolfgang Jilek, who has worked successfully since the 1970s with Aboriginal healers in the treatment of patients with alcohol problems and other psychiatric disorders perceived to have a cultural component (Jilek 1982a; see also Jilek 1978, 1982b; and Jilek and Jilek-Aall 1982, 1991). In particular, he has documented the therapeutic effectiveness of Coast Salish 'Spirit Dancing' as a treatment strategy, especially for alcoholism. In Toronto, the Centre for Addiction and Mental Health now has a small Aboriginal program that seeks to include Aboriginal healing services (Tillson 2002). However, in general the psychiatric profession in Canada has not been particularly open to Aboriginal healing approaches.

Aboriginal communities themselves have taken the lead in promoting healing for their people. A well-known case is that of Alkali Lake, British Columbia, a community that was rife with alcoholism and its attendant problems (violence, sexual abuse, suicide, etc.) that turned itself around to become almost totally alcohol free (York 1989; Johnson and Johnson 1993; see also the band-produced video *The Honour of All*). This transformation was accomplished with the assistance of a non-local traditional healer who was asked to help the community rediscover the sweat lodge and other healing approaches. The use of such visiting healers has become common in much of Canada as communities seek to revitalize their spirituality and healing where locally available knowledge and specialists are unavailable.

Throughout Canada, and especially in the west, 'healing circles' are also common. These are therapeutic sessions organized by Aboriginal people to deal with problems such as the effects of residential schools, sexual abuse, and alcoholism. In general, there has been an extensive revitalization of the sweat lodge as well, used as a general treatment approach for a wide variety of physical and mental health problems (as well as for social and spiritual purposes), an approach that also has the effect of reintegrating individuals into their cultures. As in the Alkali Lake case discussed above, in many cases the sweat lodges are being reintroduced through the assistance of elders and healers from other communities, and often other cultural traditions, the implications of which we shall discuss later in this chapter.

Slowly, over the years, federal and provincial governments have come to realize the utility of Aboriginal approaches to healing. In 1980 a report issued by the Medical Services Branch advocated for 'a closer working relationship between traditional healers and physicians' (cited in Gagnon 1989:176), and in 1983 then Minister of Indian Affairs John Munro told a National Indian and Inuit Health Conference that Health and Welfare Canada fully recognized the value of traditional Native medicine. In a submission to the Special Committee on Indian Self-Government (the Penner Report), National Health and Welfare's position was clearly artic-ulated: 'We have come to appreciate very much the relevance and the utility of traditional approaches, particularly to mental health problems – approaches which address the suicide rate, approaches which address addiction problems. We believe that in areas such as those the application of traditional medicine and native culture perhaps can be more success-ful than anything we could offer in terms of contemporary psychiatric approaches to those kinds of problems' (cited in Penner 1983:35).

In recent decades, the federal government has sometimes funded the provision of Aboriginal medical services throughout parts of Canada (Gregory 1989). Under the current non-insured health benefits program of Health Canada, the federal government will cover the travel costs associated with bringing a healer into a community, or taking a patient to a healer, provided the following conditions are met:

– the traditional healer is recognized as such by the local Band, tribal Council, or health professional
– the traditional healer is located in the Client's region/territory of residence
– a licensed physician, or if a licensed physician is not routinely available in the community, a community health professional or First Nations and Inuit Health Branch (FNIHB) representative has confirmed that the Client has a medical condition (Health Canada 2003a)

This last requirement is particularly interesting because it demonstrates how biomedicine has gained significant control over the Aboriginal healing process by empowering its practitioners not only to authorize the treatment but to do so within the context of a biomedical, not Aboriginal, conceptualization of 'medical condition.' This issue is further underscored by the fact that the FNIHB will not cover the costs for 'honoraria, ceremonial expenses or medicines,' which remain 'the sole responsibility of the client.'

Conferences between Aboriginal healers and biomedical practitioners are becoming more common, as the two groups seek to understand each other better and to facilitate collaborative relationships. One such conference was held in The Pas in 1986 (Gregory 1989). The purpose of this conference was to seek the advice and assistance of healers in the development of curricula for a new northern nursing program. In 1993, a conference of healers was held at the Regional Psychiatric Centre in Saskatoon, a federal correctional facility that offers a variety of psychological treatment programs. Healers from across western Canada attended with correctional psychologists and psychiatrists in an effort to facilitate a more traditional approach to the healing of Aboriginal offenders. Indeed, the area of corrections in general has shown slow but steady progress since the 1990s, including the opening of 'healing lodges' in Maple Creek, Saskatchewan (for female offenders), and in Hobbema, Alberta (for male offenders).

Several provincial governments have also released statements or policies pertaining to Aboriginal healing approaches. Ontario, for instance, released a policy paper on Aboriginal health in the mid-1990s in which it was stated as a fundamental principle that 'Traditional Aboriginal approaches to wellness, including the use of traditional resources, traditional healers, medicine people, midwives and elders, are recognized, respected and protected from government regulation. They enhance and complement healing, as well as programs and services throughout the health system' (Ontario Ministry of Health 1994:15). Similarly, the 1990 Health Act in the Yukon includes provisions to allow 'Aboriginal control over traditional Aboriginal nutrition and healing practices and to protect these healing practices as a viable alternative for seekers of health and healing services' (World Health Organization 2001). In both cases, though, just what 'protect' means remains unclear.

There has also been significant research into various aspects of Aboriginal healing. Much of this research has focused on the persistence of cultural health beliefs held by contemporary Aboriginal people and how this affects their strategies for seeking health care from both the traditional and the biomedical systems. Garro (1987, 1988a, 1988b, 1990), for instance, has documented the knowledge and attitudes about diabetes, high blood pressure, and other illnesses among *Anishinaabeg* (Ojibwa) communities in Manitoba. She has also described the manner in which Aboriginal healing is utilized by these people. Abonyi (2001) argues that the Mushkegowuk Cree consider diabetes to be not only a sickness but also a symptom of the colonial experience. Culture and identity figure prominently in their perception of diabetes. Renegotiating identity and revaluing culture emerged as important avenues for redressing the problem. Similarly, Waldram and colleagues (2000) have also documented how Aboriginal approaches, especially the use of herbal medicines, have been adapted for treating diabetes in an urban Aboriginal population despite an acknowledgment by patients and healers that the disease is a relatively new phenomenon.

In another study, Garro (1991) documented 468 illness case histories, of which 4 per cent involved requesting an *Anishinaabe* healer for a remedy, and 17 per cent involved requests for a diagnosis. The total of 21 per cent of illnesses that resulted in a consultation with a healer was in contrast to 48 per cent where physicians were seen. In 7 per cent of the cases, a healer was consulted without also consulting a physician. Overall, of the 61 households studied by Garro, some 62 per cent reported having visited a healer over the eight-month period of her research. She also documented the extensive use of herbal medicines by these people.

In a different vein, David Young and his colleagues have attempted to determine the efficacy of a traditional treatment for psoriasis by employing the testing and validation measures of biomedicine (D.E. Young, Swartz, Ingram, and Morse 1988). This is a difficult and politically dangerous type of experiment, since it requires the removal of the treatment from its proper cultural context and evaluation using standards other than those for which the treatment was derived.[1] Working with northern Cree healer Russell Willier, Young and his associates documented his treatment of non-Aboriginal patients; they utilized both videotape and still camera and employed biomedical practices in judging the outcome (for example, measuring the size of the psoriasis scabs). Some of the herbal medicines used by Willier were even submitted for laboratory analysis.

Herbal medicines in particular have attracted considerable attention from the non-Aboriginal world, more so than other aspects of Aboriginal medical traditions. While Willier may have been somewhat of an innovator in partnering with researchers to document his treatments, today such cooperation is far more common. In Saskatchewan, for instance, northern Cree healers have begun to work with medical researchers to examine herbal medicines for use in the treatment of hypertension.[2] And the Canadian Institutes of Health Research, through its Institute for Aboriginal People's Health, recently awarded almost $1 million to a Montreal team to study anti-diabetic plants in northern Quebec Cree territory.[3] As the complex issues surrounding intellectual property rights continue to be addressed (see Hill 2003), we can expect more of these kinds of collaborations.

From yet another perspective, Waldram (1993, 1997) has described how Aboriginal spirituality programs in prisons should be viewed as a form of 'symbolic healing': that is, a process of healing involving the identification and manipulation of culturally specific symbols (such as the sacred pipe, tobacco, sweat lodge, and sweetgrass) by elders in a manner that promotes healing among offenders. Many Aboriginal offenders are suffering from a process of despiritualization and cultural identity problems. Involvement with elders and healers helps to re-establish their spiritual and cultural identities as Aboriginal people and, in turn, not only contributes to their own healing (for instance, in resolving alcohol and drug problems) but also makes them more amenable to the messages of the biomedical/psychosocial treatment programs.

The scientific study of Aboriginal healing approaches remains contentious. There are some Aboriginal people who feel that their medicine is a gift from the Creator and that, as a result, there is no need to 'prove' its efficacy according to scientific principles. Some also continue to believe that much of this knowledge is both sacred and secret and therefore not to be subjected to critical inquiry or broadcast outside of a select group. But there are others who believe that limited scientific study is essential to having Aboriginal healing accepted by both Aboriginal and non-Aboriginal people as a viable alternative to biomedical and psychotherapeutic approaches. This, in turn, is seen as an important element in broader processes of cultural revitalization. The debate continues.

THE IMPLICATIONS OF MEDICAL PLURALISM

'Medical pluralism' refers to the practice of utilizing the medical services of more than one medical system. Research in Canada (Millar 1997) and the United States (Eisenberg et al. 1993) has demonstrated that more than one-third of each country's citizens have consulted with a complementary or alternative health practitioner; the options available to patients appear almost endless. Many Aboriginal people in Canada have access to biomedical services and alternative or complementary non-Aboriginal treatment modalities (such as chiropractic, acupuncture, homeopathy) in addition to their own healing systems. The continued use of indigenous healing after the introduction of biomedical services is a global phenomenon (see Press 1969; Schwartz 1969; Garrison 1977; Woods 1977; Asuni 1979; Waldram 1990b). The literature suggests that patients move fairly easily from one system to another, for as Welsch (1983:34) accurately notes, people move between alternative *treatments*, and not alternative systems, and according to Asuni (1979:37), 'He [the patient] will use both ... with or without the knowledge or approval of either.'

It is widely known that some Aboriginal patients will seek treatment simultaneously from a physician and an Aboriginal healer. In such instances, two cognitive processes may be at work. First, the patients' 'explanatory model' – their personal conceptualization of their symptoms, etiology, and need for treatment (see Kleinman 1980) – may include a bifurcated notion of etiology and symptomatology. In other words, they may seek out physician treatment to alleviate the symptoms and the healer to eliminate the cause. Second, they may be simply employing a shotgun approach to treatment, seeking the assistance of practitioners from both medical systems to ensure that all possible causes and symptoms are addressed. It is also known that some Aboriginal people will utilize the two medical systems in a serial fashion, seeking treatment solely from one until a certain subjective point of dissatisfaction is reached, whereupon the services of the other are obtained. In the case of chronic or problematic illnesses, this pattern can repeat itself many times over.

Kennedy (1984) has written about the extended medical history of one Okanagan (interior Salish) man as he sought treatment for leg ulcers over a sixty-seven-year period. His case is no doubt extraordinary, for during this period he utilized the services of Aboriginal healers, physicians, Chinese traditional doctors, a variety of self-treatments, and even the Shaker church. As he moved from treatment to treatment, his views of the illness (his 'explanatory model') changed. At times he thought the problem was due to poisonous plants, at other times sorcery or 'bad medicine,' and at still other times a combination of etiologies. Kennedy notes that the severity of the particular illness episode conditioned his response; he often went to physicians and hospitals when the symptoms were most severe. She also notes that the patient's adherence to the prescribed treatment of any practitioner was greatest when the explanatory model of the patient and healer were most similar.

Garro (1990, 1991) has also provided a good description of Manitoba *Anishinaabe* views of treatment and illness. She notes that there are two broad categories of illness, 'White Man's Sickness,' for which a physician's treatment is sought, and '*Anishinaabe sickness*,' for which a healer's treatment is sought. Most patients will seek out the services of a physician first when they fall ill, for, according to Garro (1991:215), 'unless there are indications to the contrary, it is generally assumed that an illness is not an *Anishinaabe sickness*.' She continues: 'People go to see physicians both because there are no costs associated with their use and because the physician's treatment is judged efficacious. Indeed, treatment by physicians is often seen as offering a higher likelihood of cure in cases that are not due to "*Anishinaabe* sicknesses." This is reinforced by the medicine man referring patients to physicians in many cases of illness which are not seen as being "*Anishinaabe sicknesses*."' But Garro emphasizes that the healers do not constitute a treatment of last resort, when the physician's treatment has failed. Rather, those individuals whom she documents as being treated by healers tended to point to features of the illness that implied '*Anishinaabe sickness*.'

The significance of medical pluralism as a treatment strategy needs to be drawn out. Pluralism actually empowers the patient, who, through the choice of medical system and practitioner, has a measure of control over his or her own health care. Likewise, the availability of significantly different alternatives further provides for choice in the event that the encounter with one system is unsatisfactory. Cultural understandings of illness and treatment are validated, since Aboriginal healing can be sought, yet the patient can also access biomedical services to treat the same problem, or a component of that problem. In effect, medical pluralism allows the patient to retain both control and the cultural context of healing. Ironically, under Canada's current health policy, access to biomedical services is often cheaper and easier than access to traditional services, an important factor in their relative frequency of use.

From the perspective of the practitioners, medical pluralism poses some problems. It would be safe to conclude that most physicians do not question their patients with regard to the use of alternative treatments; many do not even enquire if home management has been attempted. For many physicians, Aboriginal healing lacks credibility to such an extent that they regard even questions about it as ludicrous. However, if the patient is seeing or plans to see a healer, then some conflict can occur. For instance, herbal medicines and prescription drugs may negatively interact, or the healer may require the patient to discontinue medication in order to undergo a healing ceremony. The fact that a patient may be consulting within two different medical systems, without the knowledge of either, may empower the patient, but may also lead to contradictions in treatment and possible medical complications (an issue of relevance in all cases of medical pluralism).

It should be made clear at this point, however, that most Aboriginal healers have a well-defined understanding of their abilities, knowledge, and limitations. Like physicians, when confronted with a problem for which they are not 'qualified' they will make a referral, either to another healer or to a physician. Of course, in the absence of medical training, questions can be raised about the qualifications of healers to diagnose conditions requiring biomedical consultation; but similar questions can be raised about the qualifications of physicians to make referrals to healers, a practice that is becoming more common. At the heart of the matter is the need for increasing dialogue between healers and physicians, including the possibility of collaboration (which we will address shortly).

ABORIGINAL HEALING AND URBANIZATION

When many people think of Aboriginal healing, they often visualize the context of a reserve or remote community, where the healing traditions are integral parts of, and supported by, the culture. However, since more than one-third of Canada's Aboriginal people now live in urban areas (and the urban population is growing quickly), this new context needs to be addressed. Characteristically, in cities Aboriginal people from different cultural traditions live side by side with Euro-Canadians and residents from other parts of the world. Is Aboriginal healing left behind when migration takes place, or is the knowledge regarding this form of healing transplanted to the urban context? This is particularly pertinent since, in the city, Aboriginal people are surrounded by biomedical as well as alternative and complementary services and facilities.

There have been relatively few studies of Aboriginal healing in urban North America. A project undertaken by Waldram (1990a, 1990b), examined the issue of Aboriginal healing in the urban context in greater detail, in a study of health care utilization in Saskatoon. Overall, he found that traditional Aboriginal healing was maintained by urban dwellers, that socio-economic variables explained little, and that the utilization of Aboriginal healing did not detract from the use of biomedical services.

However, contrary to accepted wisdom (see Fuchs and Bashshur 1975), utilization of Aboriginal healing was not related to problems in accessing biomedical services. The most important explanatory variables were measures of cultural continuity, especially those pertaining to language. For instance, those individuals who spoke an Aboriginal language demonstrated a greater propensity to seek out Aboriginal healers and to believe in the superiority of Aboriginal healing over biomedicine for certain health problems. Hence, it was determined that urban Aboriginal people in this study continued to believe in and utilize Aboriginal medical services for reasons largely unrelated to the existence of biomedical services or problems in utilizing those services. Aboriginal healing remains important for cultural reasons, including beliefs in efficacy.

Waldram's (1990a, 1990b) study also examined issues relating to access to Aboriginal healing in Saskatoon. The study found that only a small fraction of the Aboriginal respondents knew a healer in the city, and slightly fewer than half believed they would not be able to find one if they tried. Not surprisingly, therefore, some 60 per cent responded affirmatively to the question 'Would you like to see an Indian healer available in a clinic?' Even those most firmly anchored in their Aboriginal cultures (as indicated by language variables) were supportive of this kind of formal access to Aboriginal healing. A clear need for better access was established in this study. As health care consumers, Aboriginal urban residents wanted access to a full range of medical services in the city, not just biomedical services, and they were unconcerned with the many implications that such formalization would entail (see the next section for a discussion of these issues).

By comparison, it has also been noted that the demand for access to services provided by Aboriginal healers at the Anishnawbe Health Centre in Toronto has been overwhelming (George and Nahwegahbow 1993:242). One key problem for any urban facility wishing to offer Aboriginal healing is, of course, the inherent cultural complexity found in cities. Given that Aboriginal healing is culturally based, how does one facility accommodate the many cultural traditions of its patients, including those with a strong Western cultural orientation? Generally, they don't, but rather seek to offer a more culturally generalized service that may, on one level, be suitable for their clients. At Building a Nation in Saskatoon, for example, the therapeutic model combines Aboriginal and mainstream psychotherapeutic approaches in a client-centred program that is tailored to the needs of each individual; the Aboriginal component is developed around a holistic Medicine Wheel framework that has emerged in recent years as a kind of pan-Indian pedagogical and treatment model (for example, Nabigon and Mawhiney 1996; Mulcahy and Lunham-Armstrong 1998; Weiser 1999; Tillson 2002). Even if they know little about it, many Aboriginal people have at least heard of the Medicine Wheel, and, regardless of controversies over its origins (Kehoe 1990), there is a strong inclination to accept its symbolism as inherently Aboriginal and therapeutic.

CURRENT ISSUES

There has been a great deal of discussion regarding the formalization of Aboriginal healing to make it more readily available and about the need for collaboration between Aboriginal healing and biomedicine. We will briefly detail some of the issues that this might entail.

Epistemological and philosophical issues

Although both Aboriginal healing and biomedicine seek to heal patients, there are some fundamental differences in epistemology and philosophy that inhibit formal collaboration. Aboriginal healing is based on *tradition*, which is to say that, as a medical system, it accepts that the medicines, techniques, and knowledge of the past were effective because they have been time-tested and, in many instances, shared with humans by the Creator. In a sense, while new approaches to treatment are incorporated, this medicine is primarily informed and guided by the traditions of the past. Practitioners usually gain their knowledge very slowly, so that most are relatively old and the oldest (elders) are the most revered. In turn, the accrual of new knowledge is relatively slow. While Aboriginal healing is empirical, its knowledge exists primarily within the oral tradition. There is also a great degree of individualism and idiosyncrasy in the practice of Aboriginal healing. Current users are less concerned with questions of efficacy; they have been raised with the belief that Aboriginal healing works simply because it is inherently linked with past and revered cultural traditions and because it is the 'gift' of the Creator. To question if and how a plant medicine works, for instance, would be sacrilegious – and somewhat moot. In contrast, biomedicine is positivist, based on a philosophy of scepticism. Something must be proven to work before it is accepted, and the method by which such proof is attained is scrutinized carefully. While biomedicine is also informed by tradition, it tends to be dissatisfied with the status quo and

constantly seeks new knowledge, which in turn is scrutinized and verified. This means that medical knowledge changes rapidly. Relatively
young practitioners experience a brief, but intense, period of training to
become competent, and it is often difficult for older physicians to
remain in touch with the latest medical developments. And, certainly,
no two physicians learn or retain exactly the same knowledge no matter
how consistent their training has been.

Nevertheless, a physician's knowledge is fairly standard and is
derived from both oral instruction and written texts. Further, there
remains a fixed doctrine of acceptable medical practice that ensures a
certain standard of care to which all practitioners must adhere, reinforced by provincial licensing bodies and laws. Aboriginal healers, in
contrast, generally experience no such regulation and are subject to different standards of competence that are culturally based and considerably more amorphous. While a physician who violates accepted medical
practice may be legally removed from that practice, an Aboriginal
healer who violates his or her healing traditions will be subject to more
informal mechanisms of control, such as ostracism and loss of community credibility.

The philosophical underpinnings of science render it unlikely to accept
medical systems that are not verifiable through the scientific method.
While Aboriginal healing is quite open to new ideas, biomedical science
is rigid, and hence it will either demand that Aboriginal healing be examined scientifically or else will reject it as faith or religion – that is, as inherently unscientific. The fact that spirituality is so central to Aboriginal
healing allows biomedicine more easily to dismiss it outright.

Of course, it is not appropriate to paint all biomedical practitioners
with one brush when it comes to Aboriginal healing. Many examples
exist around the country of physicians and nurses working in conjunction with Aboriginal healers in one form or another. Gregory (1989), for
instance, found that 52 per cent of the northern Manitoba nurses he
interviewed had made referrals to elders and healers, and that the Medical Services Branch had even provided some funding to bring healers
into communities from elsewhere. However, Gagnon (1989) found that
among physicians and medical students working at the Lake of the
Woods Hospital in Kenora, Ontario, as well as at the Northern Medical
Unit at the University of Manitoba, 'most ... are in favour of some form
of collaboration *but indicated a reluctance to relinquish control*' (1989:181;
emphasis added). Some 90 per cent believed that traditional healers
played an important 'psycho-social' role (but not necessarily a *medical*

role), and only 55 per cent stated that they would actually allow a healing ceremony to be held in their hospitals. Furthermore, 73 per cent stated that traditional medical practices should not 'interfere' with biomedicine. Aboriginal healing, it seems, was something to be done in the community, but not within biomedical institutions. The isolation of the physicians from the community level was apparent from the fact that only 15 per cent of them had ever referred a patient to a healer. Similar results were found in a British Columbia study, which showed that, among a sample of seventy-nine physicians, the greatest support for the use of Aboriginal healing was for health maintenance, palliative care, or relatively benign health problems; there was considerable opposition to its use for serious medical conditions (Zubek 1994). Not surprisingly, those physicians with the greatest experience in treating Aboriginal patients had the most liberal views of Aboriginal healing.

These studies are dated now, and there is much informal evidence that the situation has improved somewhat, in part as a result of increasing Aboriginal control over health care. Nurses, in particular, have proved to be quite receptive to cultural issues and the involvement of Aboriginal healers (Clarke 1997). There remains, however, a reluctance to accept Aboriginal healing as a viable option, primarily for epistemological and philosophical reasons.

The question of efficacy

A central issue to be considered here is one of efficacy. Does Aboriginal healing 'work'? We believe that this question is central to any discussion of barriers to collaboration for, as we have seen in previous chapters, there is a long-standing tradition among biomedical practitioners in particular, and non-Aboriginal people in general, of viewing Aboriginal healing as quackery. Not surprisingly, this is one question that few seem to want to address directly; non-Aboriginal people in particular fear being accused of racism if they bring up such an issue.

The efficacy of Aboriginal healing must be seen within its proper social and cultural context (Waldram 2000). Medical anthropologists have shown us that what constitutes an 'illness' is culturally contingent (including intracultural variation), and that therefore it is best to think of 'illness' as socially and culturally defined. Therefore, what constitutes an effective treatment for an 'illness' will also be socially and culturally defined. To use an Aboriginal example, victims of 'bad medicine' are 'ill' as defined by their Aboriginal cultures; whether biomedical science can discern any disease is irrelevant. The culturally appropriate means of dealing with 'bad medicine' is to seek out a healer, who will perform the necessary healing ceremonies. The patient is 'healed' in so far as the patient, and the patient's significant others, believe that the 'bad medicine' has been removed. But the issue is not as simple as this sounds, since it has been suggested that within Aboriginal healing traditions 'illness is not necessarily a bad thing' and that '[i]t is often sent to help people re-evaluate their lives' (Aboriginal Nurses Association of Canada 1993:14). This is where ideas of considerable antiquity can remain influential today. Hence, illness might be viewed as a significant indication of personal breaches of the moral order of society, simultaneously calling for proper rehabilitation of that breach and for reinforcing the norms and values of the society. The individual suffering distress may not be the same person who caused this breach, and therefore not only may different kinds of treatments be called for (one for the 'patient' suffering distress, one for the 'patient' who caused the problem), but a treatment may be seen as successful even where the patient dies. Aboriginal healing seems less concerned with prolonging life than with improving the quality of life, both in this world and in the next.

Questions of efficacy are most commonly raised with respect to the use of herbal medicines, possibly because this is one area that biomedicine can scientifically examine. But it is necessary to keep in mind that even the preparation and administration of herbal medicines is often steeped in spirituality, so that the removal of the spiritual component in a scientific search to see if a herbal preparation 'works' may violate the proper cultural context. David Young and colleagues (1988) report on an experiment with northern Alberta Cree healer Russell Willier, whose treatment for psoriasis was scientifically examined. Willier allowed one of his herbal medicines to be analysed in the laboratory (while keeping the actual ingredients secret), and some antibacterial agents were found. The overall treatment experiment was, in scientific terms, inconclusive. Willier himself was also dissatisfied with the results, which he explained were the result of the unusual circumstances in which he was required to function (that is, in an Edmonton clinic with non-Aboriginal patients who were required to faithfully administer herbal remedies in their own homes). Our point here is that biomedical scientists often fail to comprehend the cultural context of such healing and look instead for purely clinical evidence (Waldram 2000).

The question 'Does it work?' is an important one. There is substantial evidence within the oral tradition and histories of Aboriginal people of the healing of terminal diseases, especially cancer, through Aboriginal healing. Aboriginal healing traditions purport to have cures for all kinds of disorders, but it is rare indeed when these are shared with non-Aboriginal people. There is a genuine fear that non-Aboriginal people will steal the recipes for herbal medicines, for instance, and sell them for money; this is not an unreasonable fear, given that the pharmaceutical industry has a history of looking to indigenous peoples' medicines for new drugs. Few Aboriginal healers have ever allowed the scientific examination of medicines and other treatments, and scientific practitioners will not likely endorse any Aboriginal approach that it cannot verify with its own methods. Anecdotal evidence does not represent acceptable proof in science.

Validating Aboriginal healers

The biomedical and Aboriginal systems are in conflict with respect to validating both healing knowledge and practitioners. As we noted above, with biomedicine, practitioners receive formal education, must pass rigorous examinations, and must continue to practise effectively while under the scrutiny of licensing and professional associations. Canadian law protects the patient from exposure to unqualified medical practitioners and will assist patients who are harmed as a result of medical incompetence. In contrast, since Aboriginal medical knowledge is often handed down from generation to generation to individuals selected by existing healers, the validation of their knowledge is considerably less formal. Healers in the Aboriginal tradition are culturally and community validated, and those who wish to avail themselves of the healer's services follow the culturally prescribed method of requesting assistance. There are no licences and no regulating bodies. In general, individuals avoid those considered to be incompetent or known to deal in 'bad medicine.' However, even here there can be some uncertainty. For instance, Garro (1990:428) has documented a lack of consensus among *Anishinaabe* in Manitoba regarding who is a legitimate healer, who deals in 'bad medicine,' and the degree of competence in various healing specialities.

From a cultural perspective, then, community validation of Aboriginal healers can be problematic. Once we begin to talk about making Aboriginal healing more formal and more readily available, and about developing collaborative programs, the question of validation becomes even more difficult. It is not easy for most non-Aboriginal people, and even many Aboriginal people who have little traditional cultural knowledge, to distinguish true Aboriginal healers from others whose knowledge lacks cultural or community validation. Indeed, there is a whole growth industry, related to current 'New Age' trends, in promoting and selling Aboriginal healing and philosophies (Aldred 2000). Charlatanism is such a serious issue that a group calling itself the Traditional Elders Circle of the Indigenous Nations of North America passed a resolution as early as 1980 warning that many so-called medicine people lack the proper knowledge and authority to heal and carry sacred objects, such as the pipe. A key issue was the use of healing approaches for profit, often involving non-Aboriginal clients. Subsequently, the American Indian Movement passed a resolution condemning charlatans and went so far as to name specific individuals. Paramount on the list was Sun Bear, a 'plastic medicine man' who has developed his own series of books and workshops and even his own tribe of followers (Churchill 1990).

In Canada, we have recently seen a variety of travelling Aboriginal 'healers' who move from community to community in a manner reminiscent of the medicine shows of the nineteenth century. Workshops on 'traditional' Aboriginal healing have become commonplace. Two characteristics, above all, typify the individuals most likely to be involved in these activities: they are fluent in both English and the ways of bureaucracy. Many could well be graduates of Dale Carnegie or Toastmaster's courses, so compelling are they. In effect, they are successful because they can, and will, deal with bureaucracies, sign contracts to deliver their services, keep records of expenses and, above all else, tell people (Aboriginal and non-Aboriginal alike) what they want to hear. Some of these individuals may well be community-validated healers, but not all. Indeed, for some critics, the mere fact that a 'healer' would collect a fee for services rendered is a sign that he or she lacks such validation.

Aboriginal healers with cultural or community validation are more likely to speak their Aboriginal language and be, at the most, bilingual; they are also humble about their abilities. One would not normally hear a healer pronounce that he or she is in fact a healer; this is a status that is ascribed to them by others. Some are still afraid of legal prosecution, a legacy of the past. Furthermore, they operate under constraints related to their own world views, in which openly discussing their healing abilities could lead to a revocation by the Creator of the gift to heal (Aboriginal Nurses Association of Canada 1993:15).

It is not surprising, therefore, that the biomedical and Aboriginal systems find it difficult to work together. Indeed, if many healers will not even admit that they are healers (as is often the cultural protocol), then some serious cultural communication problems are evident. Allegations of charlatanism are fairly common in Aboriginal circles, even in cases involving healers whose work is actively supported by Aboriginal organizations. In the absence of clear avenues of certification, it is hard to imagine that biomedical practitioners will be able to decipher this complex cultural issue. Many have responded by simply ignoring the issue altogether when working with an Aboriginal healer, no doubt hoping that there won't be an 'incident,' while a common strategy employed by those who wish to have some formal collaboration is to hire an Aboriginal liaison and let him or her manage any crisis that might erupt. A 1990 report on health care in Saskatchewan seemed to sum up the general government approach to the matter, stating that, 'Because of the very personal nature of the medicine man's services, it would be inappropriate to suggest he become part of a highly regulated and organized health care system' (Murray 1990:210).

Legal issues

The legal status of Aboriginal healing is ambiguous, and several key questions remain unanswered:

- What legal protection is afforded to agencies that employ or enable Aboriginal healing?
- What legal protection does a healer have in his or her practice?
- What legal protection does a patient have who undergoes treatment with an Aboriginal healer?

These are pertinent issues in two important contexts: first, when a regulatory agency asserts its authority to define lawful medical practice; and second, when something goes wrong and a patient is harmed as a result of, or in conjunction with, an Aboriginal treatment. Unfortunately, there is too often a hushed silence on the allegation that Aboriginal healers 'may do more harm than good.' Medical folklore is replete with physician stories about Aboriginal patients who have suffered as a result of treatments by healers (usually seen in the context of patients who discontinue medications to undergo healing). However, only occasionally do reports surface of actual cases. The 1997 death of a leading Alberta Indian chief, who collapsed after emerging from a sweat lodge, is one of the rare examples.[4]

Embedded with these questions and issues remains the considerable ambiguity that surrounds Aboriginal healing practice itself. What, exactly, is going on when a patient consults with an Aboriginal healer? Because Aboriginal healing practice is infused with cultural and religious significance, one wonders if, in terms of the Constitution, it could be seen as an 'Aboriginal right' under Section 35. The answers to such questions will not come easily, but we believe they must be addressed before any significant change to the status quo can occur.

In an early consideration of this issue, Robb (1988) provides an interesting legal viewpoint on Aboriginal healing. In general, Robb sees the problem as one of a lack of Aboriginal sovereignty, since, under the current system, even on-reserve Aboriginal people are subject to provincial laws of general applicability, in addition to being under federal jurisdiction by virtue of Section 91 (24) of the Constitution Act. The federal Food and Drugs Act, for instance, makes it an offence to advertise or sell 'any food, drug, cosmetic, or device ... as a treatment, preventative or cure for any diseases, disorders, or abnormal physical states' as defined in the act, including alcoholism, gout, depression, diabetes, gangrene, influenza, and obesity (ibid.:135). We note that the Canada Health Act (1984) defines both 'health care' and 'medical' practitioners as those 'entitled under the law of a province' to provide the relevant services. Neither federal act discusses Aboriginal healing.

Provincial control over much of health and medical practice remains at the heart of the key issues. Robb identifies Alberta's Medical Profession Act as a problem, for it makes it an offence for anyone to practise medicine except a registered (licensed) physician. This is generally true in other provinces as well. According to Robb, the definition of 'practise medicine' is 'breathtaking in its scope,' and includes prescribing or administering any treatment, performing any operation or manipulation, applying any apparatus or appliance, or advertising (including uttering statements) with respect to 'the prevention, alleviation or cure of any human disease, ailment, deformity, defect or injury' (Robb 1988:136). In contrast, however, Ontario's Regulated Health Professions Act (1991) specifically exempts 'Aboriginal healers providing traditional healing services to aboriginal persons or members of an aboriginal community' from the provisions of the act. This legislation does not define 'traditional healing services,' or 'aboriginal,' and it is interesting to note that the exemption does not apply where an Aboriginal healer provides services to a non-Aboriginal client. Further, we wonder what it means for Aboriginal healers and patients alike to be exempted from this legislation. Do Aboriginal patients not have the legal right to be treated in a competent way by Aboriginal healers, for instance?

Separate from the question of regulated medical practice, there are criminal- and civil-liability issues. According to Robb (1988), the law allows that parents, guardians, or spouses must provide the necessities of life, including medical treatment; the courts have established that medical services in accordance with a person's faith, religion, or belief are not 'reasonable.' Various laws also define the criteria by which lawful medical practice can ensue. Clearly, these criminal provisions threaten Aboriginal healers as they currently practice. In terms of civil liability, the law states that medical practitioners are not expected to guarantee successful treatment, but they must possess the necessary skill and knowledge to practise according to accepted standards (such as those that would be expected given the locale of the practice). Clearly, there are implications for both the Aboriginal healer and the physician in any formal collaborative relationship. In effect, if Aboriginal healers are practising 'medicine' as defined in Canadian law, then they are doing so without a licence. If it is something else that they are doing, if it can be said that they are involved in a *cultural* or *religious* practice, then it seems that some legal protection, or at least a constitutional clarification, is still required. To simply rely on 'culture' to validate healing will inevitably lead to legal problems. The following example highlights this.

In 1992, the British Columbia Supreme Court issued its judgment in the case of *Thomas v. Norris* (Denis 1997). In this instance, Mr Thomas was awarded damages for 'assault, battery and false imprisonment when he was initiated into the Coast Salish Big House Tradition called the Spirit Dance.' Thomas was a member of the First Nation, but had lived off reserve for many years and did not self-identify with the Coast Salish culture. His wife at the time, believing that the Spirit Dance would heal him of his alcohol problem and repair their marriage, requested that he be initiated. According to Coast Salish custom, the collective right of the people to force an individual such as Mr Thomas to undergo Spirit Dancing, in the interests of the community at large, were paramount over Mr Thomas's individual rights. Justice Hood disagreed, stating that Mr Thomas's individual rights – in this case, guarantees against 'assault, battery and false imprisonment' – prevailed within Canadian law. Furthermore, the judge ruled that Spirit Dancing was not an 'aboriginal right' under Section 35 of the Constitution. The judge also stated of the plaintiff that, 'He lives in a free society and his rights are inviolable. He is free to believe in, and to practice, any religion or tradition, if he chooses to do so. He cannot be coerced or forced to participate in one by any group purporting to exercise their collective rights in doing so.'[5]

According to the judgment, Mr Thomas was 'forcibly seized' in 1988 and taken to the Semenos Long House of the Cowichin Indian Band. Over a four-day period, Mr Thomas was periodically 'lifted up horizontally by eight men, who then took turns digging their fingers into his stomach area and biting him on his sides.' He was given only a cup of water each day, but no food. 'At one point [the judgment stated] he was taken to a creek, stripped naked and forced to walk backwards into the water and to "go under three times."'' He was then whipped or beaten with cedar branches, hard enough to raise welts on his skin. When Mr Thomas began to suffer from a pre-existing ulcer, he was taken to hospital for treatment. The attending physician testified that he was suffering from 'dehydration and multiple contusions' in addition to the peptic ulcer.[6]

Two of the defendants in the case were elders, whose responsibility was to ensure that the initiation was properly carried out according to custom. One elder testified that it was culturally appropriate to 'grab' an intransigent potential initiate at the request of another band member and stated that they had decided to make the initiation easier for Mr Thomas in comparison to what they themselves had experienced in the past. He stated that he had personally observed the ceremony to ensure that no harm would be done; but he also acknowledged that, earlier in 1988, an initiate had actually died during the ceremony. By the judgment, the plaintiff, Mr Thomas, was awarded $12,000 in damages for 'assault, battery and false imprisonment.' Clearly, what we have here is a clash of cultures, legal traditions, and notions of individual versus collective rights.

Spirit Dancing is easily misunderstood when stripped of its proper cultural context as described in the judgment (as any biomedical or European religious practice would be). An accurate understanding of this cultural context (see Jilek 1982a), as expressed by the elders, provides a very different view of the process of initiation into the dance that Mr Thomas underwent. But, as was pointed out, Mr Thomas did not himself subscribe to this aspect of Coast Salish culture, and the courts supported his assertion that the initiation was nothing more than a kind of torture. The lessons in this case for Aboriginal healing are clear: there are inherent legal dangers, since not all Aboriginal people are equally supportive of their heritages, and contemporary Aboriginal people live within a nation with its own legal code and underlying philosophy, which are sometimes at odds with Aboriginal ways.

Another case demonstrates the precarious legal nature of Aboriginal healing. This involved an Ecuadorian shaman who was invited to an Ontario First Nation to offer healing services. The shaman instructed a diabetic community elder to stop taking her medication before and during a three-day healing ceremony in 2001. Along with many other participants, she consumed quantities of herbal medicines containing ayahuasca (brought from Ecuador) and tobacco, in a traditional Ecuadorian recipe. On the third day, the elder died of nicotine poisoning, and the shaman was subsequently charged with criminal negligence causing death. He pleaded guilty to a lesser charge of administering a noxious substance and trafficking in an illegal drug (the ayahuasca), and received a one-year conditional sentence.

It is true that both the shaman and his medicine were foreign to both Canada and the specific community, and that this was not, strictly speaking, a case about Canadian Aboriginal healing. But several aspects of the case are informative. To begin with, the shaman was using a treatment that was legal in his native Ecuador, and in his defence he submitted many letters from the Ecuadorian government, scientists, and patients (including many from the community of the elder) attesting to the efficacy of his treatments. Some patients claimed to have been cured of cancer, diabetes, and grief. But others complained that they had not been informed of the possible side effects of the treatment, and First Nations officials subsequently decided that such foreign 'traditional' treatments were never intended for their people after all. Most significant, perhaps, is that the judge in this case allowed for the lesser charge, noting that 'The court is satisfied that this was a sacred ceremony conducted by traditional healers.' Added to this were these comments by the Crown attorney: 'One of the most important things to come out is the courts have legitimized traditional medicine. However, the other important thing that has come out is that there are limits on traditional medicine and the limit is that you cannot use prohibited drugs in the traditional medicine process.'[7] This would appear to open a very wide door for the practice of Aboriginal healing in Canada. Certainly, more cases will come as the courts continue to grapple with the complex issues involved.

SOME IMPLICATIONS OF THE REVITALIZATION OF ABORIGINAL HEALING

Chapter 5 described the manner in which Aboriginal healing traditions were embedded within their host cultures. That chapter also concluded by examining the historic threats to Aboriginal healing and culture posed by government policy and church actions. It is important that we view Aboriginal medical traditions in a contemporary context, one that not only appreciates the intrinsic cultural changes that have ensued but also accepts that much non-Aboriginal knowledge is now embedded within Aboriginal medical 'traditions,' and that many Aboriginal people have little knowledge of these traditions and are inclined to rely on the biomedical system to meet their health needs.

As Aboriginal healing becomes even more popular among Aboriginal people, and as it continues to attract non-Aboriginal clients searching for alternative or complementary therapies, new challenges arise. These include

1 An increase in demand – With both Aboriginal and non-Aboriginal people searching out Aboriginal healing practitioners, the demand for their services has increased. This is especially true given that so many institutions, such as correctional facilities, hospitals, and clinics, con- tinue to scramble to bring healers on staff in efforts to provide 'cultur- ally appropriate care' to Aboriginal clients. Simply put, there are not enough healers to go around. This has resulted in a downward demo- graphic shift – 'healers' are often younger today than in the past – and controversy over the legitimacy of those claiming to be healers in order to fill employment vacancies.

2 A change in practice – With the increasing demand comes a change in how Aboriginal healing services are provided. More clients means less time to treat each person. This is particularly true with institu- tional programs. Within the correctional system, for instance, tight prison schedules force healers to offer sweat lodge ceremonies and healing circles at routinely scheduled times and within specific time parameters (Waldram 1997). Similarly, the renewed interest in Aboriginal healing by Aboriginal and non-Aboriginal people has led to the development of the 'workshop' approach to educating potential clients about the world views and symbols employed in healing.

3 The emergence of eclecticism or 'pan-Indianism' – The increase in demand, in the face of a shortage of healers, has led communities and organizations to take less rigid positions on the specific cultural tradi- tions of the healers with whom they work. When a community desires healing but has no healers, it searches elsewhere, and this often means bringing in a healer whose approach is foreign to the cul- ture of that community. In particular, we are seeing Plains Indian world views and treatment approaches being imported into other

regions of the country, sometimes added to local traditions, but some-times also in effect *becoming* the local tradition. This represents a com-munity-driven process of cultural change that has not been adequately studied.

CONCLUSION

Aboriginal healing continues to undergo revitalization, and these approaches to treatment are increasingly being recognized as appropri-ate for many of the health and behavioural problems experienced by Aboriginal people. Further, the linkage of healing and spirituality with cultural identity is evident in many healing initiatives developed by Aboriginal people themselves, as the historic processes of deculturation and despiritualization are reversed, a significant part of a broad move-ment towards the 'healing' of the Aboriginal population. Indeed, the 'healing' movement, now in full force, may represent the single most profound source for social, cultural, and health revitalization (Four Directions International 2002).

10

Self-determination and health care

The last two decades have seen enormous strides in the area of Aboriginal self-determination. What was once only a dream is, today, the accepted reality in Canada. The road to self-determination has been long and fraught with many difficulties, and there has been substantial opposition. While one of the stumbling blocks has been the problem of defining 'self-determination' in a manner acceptable to all Aboriginal groups, all provincial governments, the federal government, and Canadians in general, in recent years this political issue has been superseded by Aboriginal efforts, sometimes rather quiet, to simply gain increased control over various aspects of community life. This has characterized the self-determination movement in the area of health care as well.

Health, in general, has never received the kind of attention that other aspects of self-determination have garnered. For the most part, lip-service has been paid to matters of health care, with the demands for 'Indian control of Indian health' competing with other demands, such as for control over education and social services (especially child welfare). Logically, the urgent need to improve the economic situation of Aboriginal people has attracted the greatest attention, and one can argue that improvements in health, through changes to the health care system, are not likely to be dramatic in the absence of more basic changes in the socio-economic position of Aboriginal people. But, while economic and constitutional matters have made the headlines and occupied the Aboriginal organizations to a great extent, there have also been some interesting and significant changes with respect to health care. Our intent in this chapter is to examine some of the more pertinent aspects of the self-determination movement with a focus on the field of health and especially health care.

THE ROAD TO SELF-DETERMINATION

As we have seen throughout previous chapters of this book, Aboriginal people have retained many elements of their healing systems, and this fact alone suggests that they have also retained some measure of self-determination. Further, we must appreciate that the issue of self-determination in health care is not exclusively a recent development. Historically, Aboriginal people were not simply passive recipients of European and Euro-Canadian medical care and the culture change that often accompanied it. Such care was actively sought out when deemed necessary, but Aboriginal people retained a strong measure of control over their health care by retaining important elements of their healing systems. The case of the Six Nations (or Grand River) Iroquois, as documented by Weaver (1972), demonstrates the extent to which one Aboriginal group was willing to go to ensure local control of developing biomedical services, with initiatives dating back to the mid-1700s. In the contemporary era, other groups have achieved varying degrees of self-determination in the health area through political means largely tangential to health. The James Bay Cree provide one such example.

The Cree and Inuit of James Bay were the first groups to sign a comprehensive land claim agreement in Canada. Under the terms of the James Bay and Northern Quebec Agreement, signed in 1975, a Cree Board of Health and Social Services was established in 1978. The overall agreement has led to the development of a Cree 'regional society' in northern Quebec (Salisbury 1986), and the development of a health and social services board can be viewed as fitting within this framework. The mandate of the board is expansive, encompassing all the responsibilities of any health board in Quebec as well as the responsibility to deal directly with health and social services for the Cree. But, despite the agreement, the Cree received considerable opposition to their formation of the board, being forced to undertake legal proceedings and other political action to obtain control; and even then there was an attempt to place the Cree Board of Health under trusteeship in 1980 (Bearskin and Dumont 1991:123).

What makes the Cree situation different from that of many First Nations in the country is that the James Bay and Northern Quebec Agreement removed the federal government's responsibility for much of Cree life and transferred it to Quebec and the Cree. Hence, the Cree Board of Health became one of many such boards under the jurisdiction of the Quebec government. The Cree retained all their health-related benefits as status Indians, but these were now administered through Quebec. The board itself contained representatives from each of the nine Cree villages, representatives of the clinical and non-clinical staff, a representative from the parent governmental organization (the Cree Regional Authority), and a representative from the Department of Community Health at Montreal General Hospital, which, under the Quebec public health system then in existence, was responsible for the organization and delivery of preventive health services in the Cree region. The board oversaw the operation of a regional hospital at Chisasibi, and through it the Cree gained control over the hiring of health care staff through the village and regional levels. This meant that some strides were made towards developing more culturally appropriate health care, including the establishment of a new nursing program. But, as Bearskin and Dumont (1991:125) noted, the Cree Board of Health has been challenged by newly developing health problems, such as heart disease, diabetes, and substance abuse. The lack of availability of Cree professional staff remains an issue as well (cf Moffatt 1987). Robinson (1988:1611), while supporting the idea of Cree control of health, added that 'this control needs to be extended by the training of board members and of Native health professionals and administrators at all levels.' Somewhat surprisingly, some Cree viewed the board as a non-Cree organization, and Bearskin and Dumont (1991:125) candidly pointed out that the 'board' concept was 'a new entity' for the Cree, 'distant from the traditional organizations that the Cree are used to. So enough time must be given for the Cree to get to know how such an organization functions and to integrate it smoothly into their society.' Obviously, there is more to the issue of local control of health care than simply gaining political control.

For the Cree, the battle to gain control was a difficult one, fraught with tense negotiations with the Quebec government in particular, and accusations that sufficient funding as called for under the agreement had not been made available. The Cree situation may be more complicated, however, because of all the other social and economic changes that have accompanied the James Bay hydro project (Adelson 2000).

The success of the Cree in gaining some control over health was an important milestone in bringing the federal and provincial governments around to the more basic idea of Aboriginal self-determination. It was the federal government's new 'Indian Health Policy,' unveiled in 1979, that sparked the process of self-determination in Aboriginal health care that we see today. Central to this new policy was the belief that a simple increase in health programs and services would not result in a substantial improvement in health status. What was required was increased input by Aboriginal people themselves. Furthermore, the policy emphasized that spiritual health was as important as physical health, thus setting the stage for the re-emergence of Aboriginal healing services. In that same year, the federal government also endorsed the Alma-Ata Declaration of 1978. This declaration was signed by 134 countries, under the auspices of the World Health Organization, and reiterated the definition of health first published in the Preamble to its 1948 Constitution. This definition states that 'health is ... a state of complete physical, mental and social wellbeing, and not merely the absence of disease' (World Health Organization 1978:2), a definition that, while broad, is still popular today. Anticipating 'Health for All by the Year 2000,' the declaration endorsed the 'Primary Health Care' (PHC) movement, with a focus on the provision of basic health needs, such as safe water, nutritious food, maternal and child care, immunization, local disease control and medical services, and health education. In proposing that health be considered a fundamental human right, the Alma-Ata Declaration presented a blueprint for the development of local, community-level services with, implicitly, some measure of local control. Canada, by virtue of signing the declaration, explicitly agreed.

In 1980, Thomas Berger[1] submitted the report of the Advisory Commission on Indian and Inuit Health Consultation (Berger 1980). This may seem somewhat unusual in that the commission began *after* the announcement of the new Indian Health Policy in 1979, and hence was unable to inform the development of that policy; however, in the history of relations between the federal government and Aboriginal people, this is not so surprising. The intent of the commission seems to have been to develop a method for enacting a community consultation process as a step towards identifying the shape of the new institutions that would be required to implement the health policy. The report recommended that funds be allocated to various Aboriginal organizations 'to develop the consultative process,' and that the commission in effect be made into a permanent, Indian-controlled national health organization. The latter recommendation was not implemented, but the subsequent health transfer process appears to have benefited to some extent from Berger's detailing of community participation. Overall, the report seems to have had little impact, no doubt the result of its timing, which meant that some of its recommended initiatives were already being considered by the federal government. But such reports do add to ongoing public debate and serve to increase the momentum for positive political change. They add to the discourse.

The 1983 report of the Special Committee on Indian Self-Government (also known as the 'Penner Committee' after its chair, Keith Penner), added its voice to increasing demands for changes in Aboriginal health care. Although only a small portion of the report dealt with health matters, it emphasized the need for a more holistic approach to health care, incorporating Aboriginal approaches with biomedical and emphasizing preventive health programs. Interestingly, the report stated that 'witnesses did not specify how health care services should be provided. The emphasis was on control of the system rather than designing new systems' (Penner 1983:35). Aboriginal control, witnesses argued, should be flexible when implemented, allowing for negotiations with federal and provincial governments and agencies, as well as private enterprises, to develop an integrated model of health care services. Following on the heels of the Penner Report, in 1986 the Sechelt Indian Band Self-Government Act gave the British Columbia First Nation municipal status, including control over health services. The stage for health transfer was now set.

For registered Indians, health transfer actually began in 1982 with the 'Community Health Demonstration Program,' a plan to allow First Nations to experiment with different models of delivery and different degrees of control. Thirty-one such projects ultimately received funding. However, it became apparent that other transfer initiatives were slowed or stalled while these 'experiments' were undertaken (D.E. Young and Smith 1991:19). A critique of the program by Garro, Roulette, and Whitmore (1986:281), focusing on the experiences of Sandy Bay, Manitoba, suggests that many Aboriginal organizations asked a fundamental and quite reasonable question: Why was a 'demonstration' necessary? Furthermore, they wondered what would become of the projects when the two-year funding was terminated. Apparently, the project's objectives were not well thought out and its principles not uniformly applied. Hence, projects were funded that did not even propose the transfer of health services; in fact, only seven of the thirty-one actually dealt with the transfer issue (ibid.:282).

The Sandy Bay proposal represented a continuation of previous efforts to improve nursing and other services by hiring a health coordinator on the reserve, initiatives that were stymied by a lack of federal funding until the Demonstration Program was announced. The proposal also dealt with the transfer of health services to the First Nation, and the problems it met characterized those of many other First Nations who entered this process. According to Garro's study, the project allowed the Sandy Bay First Nation to undertake a health needs survey, to develop a local health committee, and to refine administrative policies. They were also able to initiate more prevention programs. However, there were some problems. Apparently, the community members were not easily involved in health matters, and they tended to retain a view of the nursing station as primarily a place for treatment. Furthermore, there were some problems in developing the health committee to a point where it could offer guidance to the health centre. Some progress was made in these areas towards the end of the two-year project, but obviously the short time span was inadequate in terms of mobilizing and empowering the community in the complex area of health matters. As Garro and colleagues (1986:283) note, it was the fact that the First Nation had had some experience working in health areas previously that allowed it to accomplish what it did. In general, the Demonstration Program did not allow for sufficient time for communities to hire, train, and mobilize.

In their paper, Garro and colleagues (1986:283) were quite critical of the government's approach to health transfer as indicated in the Demonstration Program. Aboriginal organizations, while consulted, were not made aware that only communities funded under the Demonstration Program would be allowed to transfer health services to local control. This was, in these authors' view, 'a breach of the consultation process proclaimed in the 1979 Health Policy,' and represented 'a unilateral decision [which] does little to engender trust and cooperation between government and Indian groups.' Furthermore, the Demonstration Program focused on the First Nation level, prohibiting a 'unified expression of Indian interests in the field of health care.' Indeed, this approach to self-determination, stressing community-level initiatives and the transfer of some federal powers, was part of the broader federal approach, one that continues to be much criticized by some Aboriginal groups.

THE INDIAN HEALTH TRANSFER POLICY

The Community Health Demonstration Program was effectively terminated in 1985. In 1986, First Nations in Canada were informed of the formation of the 'Program Transfer and Development Directorate' to direct the new 'Indian Health Transfer Policy.' And in 1988 the federal cabinet gave its approval for the transfer of federal resources to First Nations for health programs south of the sixtieth parallel. The basic premise of the policy was that First Nations could develop slowly, through stages, to the point where they ultimately obtained control over the delivery of health services. According to the federal government, the policy was developed 'after much discussion and consultation within and outside' the Medical Services Branch (Lynch 1991:173). The approach emphasized a federal perspective on self-determination, to be implemented on a community-by-community basis, though eventually accommodation would be made for regional associations of First Nations to take on health care. Similarly, while the original program envisaged only the transfer of health services, now known as the Health Services Transfer Program, by the early 1990s it had become apparent that some communities desired a slower process involving incremental control. As a result, in 1994 a new program, called Integrated Community-Based Health Services, was implemented that involved a more limited degree of control. Then, in 1995 the federal government added its final form of control over health services through its 'Inherent Right to Self-Government Policy' (Health Canada 2004). All of these initiatives fall under the jurisdiction of Health Canada's First Nations and Inuit Health Branch (FNIHB).

A brief examination of the most popular form of transfer, the Health Services Transfer Program, provides an idea of how the process unfolds and the concerns that the federal government has about the process as a whole. It begins with the Pre-Transfer Planning phase, in which the First Nation establishes a health management structure, undertakes a health needs assessment, and drafts a community health plan. A wide variety of health programs are eligible for transfer, including primary health care, dental services, and health promotion. The First Nation then enters the Bridging phase, where the FNIHB reviews the health plan, often sending it back for further development. Eventually a Memorandum of Understanding is achieved that sets out the basic terms of the funding arrangement. This constitutes the transfer agreement. The Implementation phase has the First Nation implement the health plan and deliver the agreed-upon services. Finally, the Reporting phase requires that the First Nation produce an annual report on the programs delivered, along with an audit, and undergo an evaluation every five years.

This process pertains only to First Nations people living south of the sixtieth parallel; all Aboriginal groups north of this line, in the Yukon, Northwest Territory, and Nunavut, are required to negotiate health care and other aspects of self-government with the federal Department of Indian and Northern Affairs (Health Canada 2004).

Some First Nations leaders and organizations expressed reservations about the health transfer program during its early years. In 1988, the Assembly of First Nations suggested that the program was ultimately designed to assist the government in reducing its spending on Aboriginal health, and therefore abrogated treaty rights and its fiduciary relationship to Indians (Assembly of First Nations 1988). In the wake of the government's own exercise in determining where budget allocations could be cut across all federal programs (as evidenced in the so-called Nielsen Report, see Weaver 1986), the fears of Indians that there was, indeed, a 'hidden agenda' behind the health transfer program were perhaps well-founded. In a critical analysis of the nascent health transfer program, Culhane Speck (1989) argued, along with many Aboriginal people, that the policy 'does not represent a positive departure from the past or a fundamental change in position by the federal government' with respect to health care. Particularly problematic for her were the government's continued refusal to accept a legal responsibility for Aboriginal health and what she saw as the attempt to ultimately transfer the responsibility for it to the provincial governments (as with the White Paper of 1969's proposals to terminate Indian 'status' and turn over program administration to the provinces, a change First Nations have generally resisted). Culhane Speck even argued that the transfer policy was inherently assimilationist, parroting the government rhetoric of 'self-determination' while unilaterally diverging from the Indian meaning of the concept. This critique was advanced by Georges Erasmus, among others, at that time as well. At a national conference in 1989, Erasmus, then national chief of the Assembly of First Nations, argued that 'it is not possible to consider health transfer in isolation from all other developments taking place in Indian communities' (DNHW, *Health Transfer Newsletter*, Special Issue 1990:2). In fact, the whole idea of the 'transfer' or devolution of any services to First Nations did not fit with Erasmus's view of self-determination, focused as it was on having the 'inherent' right to self-government accepted in the Canadian Constitution. However, he was forced to accept that those First Nations that saw health transfer as a way to meet their own needs and goals had a right to participate. The chief of the Mathias Colomb First Nation in Manitoba perhaps spoke for many others when he noted that, 'Overall, this policy direction had been criticized as an attempt to abrogate treaty rights and have Indian people administer their own misery. Nevertheless, we entered the transfer process – but with our eyes wide open. We saw transfer as a way to achieve some of our objectives and we felt we could look after ourselves in dealing with the government' (Connell et al. 1991:44).

Indeed, it quickly became apparent that many First Nations were willing to run the health transfer gauntlet; by the fall of 1989, fifty-eight Pre-

Transfer projects were underway, involving 212 Indian communities across the country (DNHW, *Health Transfer Newsletter*, Fall 1989:1). Most were in the earliest stages, but their numbers were clearly indicative that this was one initiative that many First Nations were willing to take seriously. Some opposition still remained, however, including that offered by the Union of Ontario Indians and the Assembly of First Nations, who continued to argue that the health transfer process was an abrogation of the federal government's responsibilities for Indian health.

The 1989 health transfer conference also brought calls from Indian delegates to remove some of the constraints built into the process. The two-year limit on funding for the development of Community Health Plans and the limited funding for health needs assessments were two areas that generated much discussion. Staff training also required greater funding. There were also calls for giving First Nations the opportunity to take control of existing Medical Services Branch (MSB) facilities, such as the Sioux Lookout Zone Hospital, as part of the transfer process (although these hospitals would ultimately be phased out). All of these concerns were eventually acted upon by the federal government

By the fall of 1990, eight transfer agreements had been signed, and some 67 First Nations were involved in Pre-Transfer planning. These agreements were signed with both single First Nations and larger tribal councils representing multiple First Nations (D.E. Young and Smith 1991:20). The next decade would see an explosion in the involvement of various First Nations communities and regional authorities in the health transfer process. By the end of 1992, there had been twenty-three transfer agreements signed, representing 71 different First Nations in British Columbia, Saskatchewan, Manitoba, Quebec, Newfoundland, and New Brunswick (DNHW, *Health Transfer Newsletter*, Winter 1992:5). As of March 2002, of the 599 eligible First Nations communities, 284 or 47 per cent had signed a Health Services Transfer Agreement. Of these, 61 per cent were multi-community transfers and 39 per cent were single-community transfers. In contrast, only 12 communities had entered into self-government agreements that included health transfer. The Integrated Community-Based Health Services version was more attractive, with 151 communities involved. Finally, an additional 41 communities were in the Pre-Transfer phase. Overall, a very significant 81 per cent of eligible communities could be said to be actively involved in the health transfer process in some manner. It is evident to many that this is a tremendously successful program, despite stumbling blocks and logistical problems along the way. Nevertheless, despite this success, the transfer process has not been embraced equally in all regions of the country. For instance, the proportion of communities that had signed a Health Services Transfer Agreement by 2002 (46 per cent) ranged from 79 per cent in the Quebec region to only 7 per cent in Alberta (Health Canada 2002). As we shall see later in this chapter, criticism of the process continues to be expressed, with some arguing that health transfer simply represents the downloading of costs to the local health authorities (Jacklin and Warry 2004).

MÉTIS EXPERIENCES WITH SELF-DETERMINATION

As has been made clear throughout this volume, the anomalous position of the Métis within Canadian society has not only made it difficult for us to obtain good information about them; it has also made it difficult for them to advance their cause for self-determination, in the area of health care and other areas as well. There are only a few federal level health programs that include the Métis, and the federal government generally seems interested in Métis self-determination primarily when federal lands or other resources are at risk. In Canada's northern territories, specific Aboriginal status seems largely irrelevant to the availability of health services, and the Métis receive the variety of benefits subsumed under the south's non-insured health benefits program; however, south of the sixtieth parallel the Métis fall squarely within provincial jurisdictions, and the provinces seem even less keen about Aboriginal self-determination than the federal government. With the exception of the Métis Settlements in Alberta, most Métis do not have the benefit of a collective land base or reserves, and this renders self-determination initiatives more difficult.

Not surprisingly, then, Métis control over health services is considerably farther behind that of the First Nations (Lemchuk-Favel and Jock 2004). This is tempered, however, by the fact that the Métis are treated the same as other provincial citizens, able to utilize health services according to relevant provincial policies that apply to other citizens. This may explain why self-determination in the area of health seems to be less of a priority among the Métis, especially when viewed alongside the lack of a collective land base and other rights that First Nations seem to have. For instance, at a 2002 meeting sponsored by the Métis Centre of the National Aboriginal Health Organization and the Métis National Council, Métis leaders and health professionals described the jurisdictional issues facing the Métis primarily in terms of the lack of clear hunting and fishing rights and its negative effect on the 'traditional diet and diabetes' of Métis people, rather than in terms of a lack of self-determination in the area of health services.[2]

Nevertheless, many provincial Métis associations have made efforts to increase control over the delivery of specific services to their Métis members, often appealing to the need for culturally appropriate services. A good example is the Métis Addictions Council of Saskatchewan, Inc. (MACSI), a program under the auspices of the Métis Nation of Saskatchewan but incorporated within the province as a non-profit organization and a registered charity. MACSI is governed by a board of directors, and each Métis regional council in the province has the authority to appoint a representative to this governing body. It was established in 1969 to provide alcohol and drug abuse rehabilitation programs to both the Métis and the off-reserve Indian population, while remaining open to all citizens of the province. This latter point is significant in that it demonstrates how many Métis programs tend to be less segregated than those designed by First Nations. A 1997–8 review of data on inpatient, outpatient, detoxification, and long-term residential facilities operated by MACSI and funded by Saskatchewan Health indicated that only 53 per cent of the clients across all these programs were Aboriginal. Further, the majority of Aboriginal people utilizing MACSI inpatient and outpatient services were treaty Indians, perhaps a reflection of the more urban nature of MACSI services (MACSI's main program centres are located in Prince Albert, Saskatoon, and Regina).[3] As an agency funded by the Saskatchewan government, however, MACSI is subject to periodic audits, and one such audit found that certain funds were inappropriately used between 2001 and 2004. As a result, the province appointed an interim director to take charge, and all the members of the MACSI board were replaced.[4]

A different situation is presented by the Métis Settlements of Alberta. These settlements, formerly known as 'Colonies,' were established in 1930 as land bases for the province's Métis population. Eight of the original twelve settlements remain. Legislation has established them as de facto municipalities within Alberta, and therefore the province has taken the lead role in working with the residents to develop all relevant infrastructure and services. In 1998, a project called 'Health for All' saw the development of a collaborative effort between the provincial Lakeland Regional Health Authority and four of the settlements, to deal with Métis health issues. The main focus of the project was to change the manner in which health services were delivered to the four relatively remote communities by adding the position of settlement nurse to the existing teams of public health, home care, and medical service providers from outside who made periodic visits. The governing structure of the project included an Aboriginal health council and a steering committee consisting of representatives from the four settlements.

A variety of outcomes were noted for this project. Among these, an improved capacity of the local population to take care of their health needs was paramount. Health issues were also brought forward onto the political agendas of the settlements, creating a new awareness of these problems that had not been highlighted in the past. Anecdotal information also suggests that there has been an overall improvement in health status. It was the participation of the local people in the governance of the program that was key, in so far as they were able to identify issues and priorities. Finally, relationships with the regional health authority improved dramatically.[5]

THE IMPACT OF HEALTH TRANSFER

The health transfer process cannot be viewed separately from the broader process of increasing self-determination for Aboriginal people in Canada. Health services, along with education and social services, are the three areas in which the greatest strides have been taken. Nevertheless, it is logical to ask if the overall health situation has changed as a result of the health transfer process, a particularly pressing question given the widespread ill health that we have already documented. In asking this question, however, we must accept that including health transfer within the currently popular 'health determinants' framework does not render analysis any less difficult (Health Canada 2003e). This framework suggests that a myriad factors affect the health of individuals and communities, and it is virtually impossible to isolate those related to transfer from all the others in order to produce a verifiable causal statement. In this section, we will look at the available evidence on the impact of health transfer.

The William Charles First Nation, located at Montreal Lake in Saskatchewan, was the first to obtain control of health care under the transfer policy. The First Nation consisted of a total membership of 1,800, with close to 800 living on the reserve located 100 kilometres north of Prince Albert. In 1984, the First Nation commenced a feasibility study for a new health facility on the reserve, in conjunction with the Medical Services Branch. The study indicated that the living conditions on the reserve were poor: only five houses had running water and proper sewage disposal, and most were overcrowded. Economic conditions were also poor, with most families reliant on welfare for at least part of the year. There was a serious alcohol and drug abuse problem, and family violence and sexual abuse rates were high. The people suffered from high rates of respiratory diseases, as well as gastro-intestinal diseases and skin infections. The study also documented a lack of health care knowledge and poor self-care, and there was a lack of reliable medical services. The community was serviced by a half-time nurse and two community health representatives. Three individuals worked in addictions. For most medical treatment, residents travelled to the city of Prince Albert, an hour or so away (M. Moore et al. 1990:153–4; Bird and Moore 1991:47).

The study determined that there was a need for a new, primary health care facility under First Nation control, with better access to physicians and nurses so that health care could be delivered to the people, rather than the people having to travel to health care facilities in Prince Albert (in 1984, travel costs for medical reasons were $236,000). The First Nation's actions on this front actually pre-dated the Health Services Transfer program, and therefore there was some foot-dragging by the federal government. But, in 1987 the Medical Services Branch accepted the First Nation's proposal, and the parties entered into the negotiating (now known as Bridging) phase.

According to those First Nation representatives involved, 'the negotiation process was very stressful, partly because such detailed agreements had never been drafted before in Canada and all parties were learning as we went along' (Bird and Moore 1991:47). The transfer agreement that emerged from these negotiations was comprehensive and demanding. For instance, it committed both the federal government and the First Nation to ensuring that the quality of health services would not diminish under the First Nation's control, and it allowed the federal government to 'intervene to stabilize the health service in times of emergency or institutional difficulty' (ibid.:48). Nevertheless, both parties were committed to working together to achieve the aims of the health plan. Not surprisingly, the agreement also noted that it did not prejudice treaty rights and future claims (the First Nation taking the position that health care is a treaty right).

After three years of planning, the new William Charles Health Centre was opened on the Montreal Lake reserve. The health centre was designed to provide a wide array of services. Many of these services were educational and preventive in orientation, including school-based health education; immunization programs; alcohol education, referral, and follow-up; pre-natal health education; and health promotion and education for chronic disease patients. The new centre also provided more consistent medical treatment, calling for a physician to visit the community one day each week, a dentist once a month, and full-time community nursing services (M. Moore et al. 1990:154). The original hope to formally include Aboriginal healing services was put on hold while the health centre personnel investigated the legal implications of such action.

Within a few years of the transfer, anecdotal information and the observations of health centre staff suggested that there had been some important changes. In general, the First Nation's members had come to feel more secure about their health, as a result of having better qualified personnel available on a more regular basis. Emergencies that would have required evacuation to the city were now more likely to be handled at the community level. In some cases – with childbirth and coronary attacks, for example – the availability of immediate medical service made a critical difference. The educational component of the centre enabled more people to attempt home management of minor illnesses (especially of children by parents) and reduced the number of after-hours calls at the nursing station. Some elders, who previously had tended to avoid the nursing station and city medical facilities, had become more comfortable with the services provided at the centre, including the ability to use their Cree language; as a result, more elders were amenable to periodic medical examinations. Indeed, according to M. Moore and colleagues (1990:157), cultural and linguistic compatibility were essential ingredients in the health centre's success:

The feeling of just being a number in a 'White' medical clinic where English is the only language has been replaced by being served by people who know the name, family members, customs and language of the Elders. People living on a trapline with no washing facilities can come directly to the health centre knowing they are welcome and that staff are accustomed to seeing people in such circumstances. Instead of feeling a sense of shame and uncomfortable visibility, people feel at home. Translation is never a problem as all but three staff speak Cree, and many translators are available.

Preliminary reports also indicated that the number of immunizations of children increased substantially after the centre was opened. Further, an examination of patient charts for the first quarters of 1989 and 1990 suggested that some changes in health status may also have ensued. For instance, whereas there were fifteen hospital admissions for ear infections during the year prior to the opening of the centre, in this period in 1989–90, there were none. There was also some suggestion that hospitalizations for upper respiratory infections had declined. However, these data were obviously incomplete. The perceptions of the nurses nevertheless suggested that, while the centre received a 'backlog' of patients when it first opened (individuals who had been reluctant to seek care under the former system), after a year there was a noticeable decline in admissions of acute cases and a corresponding increase in the numbers of those seeking treatment at earlier stages of illness. Health centre physicians also noted a decline in emergency outpatient visits (M. Moore et al. 1990:161).

The creation of the William Charles Health Centre, and the transfer of control over health care to the First Nation, resulted in an important shift in community attitudes and practices. According to M. Moore and colleagues (ibid.:163), this represented the more 'intangible' benefits of the transfer process:

Before the health centre, the community fabric was disintegrating. Residents lived in considerable fear, isolation and despair. The relations among health service providers and other community services reflected this isolation as well as contributed to it. The staff and to the lesser extent the health committee have begun to recreate the sense of community. They have discovered ways to support each other and work together, yet maintain separate identities. They provide a role model for the concept of community for the people whom they serve ... It is perhaps this element of the spirit that causes the health centre to be seen as a 'community centre' ... People have a greater sense of 'belonging' – an element that has been missing.

The Eskasoni First Nation in Cape Breton, Nova Scotia, represents a different and more recent example of the transfer process. In 1999, the community of 3,200 Mi'kmaq took over control of primary health care on the reserve in an effort to reduce the high rates of mortality and morbidity resulting from alcohol and substance abuse, respiratory problems, heart disease, and diabetes. Addiction to prescription drugs was also a problem. Access to medical resources was not an issue; in fact, community residents had quadruple the number of annual physician visits in comparison to the provincial norm, in part because of the federal government's requirement that a physician provide a prescription for over-the-counter medications covered by the non-insured health benefits program (Health Canada 2003e). The problem was deemed to be within the purview of the health services that were delivered to the community. In particular, three areas were determined to be in need of the greatest effort: pre-natal care, diabetes management, and prescription drug abuse (Lemchuk-Favel and Jock 2004).

Collaboration with Dalhousie University in conjunction with the federal and provincial governments was especially important in the development of the new primary health care program. In particular, Dalhousie recruited salaried physicians to replace the fee-for-service practitioners who had been providing medical services, and with the cooperation of the First Nation made the community a medical teaching and research site. It was argued that the salaried medical staff would be better able to deal with a community experiencing chronic health problems because there would be fewer time pressures on the clinicians. Further, such a situation would allow for greater involvement in preventive health care, patient assessment, and case management of patients with complex needs (Health Canada 2003e). While a new health centre was constructed, jurisdictional issues meant that the building would feature two interconnected wings, one for the federal staff and one for the provincial. Despite this fractured appearance, the new program actually served to improve the integration of the various health services provided to the community.

An evaluation of the program after only eighteen months suggested that some important changes had occurred. The number of physician visits per resident declined from eleven to four per year, and the number of patient visits to the hospital emergency department declined by 40 per cent. The costs of medical transportation declined from $545,000 in 1997 to $370,000 in 2001. It was suggested that many of these changes were due to the increased access to a multidisciplinary health team available five days a week, compared to the earlier situation of clinical services available only three times a week (Health Canada 2003e; Lemchuk-Favel and Jock 2004). Pre-natal care improved as well, as most pregnancies (96 per cent) were now followed throughout the entire course of pregnancy and post-natal care. Finally, there was a decline in the issuing of prescription medications, especially antibiotics, antihistamines, and cough medicines.

Several issues did arise subsequent to the development of the integrated primary health care centre. Collaboration between the federal and provincial staff proved difficult to develop in practice, particularly in the early days, although there is some suggestion that this has improved over time. It has also been noted that since the province would fund primarily physician services and not the other kinds of services needed in a multidisciplinary model, the health centre appeared top heavy (with a ratio of three physicians to one nurse). The provincial hospital system saved a substantial sum as a result of the decline in visits by Eskasoni residents, but there was no mechanism in place to allow these savings to be transferred to the funding of the other aspects of the integrated health care plan, such as substance abuse and mental health (Health Canada 2003e; Lemchuk-Favel and Jock 2004).

These two examples outline some of the ways in which communities have benefited through the health transfer process. The limited research that has been done on the consequences of health transfer has, for the most part, demonstrated important qualitative changes. These would include an increase in awareness of health issues; a higher priority for health issues on the political agenda; the development of health care services tailored more specifically to the linguistic and cultural needs of communities; improvement in the integration and coordination of disparate health services; and a decline in the usage of medical services (Health Canada 1999). Absent, for the most part, has been research linking changes in health status to health transfer. In particular, there seems to be an unwritten assumption that health transfer necessarily leads to an improvement in health. We would suggest that this remains an open question, since local control of health cannot be seen in a vacuum, as separate from the other political, social, economic, and cultural issues that vie for attention in communities.

Generally, what we have not seen is research into the community level processes leading up to and following health transfer. These are not always smooth processes, and the opportunities that transfer brings are sometimes balanced, even nullified, by local level complexities. We are reminded that health is political, as Adelson (2000) has pointed out in her analysis of recent developments among the James Bay Cree, and that analysis of the health control movement must comprehend the political environments in which the process unfolds and the political consequences that ensue when transfer is complete. Warry's (1998) study of the process of health transfer among the North Shore Tribal Council in Ontario is one of the best, and most detailed, examinations of what was going on at the community level as transfer was discussed, negotiated, and implemented. Personality conflicts, internal political struggles, and setbacks resulting from periodic elections that often saw significant changes in local leadership all had an impact on the shape of the transfer process. Local level fears that the council would consolidate its power through health transfer betrayed an underlying suspicion of new political mega-organizations that had no real traditional counterpart. While it is true that, prior to colonization, Aboriginal peoples had 'control' over their health care systems, contemporary control over complex biomedical, psychotherapeutic, and even revamped 'traditional' services remains a far more complicated process and one for which there is no real precedent.

SELF-DETERMINATION AND HEALTH STATUS

As noted above, there has been little research done on the impact of health transfer on community level health status, and many accept on faith that health will improve with local control or, at worst, will not deteriorate. A study that has generated an enormous amount of attention looked at the issue from a different angle. Chandler and Lalonde (1998) examined the data on youth suicides in British Columbia between 1987 and 1992 and then undertook comparative analysis of the data. Not surprisingly, the data demonstrated that the Aboriginal suicide mortality rate was substantially higher than the non-Aboriginal rate, often six or seven times higher in specific years. What makes this study valuable, however, is not this recitation of well-known epidemiological trends but rather the manner in which specific Aboriginal deaths were linked to specific factors extant in those communities. In particular, the explanatory power of this approach made it apparent that some Aboriginal communities had very high suicide rates while others had very low rates. The researchers identified six 'cultural continuity factors' by which they could categorize communities:

(a) evidence that particular bands had taken steps to secure aboriginal title to their traditional lands; (b) evidence of having taken back from government agencies certain rights of self-government; (c) evidence of having secured some degree of community control over educational services; (d) police and fire protection services; and (e) health delivery services; and finally, (f) evidence of having established within their communities certain officially recognized 'cultural facilities' to help preserve and enrich their cultural lives. (Ibid:209)

Certainly the classification of communities in this manner was innovative, if somewhat subjective.

The results of this study created considerable interest. The lowest youth suicide rates were found in communities that had been 'especially successful in their negotiations with federal and provincial governments in having further established their right in law to a large measure of economic and political independence within their traditional territory,' or 'self-government' (Chandler and Lalonde 1998:209). The other factors, or 'markers,' were then ranked in this order: education, land claims, and health services; cultural facilities; and, finally, police and fire services. After summing up the number of 'markers' present in each community, the researchers were able to assign a score of 0 to 6 and compare these scores to the youth suicide rates. Not surprisingly, a strong inverse relationship was evident: the higher the number of factors present, the lower the suicide rate. Indeed, communities with none of the factors averaged almost 140 suicide deaths per 100,000, in contrast to communities where all six factors were present, where the suicide rate was virtually nil.

What do these results mean? We believe that it is a mistake to become too caught up in the authors' argument that 'cultural continuity' as measured by these six factors represents a protective factor, a 'hedge against suicide.' They admit that conceptualizing cultural continuity is problematic; they also note that in many ways what they are talking about is less continuity with an unbroken cultural past and more the 'steps being taken by First Nations communities to protect and rehabilitate the continuity of their own culture.' These steps, we suggest, must be seen within the very contemporary context of late twentieth- and early twenty-first-century Canada; it is difficult to draw the conclusion that running a fire or police service, or a health clinic, speaks to any concrete past cultural practice. These are very modern institutions that operate within a broad context of regional, provincial, and national regulations, and that draw on technology and organizational structures that are quite new and constantly changing. Rather, what we see in this study is the importance of self-determination and community vitality within this contemporary context. A community with all six factors will be very busy indeed. There will be substantial employment available in running the various institutions and programs and many community committees acting in an advisory capacity. People in these communities likely have more meaningful lives. Initiatives are generated from within and sustained by local people rather than imposed from the outside and carried out by non-residents or non-Aboriginal people. Young people are able to see real career options available in their communities. Even still, it is possible that the real explanation for these positive results lies in the relative strength and social cohesion of the communities prior to engaging in the self-determination process. Specifically, why have some communities been inclined and able to gain control over various sectors of community life while others have faltered? The explanation for both self-determination success and low suicide rates, therefore, may lie with yet-to-be-determined factors, factors that refute any effort to make a simple causal connection between self-determination and suicide.

EDUCATION, TRAINING, AND RESEARCH: THE KEYS TO SELF-DETERMINATION

Enormous strides have been made in the last decade towards improving access to health careers for Aboriginal people and building among Aboriginal people the capacity to undertake health-related research. Both of these developments are integral to Aboriginal self-determination, as they serve to lessen dependence on the non-Aboriginal people who tend to dominate in both areas and further allow for Aboriginal people to identify the issues, priorities, and solutions that they feel are appropriate to their unique circumstances throughout the country.

Not surprisingly, there remain relatively few Aboriginal health professionals in Canada, but this situation is changing. One 1991 source placed the number of practising Aboriginal physicians at between eighteen and twenty-five in Canada (Stephens 1991:136); but by 1996 the number was estimated to be sixty-seven, with thirty-three more in medical school (Lemchuk-Favel and Jock 2004). Many medical schools have recognized the need to increase the number of Aboriginal students studying medicine, and have also recognized that many potential students face a disproportionate burden in attempting to gain entrance to and graduate from medical school. It is now common to find spaces reserved for qualified Aboriginal students to enter first-year medical programs, and many schools have developed academic support programs and have introduced Aboriginal content into their curriculum.

The University of Alberta is a good example. As early as 1988 the university developed its Office of Aboriginal Health Care Careers Program, with the goal of increasing the number of Aboriginal medical practitioners. By 2001, the university had graduated twenty-three Aboriginal physicians, five dentists, eleven dental hygienists, and three medical laboratory technicians. The program identified three elements to its mandate: to recruit Aboriginal students; to develop support services to help students once in the program; and to introduce Aboriginal health issues, including Aboriginal healing, to non-Aboriginal faculty and staff. Places are not restricted to Alberta residents, and the university recruits from all across the country, although any seats specifically reserved for Aboriginal students can be restricted to Alberta residents. The number of reserved places is not large – up to two in any given year in the medical doctor program – but Aboriginal students can elect to apply to the general admission program instead. All students must meet the same prerequisites for admission, including a personal interview, but in the latter case an Aboriginal representative is included on the interview committee.[6]

Another impetus for the development of health careers programs came with the formation of the Indian and Inuit Nurses of Canada (IINC) association in 1975. A core group of forty met to form the association, working from a list of eighty such individuals developed only with a great deal of work. The road to achieving acceptability was difficult, as it seems all cases of self-determination have been. The association was discouraged by the federal government, and 'a national Indian political group' blocked one early federal funding initiative (Cuthand Goodwill 1989:119). When funding was obtained from the Native Women's Program of the Secretary of State, one program officer objected to the fact that the first chair of the association was male. Later, in the early 1980s, the Medical Service Branch began to fund the association, putting it on a more secure footing.

The IINC is now known as the Aboriginal Nurses Association of Canada. The association has many broad objectives, including

- To act as an agent in promoting and striving for better health for the Indian and Inuit people; that is, a state of complete physical, mental, social and spiritual well-being.
- To conduct studies and maintain reporting, compiling and publishing of material on Aboriginal health, medicine and culture.
- To encourage and facilitate Aboriginal control of Aboriginal health, and involvement and decision making on matters pertaining to health care services and delivery.
- To develop and encourage courses in the education system on nursing, the health professions, Aboriginal health and cross-cultural nursing.
- To actively develop a means of recruiting more people of Aboriginal ancestry into the medical field and health professions.[7]

Of particular note is the willingness of this association to address sensitive issues, such as alcohol abuse, family and sexual violence, and

Aboriginal healing in the contemporary context. Further, when the health transfer process started to gain momentum, the association and its members played important roles at the community level in assisting communities to undertake their research, establish their health plans, and negotiate the transfer process.

The Aboriginal Nurses Association was also instrumental in the development in 1984 of the federal government's Indian and Inuit Health Careers Program (IIHCP). This program was designed 'to encourage and support Indian participation in educational opportunities and provide a learning environment designed to overcome many of the social and cultural barriers that culturally inhibit the Native students' educational achievement' (cited in D.E. Young and Smith 1991:35). It provides bursaries and scholarships, as well as funding for professional development (such as conferences), job training, and community educational initiatives. Funding has also been made available for daycare and cultural activities, including elders' services, associated with health care institutions. In 1998, the federal government transferred the program to the National Aboriginal Achievement Foundation (NAAF), to be administered alongside several other programs for Aboriginal post-secondary students. This was done, according to the federal government, to transfer more control and ownership of health programs and services to First Nations and Inuit people.[8] In 2003–4, the NAAF managed a health careers budget of more than $540,000.[9]

Many universities and colleges in Canada have developed programs to promote Aboriginal nursing education and Aboriginal health issues. Some are open to all, while others are open only to Aboriginal students. The National Native Access Program to Nursing (NNAPN), for instance, began in 1985 at the University of Saskatchewan. Funded initially by the Medical Services Branch, the program began as a pre-nursing program designed to help Aboriginal students gain admission to university (degree) nursing schools. Students normally obtained a conditional acceptance to a nursing school in Canada and then attended a nine-week spring course at the University of Saskatchewan campus. Individual students were given the opportunity to experience the university environment, upgrade skills and knowledge, and learn about study skills, exam writing, and library research. Clinical observations and fieldwork also provided the student with some idea of what it meant to be a nurse. Upon successful completion of the course, the students moved on to their individual nursing schools to enter the nursing program. The program has achieved an excellent success rate to date. Beginning with just eleven students in 1986, by 1993 some ninety students had taken the program, 73 per cent of whom were subsequently recommended to continue in nursing. By the fall of 1992, of those who had completed the program, four students had completed their Bachelor of Science in Nursing (BSN) degrees, two had completed Registered Nursing (RN) degrees, and four had completed degrees in other areas. Overall, forty-six students who had completed the program were still attending college or university (including nineteen in a BSN program).[10] In 1998, the program evolved into a component of the Nursing Education Program of Saskatchewan (NEPS), by which time 196 students had experienced the spring program. The NEPS program seeks to increase the number of Aboriginal people in the 'healing' careers by facilitating recruitment and retention of Aboriginal nursing students at the University, including offering academic, personal, and cultural counselling services.[11]

For many years, the backbone of Aboriginal health services was the Community Health Representative (CHR) program. The CHR program dates back to the early 1960s and has undergone significant changes since then. It was originally intended as a means of providing support to the non-Aboriginal nurses who dominated the provision of Medical Services Branch health services and as a liaison mechanism between the nurses and the community. In the early years, however, CHRs received relatively little training and tended to be marginalized within the context of nursing services by, for instance, being restricted to such activities as clerical work and community sanitation initiatives. The program clearly smacked of tokenism, since at the time there were no efforts to train Aboriginal people for the more advanced medical positions. More recently, however, CHR training has improved, to the point where CHRs provide clinical services in smaller communities without resident nurses. As part of the health transfer initiative, the role of CHRs has been redefined to some extent, moving more towards community health and education activities. In 1992, the National Indian and Inuit Community Health Representatives Organization (NIICHO) was formed to

- upgrade the quality of health care of Indian and Inuit people to the standard enjoyed by the rest of the population of Canada.
- provide a forum for CHRs to communicate and exchange information with each other on various community health initiatives and on the improvement of the CHR program at national levels.
- create and promote awareness and understanding of the CHR program in Canada.[12]

Through this organization, CHRs have an advocacy and educational association that advances their interests and provides advice to various levels of Aboriginal and non-Aboriginal government on health policy initiatives.

There are other programs as well; while space constraints limit our discussion in this area, it should be clear at this point that there are many special, Aboriginal-oriented, professional and health career programs in Canada. While most are relatively recent, we are seeing the effects as Aboriginal professionals graduate and enter the workforce. Developing parallel to these educational and professional initiatives has been a revolutionary change in how Aboriginal health research is conducted in this country, one in which Aboriginal people now have a firm hand on the direction and priorities of that research as well as the manner in which it is undertaken.

The most significant development in Aboriginal health research has been the formation in 2000 of the Institute for Aboriginal People's Health (IAPH) as a component of the Canadian Institutes of Health Research (CIHR). The overall goal of the IAPH is to 'support research to address the special health needs of Canada's Aboriginal people' with an eye towards improving overall health status.[13] Research in this case, as with the CIHR more generally, includes a broad array of activities, from biomedical inquiry, clinical trials, and health determinants research to health promotion and the development of culturally appropriate health services. Ethical issues with respect to Aboriginal health research are also important.

In effect, the IAPH was mandated to develop and promote a national Aboriginal health agenda, and its impact to this end has been profound. A key means by which the IAPH has influenced Aboriginal health research has been through its Aboriginal Capacity and Developmental Research Environments (ACADRE) program. This initiative was realized in 2001 when the first four ACADRE centres were approved at the universities of Alberta, Manitoba, and Ottawa, and at the Saskatchewan Indian Federated College, now the First Nations University of Canada (FNUC). Subsequently, ACADREs were approved for Laval, University of Toronto/McMaster University, University of British Columbia, and Dalhousie University, and the FNUC ACADRE now includes the universities of Saskatchewan and Regina in the Indigenous Peoples Health Research Centre. The general mandate of these centres was explained as follows: 'Each centre must include a volunteer advisory board with majority membership being from the aboriginal community, facilitate development of aboriginal health researchers at all career stages and provide training opportunities for students, and facilitate health research capacity development in aboriginal communities and organizations.' Each centre was to receive up to $12 million over a six-year period, with a heavy emphasis on student training.[14]

The development of the IAPH and its ACADRE centres is significant in that they have become very influential in terms of who gets funded to do Aboriginal health research and what topics will be studied. Clearly, these initiatives are important in taking Aboriginal self-determination in a new direction, moving beyond the delivery of services to the much broader issues encompassed within the research and training mandate of CIHR. The IAPH stands as a testament to the realization, on the part of Aboriginal people, that health research is as important as health services delivery for improving health and well-being. It remains to be seen whether this new focus on Aboriginal health research will bring truly significant changes.

A couple of other developments in the area of health research are also noteworthy. In 2000, the National Aboriginal Health Organization (NAHO) was formed.[15] The objectives of this Aboriginal-governed organization are as follows:

- to improve and promote health through knowledge-based activities;
- to promote understanding of health issues affecting Aboriginal Peoples;
- to facilitate and promote research and develop research partnerships;
- to foster participation of Aboriginal Peoples in delivery of health care; and
- to affirm and protect Aboriginal traditional healing practices.

To achieve these objectives, two NAHO initiatives are particularly noteworthy. First, in 2001 the First Nations Centre was formed, with a mandate to facilitate the collection and dissemination of Aboriginal health knowledge. Its activities include coordination of the First Nations Regional Longitudinal Health Survey, to collect health data, and the annual issuing of the Report Card on the Health of First Nations. The First Nations Centre is guided by a Governing Committee composed of representatives from the Assembly of First Nations Health Secretariat, among others. A parallel organization under NAHO is the Métis Centre, dedicated to improving the health of Métis people in Canada, and in the north, the Ajunnginiq Centre, with a focus on the Inuit. The latter two centres are also overseen by governing committees consisting of Aboriginal people.

The second noteworthy accomplishment of NAHO has been the development of the *Journal of Aboriginal Health*, the only such journal in Canada. The journal's primary target audience are Aboriginal people themselves, including traditional healers, as well as scholars and researchers in the field. The first issue was produced in 2004; subsequent issues can be found on the NAHO website.

Another major development in the area of health research has emerged through the research program of the Aboriginal Healing Foundation (AHF). This foundation was established after a recommendation in the report of the Royal Commission on Aboriginal Peoples, with the purpose of vetting and funding healing and treatment projects that focused primarily, though not exclusively, on the intergenerational impacts of residential schools. By early 2004, the AHF had issued 1,343 grants, worth more than $375 million, to projects all across Canada.[16] Research was an important component of the AHF's mandate, and this includes not only research on and evaluation of the funded projects themselves but also the production of background and policy papers on topics such as fetal alcohol syndrome, suicide, and sexual abuse, as well as sexual offending.

These two initiatives, NAHO and the AHF, continue to demonstrate the importance of research in establishing an Aboriginal health agenda in Canada. They represent a new wave of self-determination initiatives because they transcend communities and regional authorities, seeking to tap into fast-moving developments in the information technology field and thereby empowering Aboriginal people through knowledge generation and dissemination, all the while under the guidance of predominantly Aboriginal boards and governing structures.

CONCLUSION

The process of self-determination in health care is irreversible, linked as it is to the broader struggle for self-determination of Aboriginal peoples in general. It is no longer a new process, and the evidence to date suggests that some significant changes are occurring. Aboriginal control over health care does not mean a complete rejection of biomedical and psychosocial treatment programs and methods. Rather, where possible, these are made culturally more appropriate, and Aboriginal approaches to healing are brought in to augment, but not necessarily replace, biomedical approaches.

Nevertheless, control over something as potentially serious and costly as health is not without its problems. Funding remains a perennial problem; all programs have experienced shortages, and funding seems to be becoming more difficult just as progress is being made. Mistakes in policy and practice continue to be trumpeted in local and national media, challenging Aboriginal-run programs to exceed the standards established in mainstream programming, where, these media reports would seem to suggest, nothing ever goes wrong.

Whether self-determination has led to any significant change in health status is another matter, one that the lack of data prevents us from addressing. While the issues of *control* over health care and *improved health status* are intertwined in the discourse, they are somewhat separate in practice. The issue of control is within the realm of the political, and represents the legitimate aspirations of Aboriginal peoples to have control over the delivery of health services within their communities, and control over the research that informs health policy. We do not argue with this process. But it is assumed that improved health status will follow logically from such control. We believe the issue is more complex than that. From a research perspective, we encourage concrete studies on the efficacy of Aboriginal-controlled treatment and education programs. We do not accept the view, expressed in some quarters, that such research is unnecessary, for to do so is to accept, on faith alone, that Aboriginal control is the only answer to the problem of Aboriginal health. However, the point of such research would be not to undermine Aboriginal initiatives by pointing out the failures but to generate rigorous information on what works and what does not – best practices, as it were – with an eye to increasing the extent to which self-determination improves community health. Research would also demonstrate the need for initiatives in other areas, such as employment and economic development, that have a significant bearing on health. As confidence grows and the fear of criticism or, worse, program termination, becomes remote, opportunities for this kind of research will continue to open up. Important strides are being made in this area as we write, such as with the AHF's mandate to monitor and evaluate the healing projects that it funds. Such research will only contribute to improving the overall health status of Aboriginal people.

11

Conclusion

This book is an account of health and health care among the Aboriginal peoples of Canada, written from the perspective of researchers working in an academic context, and based mostly on published sources that represent issues deemed significant mostly by historians and medical and social scientists working in the area of Aboriginal health. In the last ten years, since the first edition of this book was published (1995), there has been an explosion in Aboriginal health research, fuelled by organizations such as the National Aboriginal Health Organization (NAHO), the Aboriginal Healing Foundation (AHF), and especially the Institute for Aboriginal People's Health (IAPH) of the Canadian Institutes of Health Research (CIHR). In this final chapter we review and summarize important themes and key findings from this research, emphasizing changes in patterns of health and disease, the place of medicine within Aboriginal cultures, and the relationships between politics and health policies. Perhaps more importantly, we attempt to take stock of the field and suggest areas where research is strongest and, significantly, where it is weakest.

We began this book with a general and necessarily oversimplified overview of Aboriginal history in Canada, with descriptions of the different Aboriginal geopolitical and cultural groups at the time of contact, the social and cultural changes since contact, the political and constitutional relationships with non-Aboriginal Canadians and the Canadian state, and current socio-economic conditions. Such background information is critical for the beginnings of an understanding of Aboriginal health and health care, particularly for the non-specialist. Beyond the obvious and well-known need to understand the historico-cultural context of health, it is vital to appreciate that the concept of 'Aboriginal health' is itself a convenient but ultimately false representation of the problem at hand. It masks the rich diversity of social, economic, political, and environmental circumstances that give rise to significant variation in health problems and healing strategies in Aboriginal communities. If nothing else, this survey should make it clear that health and health care patterns show extensive variation across the country, despite the tendency for national, regional, and provincial databases to create the impression of widespread trends and homogeneity of experience. Clearly, we need to know more about the basis for health and disease in individual communities and to get beyond traditional epidemiological measures to encompass the perspectives and concerns of Aboriginal people in the communities whose health status is being assessed.

Despite the limitations of the available evidence, a historical epidemiological approach to the problem shows how the health status of Aboriginal people has changed over time. Venturing into ideas about the distant past is difficult, owing to the scantiness of the information, even without the pitfalls associated with constructing images of health and disease from fragmentary remains from thousands of years ago. Although it is widely believed that Aboriginal people in the North American continent enjoyed good health prior to contact with Europeans, unequivocal data are generally lacking, apart from sparse palaeopathological specimens, biased observations of early explorers and traders, fading oral traditions of Aboriginal people, and inappropriate extrapolations from contemporary hunter-gatherer societies. This has not deterred scholars from attempting to reconstruct the population size and structure of pre-contact populations, their nutrition and diet, and their disease patterns. In view of the subsequent tragic, post-contact state of affairs, when recurrent epidemics and famines struck Aboriginal populations with devastating impact, it is understandable that the idea of a halcyon age has remained popular. Nevertheless, it is quite evident that health problems in past populations varied, reflecting the socio-environmental conditions in which people lived and to which they responded. To suggest that there was a single health profile for pre-contact Aboriginal communities would be to deny that Aboriginal populations were as demographically and epidemiologically dynamic and capable of adjusting to their environments as populations elsewhere in the world. Certainly, epidemiological profiles have shifted in the post-contact period, and there is no reason to suspect that they were static and unchanging prior to the arrival of European explorers and settlers.

There is powerful evidence, however, that epidemics of infectious diseases played a special role in the relationship between newcomers and

Aboriginal people in North America from the fifteenth century onward. Conditions were created that allowed indigenous and newly introduced diseases to flourish, particularly after the invention and implementation of the reserve system in the late nineteenth century. The introduction of new diseases followed well-established trade routes and settlement patterns, criss-crossing regions in some cases, and burning out locally in others. Epidemics were not simply medical events but had far-reaching consequences for Aboriginal societies and the relationships between Aboriginal and non-Aboriginal people. In some cases, whole communities were decimated, often resulting in the merging of bands or the assimilation of one by another. Epidemics spurred on community break-up and migration, which sometimes spread the disease farther and occasionally encouraged intertribal warfare. Among the survivors, the loss of a significant number of community members altered leadership roles and disrupted the existing social structure. Traditional belief systems were unable to account for the new disasters, let alone counteract them. The weakening of tradition paved the way for the onslaught by European Christian missionaries. Still, relatively little is known about the health and disease histories of particular communities or reserves, so that the picture of health and disease up to the Second World War can be drawn in only the broadest of strokes. Once again, the lack of detail tends to create the illusion of a uniform quality to the health and disease experience. During this time the 'Indian problem' became medicalized, and fears about the spread of diseases from First Nations to non-Aboriginal communities shifted the blame for ill health back onto Aboriginal communities themselves.

Epidemics, especially tuberculosis, provided the impetus for the Canadian federal government to initiate and organize health services for Aboriginal people. Increased surveillance and new health initiatives helped to contribute to a dramatic decline in many infectious diseases in the post-Second World War era. But in their place, new epidemics of chronic, non-communicable diseases on the one hand (such as heart disease, hypertension, obesity, and diabetes), and injuries, violence, and the so-called social pathologies on the other hand, have come to the fore in biomedical categorizations. Regardless of whether infectious diseases or social pathologies predominate in epidemiological profiles, we must not lose sight of the fact that biomedical definitions of health and disease are inextricably linked to larger structures of authority and power. The ability to define and then survey such parameters as 'health status' carries with it the power to construct institutions of healing that prescribe, proscribe, and regulate behaviour. The creation of the image of Aboriginal communities as socially pathological, as 'desperate, disorganized and depressed,' provides, in turn, a rationale for policies of paternalism and dependency (O'Neil 1993). Clearly, contemporary researchers need to conduct their work in a manner that achieves a more proper balance between the investigation and reporting of health issues and those aspects of Aboriginal life that are positive, healthy, and fulfilling.

It is important to recognize that, prior to the arrival of Europeans, there were already in existence various Aboriginal medical systems, each with its theories of disease causation, its categories of practitioners, and its diagnostic and therapeutic techniques. Medicine was closely integrated with other aspects of Aboriginal culture and was often indistinguishable from spirituality. The response of biomedicine, the church, and the Canadian state towards traditional Aboriginal health care systems has ranged from dismissal (as hocus-pocus, witchcraft, unscientific, and at best placebo therapy) to outright suppression. While self-care and care by indigenous practitioners were the main sources of health care before European contact, external agents such as traders and missionaries soon provided medical assistance in times of hardship. Such care was offered both for compassionate reasons and to enhance the health of the enterprise, be it the collection of furs or the conversion of souls. In any event, from the outset, political authority was enacted through health surveillance, policy, and practice at the community level, undermining Aboriginal medical systems and driving many underground. There are healthy signs of a strong resurgence of traditional medical practice, and instances can be found of collaboration between Aboriginal healers and biomedical institutions and practitioners, particularly in mental health. But what we today still refer to as 'traditional' medical practice has been altered in response to the many pressures of European contact and subsequent cultural change, and it is essential that researchers not romanticize these approaches to health and treatment. They must be understood within a contemporary context, in which treatment success is balanced with failure, in which healers employ biomedical knowledge and discourse alongside knowledge passed down through generations, and in which treatment continues to be considerably idiosyncratic and resistant to enquiry. Nevertheless, it is clear that 'traditional' Aboriginal healing, with its attendant base in spirituality, continues as an essential cornerstone of Aboriginal cultural revitalization.

The idea that the federal government has a responsibility for Aboriginal health care slowly emerged towards the latter part of the nineteenth century, with Euro-Canadian settlement of the west and the signing of the treaties. As part of the bargain in exchange for the Indians' land, the Canadian government offered cash, farming implements, schools, and medical care. Medical care was considered something that could entice the Indians to submit to, or at least not obstruct, non-Aboriginal settlement. What passed for medical care – 'a medicine chest' – was mentioned in only one treaty, Treaty Six (1876), which covered central Saskatchewan and Alberta. Is the medicine chest simply a wooden box with a few medicines and bandages? Or is it a metaphor that represents the complete array of modern medical technologies and facilities, such that the 'chest' grows and is upgraded as medicine itself advances? Court cases have been fought over this interpretation. Before the issue could be resolved once and for all, it was overtaken by events: universal hospital insurance and, later, medical care insurance, established in Canada from coast to coast, rendered the issue of who pays largely irrelevant. Much of the debate today tends to centre on a set of medical services referred to as non-insured services that the government consistently tampers with, to the consternation of many Aboriginal groups.

The forerunner of today's multimillion-dollar Aboriginal health service began to take shape only towards the end of the nineteenth century, but a chief medical officer was not appointed in the Department of Indian Affairs until 1904. The early years of the Indian health service were marked by internal political struggles and severe budgetary con-straints, indicative of the lack of commitment of the federal government to health issues, despite rhetoric to the contrary. In the immediate pre-Second World War years, there were many reports of severe hardship, of near starvation and malnutrition, and of uncontrolled epidemics in many Aboriginal communities. It was not until after the Second World War that Indian and Northern Health Services expanded by leaps and bounds, in terms of budget, staff, and facilities. Transferred from the Department of Indian Affairs to the newly established Department of National Health and Welfare, it provided increased services under a post-war social policy dominated by government intervention in the health and social sectors.

Over the past two decades, the debate on Aboriginal health care has shifted from questions of 'Who gets the service?' and 'Who pays for it?' to the question of 'Who controls it?' Increasingly, health care is seen as part of the broader political process of self-determination. 'Devolution,' once the buzz-word in government circles, has transformed into actual Aboriginal control over health services throughout much of the country, especially for First Nations. Scepticism over the health transfer process has given way to enthusiasm, even if there remain some significant areas of contention. Across the country, implementation of the transfer of control has taken many forms, with varying degrees of success. One of the important consequences of the shift of control from external agencies to the level of the community is the emergence of community-based health assessment research, controlled at the local level. We can continue to expect a number of significant consequences for understanding Aboriginal health issues to emerge from this jurisdictional realignment: increasing incorporation of Aboriginal definitions and perceptions of health and illness, a more holistic view of health that reflects Aboriginal cultures and traditional ecological knowledge, and the generation of a variety of disease profiles, as health research becomes more closely oriented towards the social, spiritual, economic, and political needs of specific communities. Research, now emerging, is suggesting that in some contexts self-determination is proving healthy for Aboriginal peoples. However, as in the larger society, politics and health are sometimes in conflict, and part of the self-determination process involves working through these conflicts. Despite unequivocal evidence that Aboriginal people are suffering a variety of health problems due to tobacco smoking, for instance, in some regions of the country First Nations have asserted their rights to control health policy on the reserve and therefore are rejecting provincial bans on tobacco use in public areas. Some First Nations also actively promote the on-reserve sale of cheap cigarettes to both reserve members and those from surrounding non-Aboriginal communities. The response of the federal and some provincial governments to counter the cross-border cigarette smuggling activities engaged in by some First Nations by reducing tobacco taxes during the mid-1990s has led to an overall increase in tobacco consumption among Canadian teens. Many First Nations also see casinos as a quick way to redress the effects of colonialism and hasten economic development, without carefully considering the health and social impact that gambling might have on community members. It would be fruitful for a new research agenda to explore self-determination in all its dimensions, positive and negative, in order for us to work to develop even better health policy in an increasingly complex health policy environment.

In examining Aboriginal health and health care, then, it is important to move beyond simplistic explanations. In the past, there have been attempts to link Aboriginal health status to cultural or biological factors, to, in effect, 'blame the victim' for his or her problems. This has been the case with previous scourges, such as tuberculosis, and with more contemporary problems, such as alcoholism and HIV/AIDS. But simple biological and cultural arguments fail to adequately explain health and health care issues among Aboriginal people in Canada today. A complex interdigitation between socio-economic and political factors, including broader historical and local circumstances, explains to a greater degree the current situation than do either cultural or biological factors alone.

An approach that stresses the political economy of health seems most appropriate, given the status of Aboriginal people as indigenous, colonized minorities in their homeland. This approach should address issues of culture and biology, but should also carefully investigate historical events and policies, as well as socio-economic factors and the nature of the Canadian state and Canadian society. In so doing, we not only see the victimization of Aboriginal peoples through colonization, loss of lands, and various forms of racism, but also see Aboriginal people as individuals reacting to an oppressive situation and acting to improve their lot. Any approach that fails to consider Aboriginal people as active in response to their colonial situation, rather than simply as passive victims, will fail to comprehend not only past changes in health status and health care, but also, and more importantly, the future direction that will be taken in these areas. But we must also appreciate that colonialism is more than four centuries old in Canada, and there have been vast changes as a result. We need to understand colonialism but not be restricted by it. Health research needs to appreciate the contemporary context in which Aboriginal people live, in which immediate problems such as employment and housing, while linkable to the process of colonialism, require very contemporary solutions.

With increasing self-determination, the actions of individual Aboriginal groups and organizations run by them now play a greater role in our understanding of health and illness. Aboriginal people, like all groups, have always had considerable agency in the area of health, and researchers are documenting more and more the impact of both healthy and unhealthy personal behaviours and Aboriginal health policies at the individual and community levels. As more Aboriginal health researchers enter the arena, it is becoming more common for them and their non-Aboriginal counterparts to join forces and, with some degree of courage, point out that ill health today cannot always be blamed on history and contemporary structural inequalities. Even without changes to the status quo, there are still things that can be done to improve health status.

We join with those who, focusing on health more than on politics, argue that only through *critical* inquiry, including the study of Aboriginal initiatives, can better health be achieved. It is likely that the health situation of Aboriginal people in Canada will continue to improve in the future, particularly if attention is paid to several specific areas.

In all aspects of health research, administration, and clinical service delivery, a public health perspective must be adopted, one that is devoid of moral or racial undertones and that refrains from viewing Aboriginal people as culturally crippled. The cooperation of health professionals, both Aboriginal and non-Aboriginal, is needed to ensure that proper health education messages are received and acted upon at the community level. Associated with this is the need to make health knowledge readily available to Aboriginal individuals and health and political organizations, so that informed personnel and organizational changes are made. There continue to be problems both in the communication of sometimes highly technical research results and in the development of effective health education programs. More and more, the ability of researchers to undertake their work is being tied to their inclination and ability to make that research directly relevant to Aboriginal health consumers.

There must be a greater sensitivity to contemporary Aboriginal cultural diversity on the part of non-Aboriginal biomedical practitioners and researchers, especially to linguistic barriers and the problems engendered by the life circumstances of some Aboriginal people. Training for cultural competence is needed and is best provided by the elders, traditional healers, and other individuals designated by the specific communities where a biomedical practitioner is hired to serve. Realistically, such training will only benefit individuals who are willing and able to see beyond the blinders created by ethnocentricity and membership in an elite sector of Canadian society. That being said, however, researchers and health practitioners must appreciate that there is no single Aboriginal culture in Canada, that there is no singular Aboriginal experience, and that many Aboriginal patients find current biomedical services and approaches to be 'culturally appropriate' and preferable to so-called traditional services.

We also need to better understand the meaning of health, being healthy, and healing for Aboriginal people today. Healing, in particular, has become a ubiquitous process, but about which there has been little detailed, critical research. Similarly, a recent emphasis on understanding social capital and resilience among Aboriginal groups offers a great deal in our efforts to understand what makes a people, a community, and an individual healthy rather than ill. From this knowledge, better preventive programs can emerge that transect the levels of individual, family, and community.

Aboriginal people continue to need increased opportunities to enter and succeed in the various health professions, including health research. Entrance equity programs at colleges and universities and employment equity policies at places of employment must continue to be developed. The emergence into these fields of Aboriginal people in recent years has resulted in a profound shift in both research and caregiving, and more changes are on the horizon as the pool of Aboriginal health professionals continues to expand.

Finally, and most importantly, there remains a need for an overall general improvement in the socio-economic status of Aboriginal Canadians. This huge task, which will require structural changes to the broader Canadian economic and political milieu, is generally considered to be beyond the parameters of health research and service delivery.

In the end, we remain optimistic that the health status of Aboriginal people will continue to improve, but only through coordinated action on the research and service delivery fronts, and only in conjunction with continuing changes to the political and socio-economic landscape in Canada.

Notes

CHAPTER 1 An overview of the Aboriginal peoples of Canada

1 It is important to appreciate that the census failed to achieve a comprehensive coverage of the target Aboriginal population. Enumeration was not completed or was interrupted on thirty Indian reserves and settlements, accounting for approximately an undercount of between 30,000 and 35,000 people. The data for incompletely enumerated reserves and settlements, are not normally included in statistical tabulations. Beginning with the 1986 census, respondents were permitted to report multiple ethnic origins. Note that there are separate questions on Aboriginal 'origins' as well as 'identity,' with the latter being numerically smaller in size. More detailed breakdown of both the Aboriginal origins and identity populations can be obtained from detailed tables (Cat. No. 97F0011XCB01001) and the narrative report *Aboriginal Peoples of Canada: A Demographic Profile* ([Cat. No. 96F0030XIE2001007) from the 2001 census in Statistics Canada's website (www.statcan.ca).

2 The number of language families that can be identified in the Americas is itself controversial. Regna Darnell (1986:22) cautions that 'there can be no single answer to the question of how many indigenous languages and language families there are in Canada,' depending on the sufficiency of the linguistic data analysed and the classification model that is used.

3 Mitochondrial DNA analysis has been applied to the analysis of population movements worldwide. It is useful for studying human migration because it is only inherited from mother to daughter and therefore eliminates the recombination of genes between fathers and mothers that complicates the evolutionary picture when nuclear DNA is studied. The structure of the mtDNA molecule is well understood, and all of its nucleotide posi-

tions and coding loci are known. Any changes in it arise from mutations inherited through the maternal line, and it also mutates at a relatively fast rate compared to nuclear DNA. This makes it possible to distinguish populations that separated over relatively short periods of time, such as thousands of years. It is easily recovered from ancient bones and teeth, as well as from living people, and it exists in high numbers of copies, facilitating laboratory analysis. That said, mtDNA is just one genetic marker, and the results of this type of research cannot be expected to stand alone in the absence of other lines of genetic evidence. Unfortunately, nuclear DNA is very difficult to recover from ancient human remains, an issue that will be taken up in the next chapter.

4 This conclusion is based on the study of variation in mtDNA 'haplogroups.' These haplogroups are characterized by unique combinations of genetic sequences that distinguish them from each other. Five mtDNA haplogroups (A, B, C, D, and X) account for 95 to 100 per cent of mtDNA among indigenous people of the Americas and are understood to represent the major founding mtDNA lineages (Schurr and Sherry 2004:421). The origin of haplogroup X has prompted a great deal of controversy. At one time, speculation arose that haplogroup X might provide evidence for a pre-Columbian European presence in the Americas, speculation that was fanned by popular and incorrect representations of Kennewick Man (dated to about 9,500 years ago) as having a morphology more closely aligned with people from Europe than Asia. This misconception has been put to rest. Haplogroup X is widespread among Native Americans, reaching its highest frequencies, about 20 per cent, among some Algonquian groups. The closest affinities of this mtDNA haplogroup appear to be with south-central Siberia, not Europe (Eshleman, Malhi, and Smith 2003:11).

5 The site of Monté Verde, Chile, dates to about 12,500 years ago, prior to archaeological evidence for the Clovis culture, which occurred later, around 11,500 years ago.

6 Several surveys of pre-contact and early post-contact Aboriginal cultural formations exist; see, for instance, McMillan and Yellowhorn (2004) and Morrison and Wilson (2004).

7 Of course there had been Aboriginal efforts prior to this to mobilize politically. For instance, in the first half of this century, Métis activist Jim Brady and Indian leaders such as John Tootoosis and F.O. Loft spent considerable parts of their lives involved in political organizing. See Dobbin (1981) on Brady, and Sluman and Goodwill (1982) on John Tootoosis, as well as Meijer-Drees (2002) on the development of the Indian Association of Alberta.

CHAPTER 2 Health and disease prior to European contact

1 There is undisputed archaeological evidence for human occupation in North and South America at the close of the Pleistocene, roughly 11,000 years ago, but some sites such as Meadowcroft Rockshelter in Pennsylvania may be 20,000 to 12,000 years old (Hoffecker et al. 1993). Some scholars disagree (Goodman 1981), while others seem convinced by the evidence (Thornton 1987:6–8). Molecular genetics studies suggest the earliest occupation dates to 20,000 to 15,000 years ago (Schurr and Sherry 2004).

2 Blastomycosis is a chronic respiratory disease caused by the soil fungus *Blastomyces dermatidis*.

3 Although Jackes (1983) makes a case for smallpox diagnosis from ossuary remains.

4 'Emerging diseases' is a term that refers to diseases that have recently appeared in a population and are rapidly expanding their range. They are associated with increased cases of disease. Some examples are HIV/AIDS, dengue fever, and hantavirus.

5 See J.E. Anderson 1969; Hartney 1981; Jackes 1986, 1988; Katzenberg 1989; Katzenberg et al. 1993; Molto and Melbye 1984; Pfeiffer 1984, 1986, 1991; Pfeiffer and King 1983; Saunders 1988; Saunders and Melbye 1990; Schwarcz et al. 1985; Southern 1990; Saunders et al. 1992; Williamson and Pfeiffer 2003.

6 Stable carbon isotope analysis provides evidence of the ratio of C_3 to C_4 plants in the diet. It has been instrumental in detecting plant domestication in northeastern North America. Because maize follows the C_4 photosynthetic pathway, its presence can be detected in bone through its distinctive carbon isotope signature, which differs from that of the C_3 plants that make up most of the indigenous plant cover in the temperate zones. The shifting ratios of C_3 and C_4 plants can be detected in bone and provide evidence of the transition from a diet of almost exclusively C_3 plants to one that includes increasing amounts of the C_4 plant maize (Katzenberg 1992, 2000).

7 The Moatfield site, a Middle Iroquoian ossuary pit, was accidentally discovered in 1997 during the renovation of a public soccer field. The excavation was conducted by Archaeological Services Inc. according to the wishes of the Six Nations Council of Oshweken. The remains of approximately eighty-seven people, most of whom were adults (58) were discovered and reburied, except for a small sample that, with the permission of Six Nations, was kept for analysis.

8 A salvage excavation was undertaken in 1987 when it was discovered that most of it would have been destroyed by a housing development (Katzenberg, Saunders, and Fitzgerald, 1993).

9 William Sturtevant noted that other Aboriginal populations, such as in Australia, also suffered from introduced European diseases after contact, despite the lack of a 'cold screen' (personal communication, cited in Thornton 1987:40).
10 A chronic lung disease resulting from long-term inhalation of smoke from burning seal oil.
11 This is significantly less than the average 26 per cent of carious teeth for prehistoric and contact Canadian populations (Patterson 1984, cited in Cybulski 1990).

CHAPTER 3 Contact and disease

1 See Cook and Borah 1971; Borah 1976; Meister 1976; Helm 1980; Dobyns 1983, 1984, 1989; Hurlich 1983; Krech 1983a, 1983b; Crosby 1986; Ramenofsky 1987; Decker 1988; Snow and Lanphear 1987; Thornton, Miller, and Warren 1991; Ray 1976; Reff 1991; Verano and Ubelaker 1992; Herring 1994; Boyd 1999; Lux 2001; and F.P. Hackett 2002.
2 Henige (1990:185) dubs advocates of this perspective the 'High Counters' and takes them to task for, among other criticisms, assuming without evidence that introduced diseases automatically became epidemic and depopulating.
3 These estimates are based on depopulation ratios twenty to twenty-five times the nadir populations, derived from Dobyns's (1983) estimates of mortality from infectious disease epidemics – a seriously flawed methodology (Henige 1990; Herring 1992).
4 Some good illustrations of this approach can be found in Dobyns 1966, 1983; Helm 1980; Roth 1981; Joraleman 1982; Ramenofsky 1987; McGrath 1988; Thornton 1987; Thornton et al. 1991; Ubelaker 1988; Snow 1992; Storey 1992; and Whitmore 1992.
5 Archaeological evidence suggests that their direct ancestors, and those of the Innu of Labrador, had met and traded with Norse explorers and immigrants around AD 1000 (McGhee 1992:13).
6 The most important resources included various species of seal, seabirds, migratory birds, salmon, and caribou (Tuck and Pastore 1985:72–4).
7 Each of the known pre-Beothuk extinctions occurred in the absence of an invading population, and at least a century separates the disappearance of one group from the appearance of the next in the archaeological record. The Indians of the Maritime Archaic disappear from the archaeological record around 3,200 years ago; the Groswater Palaeo-Eskimos appear to have died out around 2,100 years ago, as did the Dorset Palaeo-Eskimos by about AD 500 (Tuck and Pastore 1985:70–2).

8 Upton (1977:134) arrives at a population range at AD 1500 of 1,123 to 3,050 in this way and settles for a final estimate of 2,000 Beothuk at contact.

9 Robert Boyd's (1999) study, *The Coming of the Spirit of Pestilence*, offers a carefully considered analysis of oral tradition, historical documents, and skeletal remains and the light that they shed on the impact of introduced diseases on the Northwest Coast from the eighteenth to the nineteenth centuries.

10 The epidemic areas are the North Coast, Wakashan, Inland Waters, Olympic, South Coast, and Interior Valleys (Boyd 1999:2, 263–8).

11 The relationship between diet and disease is underscored by V. Miller's (1976, 1982) interpretation of Mi'kmaq post-contact history. Miller's reading of the earliest accounts of travellers, adventurers, and Jesuit priests led her to postulate that a change in seasonal subsistence activities produced debilitating food-borne diseases and malnutrition among the Mi'kmaq. Reliance on European foods appears to have been linked to fatal autumn and winter outbreaks of pleurisy, quinsy, and dysentery. Epidemics of dysentery broke out after the ingestion of contaminated traded foods, and a pattern of summer gorging and alcohol consumption may have contributed to fall outbreaks. Instead of carrying out the normal activities of gathering and preserving meat and plant foods for winter, the Mi'kmaq were said to have spent the summers waiting on the coast for European ships. All this led to a winter diet heavy on dried trade foods such as hardtack. European and Mi'kmaq sources cite an increase in lung, chest, and intestinal disorders, particularly in winter (V. Miller 1976:123).

12 As discussed in chapter 2, tuberculosis has a long history in the Americas well before the arrival of Europeans. There are early, scattered reports of scrofula, consumption, and phthisis that suggest that the disease was quite common (Graham-Cumming 1967). Scrofula, or glandular tuberculosis, is among the first diseases noted by Jesuits in 1633–4, and tuberculosis appears to have been widespread among the Montagnais by 1637 (Thorpe 1989:61). Other accounts suggest that Indians along the Hudson Bay and James Bay coasts were exposed to English and French rife with tuberculosis some 200 years earlier than their counterparts in the interior (Hurlich 1983). Graham-Cumming (1967:130) suggests that eastern Indians had been exposed to tuberculosis for so long that by the last quarter of the nineteenth century the disease had become endemic and probably no more prevalent among them than among non-Indians in comparable living conditions. Certainly, there is compelling evidence that by the mid-1800s tuberculosis was already endemic in the Moose Factory region of northern Ontario (Herring and Hoppa 1999).

13 Reserves began to be feared as sources of infection as Aboriginal people themselves were believed to be on the verge of extinction (Kelm 1998, 2005).

CHAPTER 4 Aboriginal peoples and the health transition

1 It is now recognized that some chronic diseases are in fact caused by micro-organisms: for example, cancer of the cervix in women is caused by the human papillomavirus, and stomach ulcers by the bacterium called *Helicobacter pylori*. Some other diseases are also suspected to have some infectious origins, and future research will likely uncover more. While chronic diseases are not 'contagious,' one can argue that behaviours such as smoking, diet, and physical activity can certainly be passed on from person to person – for example, among peer groups or within families.

2 It is internationally agreed that a BMI of 30 and higher is considered to be 'obese,' while a BMI of 25.0 to 29.9 represents 'overweight.'

CHAPTER 5 Medical traditions in Aboriginal cultures

1 In this book, we use the terms 'medical' and 'healing' interchangeably, as both are common in the literature and efforts to define each precisely as somehow distinct from the other have been fruitless. The same holds true for distinctions between 'healers' and 'doctors.'

2 A 1992 study by Hultkrantz attempts a wide-ranging discussion of the healing traditions of Aboriginal peoples in North America but suffers from the need to overgeneralize for any given culture area. The lesson, clearly, is that individual healing traditions require in-depth, singular treatment.

3 It should be stressed here that within Aboriginal medical systems, the distinction between 'natural' and 'supernatural' is not the same as it is in Euro-Canadian cultures and the Western scientific tradition. The term 'supernatural' is somewhat inappropriate to the description of Aboriginal spirituality.

4 See, for example, www.Lakotaherbs.com.

5 In accepting the view that Aboriginal healers are pragmatic in their use and manipulation of such symbols, we may appear to be at odds with the views of many respected healers past and present, who state unequivocally that the power to heal comes from the Creator. However, it is our view that all medical systems are inherently systems of both belief and knowledge working in tandem to heal the patient and restore balance to the society. Some Aboriginal healers today speak freely of their use of key symbols in their healing activities (see Waldram 1997).

6 One of the authors (Waldram) has participated in various Aboriginal healing ceremonies in which some participants have observed small lights, which they believed were the spirits. These ceremonies took place in environments of complete darkness.

7 Here we are adopting the broad understanding of the concept of surgery, as outlined by Fortuine (1985:23), referring to 'methods beyond the usual cutting, piercing, or suturing, such as manipulation of fractures, massage of body organs, and the care of wounds, this last being traditionally in the domain of the surgeon.'

8 (S.C. 1884. c.27. [47 Vict.]).

9 Note the comparison between the ritual biting of the tamananawas ceremony and that of the spirit dancing that was the target of legal action in 1992; see the next chapter for a discussion of the latter.

10 (R.S.C. 1886, c.43, S.114).

11 In their biography of Plains Cree leader John Tootoosis, Goodwill and Sluman (1984:84) recount his view that Chief Piapot was imprisoned in Regina, allegedly for drinking (despite his claims to be an abstainer); Chief Piapot, according to Tootoosis, believed he had been arrested because of a 'Rain Dance' that he had allowed and that involved piercing.

12 (R.S.C. 1906, c.81, S. 8).

CHAPTER 6 Traders, whalers, missionaries, and medical aid

1 It should be noted, however, that the concept of vaccination was known in China and the Middle East before it reached Europe and Western medicine.

2 Edwards (1980:5–6) explains that 'Turlington's Balsam of Life' dated from the fifteenth or sixteenth century and was alleged to cure at least thirty different ailments, including gout, rheumatism, coughs, colic, and other stomach problems.

CHAPTER 7 The emergence of government health services

1 T.K. Young (1979, 1988b: 39, 101) has published data emanating from reports of two northern Ontario physicians on contract to the government, Dr Hanson for the Treaty Three area in 1887, and Dr Meindl for Treaty Nine in 1905. Their account books provide a glimpse into the conditions of their work and the kinds of medical problems they encountered.

2 We are indebted to Mellisa M. Layman, whose research into the rations program forms the backbone of this presentation.

3 Graham-Cumming (1967:118) reports that, 'It is a striking commentary on the state of affairs towards the end of the nineteenth century that when, in an attempt to stop the spread of the disease through the Indian Schools, the Department of Indian Affairs issued an order banning from school any child found to be infected, the ban was found to be impractical because hardly one

child could be found not to be infected. In practice the ban was applied only to children severely ill, otherwise the schools would all have been empty.'

4 A contemporary of Dr Stone, Dr Wall wrote in his 1926 report on the health of the Indians in the Cochrane, Ontario–La Tuque, Quebec region of the 'expectoration menace ... the universal Indian habit of free expectoration within the homes,' a habit he believed easily facilitated the spread of the tuberculosis bacterium Dr. Wall's report has also been published in *Native Studies Review* 5(1): 257–74.

5 The circumstances surrounding the death from tuberculosis of a young Copper Inuit woman from Jenness's adopted family are movingly and painfully portrayed in the film *Coppermine* (Harper 1992).

CHAPTER 8 The organization and utilization of contemporary health services

1 The causes of the demise of these university programs are varied and complex, including decline in institutional interest, contractual disputes with the government, and lack of appreciation of the 'added value' of university involvement by regional health authorities and communities.

CHAPTER 9 Aboriginal healing in the contemporary context

1 See, for instance, the critical evaluation of studies of 'ethnomedicine' by Anderson (1991) for a discussion that pertains to some of these issues.

2 University of Saskatchewan news release, 'New U of S Research Group to Study Heart-Healthy Benefits of Traditional Aboriginal Medicine.' www.usask.ca/events/news/articles/20040621–3.html.

3 *National Post* 7 June 2003, A16.

4 Saskatoon *Star-Phoenix* 31 Oct, 2004, A10.

5 *Thomas v. Norris et al.* (1992), 2 C.N.L.R., 162

6 Ibid., 142–4.

7 *National Post* 26 April 2003, A4.

CHAPTER 10 Self-determination and health care

1 Berger was a former B.C. Supreme Court judge who spearheaded the landmark Mackenzie Valley Pipeline Inquiry in the early 1970s, and who has been, and continues to be, involved in many prominent legal actions on behalf of Aboriginal groups.

2 National Aboriginal Health Organization, 'The Métis Centre Approach to Métis Health Study.' Accessed at www.naho.ca/MHC_Site. 18 Nov. 2004.

3 Métis Nation of Saskatchewan, 'Métis Addictions Council of Saskatchewan.' Accessed at www.metisnation-sask.com. 18 Nov. 2004.

4 Saskatchewan Executive Council News Release, 'Government Accepts Recommendations on Métis Addictions Council. October 29, 2004.' Regina: Government of Saskatchewan. Accessed at www.gov.sk.ca/newsrel/2004/10/29-669.html. 16 Nov. 2004.

5 Matthias Enterprises (2000). 'Evaluation of the Health for All Project in the Lakeland Health Region. Final Report.' www.health.gov.ab.ca/about/phc/projects/LakelandMetisIndependent.pdf.

6 Available at www.med.ualberta.ca/education/aboriginal.cfm.

7 Available at www.anac.on.ca.

8 Available at www.hc-sc.gc.ca/english/media/releases/1998/98_82e.htm.

9 Available at www.naaf.ca/health.html.

10 Personal interview with Claire McNab, National Native Access Program to Nursing, University of Saskatchewan, by James Waldram, 18 Feb. 1993.

11 Available at www.usask.ca/nursing/napn.

12 Available at www.niichro.com.

13 Institute of Aboriginal People's Health, 'Five Year Strategic Plan.' www.cihr-irsc.gc.ca/e/9188.html.

14 Available at www.cihr-irsc.gc.ca/e/27071.html.

15 Available at www.naho.ca.

16 Available at www.ahf.ca.

References cited

Abonyi, S. 2001. 'Sickness and Symptom: Perspectives on Diabetes among the Mushkegowuk Cree.' PhD diss., McMaster University, Hamilton.

Aboriginal Diabetes Initiative. 2000. *Diabetes among Aboriginal People in Canada: The Evidence*. Ottawa: Health Canada.

Aboriginal Healing and Wellness Strategy. 2003. *Annual Report 2002–2003*. Toronto: Government of Ontario.

Aboriginal Healing Foundation (AHF). 1999. *Annual Report*. 1999. Ottawa: Aboriginal Healing Foundation.

– 2003. *Aboriginal Domestic Violence in Canada*. Ottawa: Aboriginal Healing Foundation.

Aboriginal Nurses Association of Canada. 1993. *Traditional Aboriginal Medicine and Primary Health Care*. Submission to the Royal Commission on Aboriginal Peoples. Ottawa: Aboriginal Nurses Association of Canada.

Achterberg, J. 1985. *Imagery in Healing: Shamanism and Modern Medicine*. London: Shambhala.

Adair, J., W. Deuschle, and W. McDermott. 1969. 'Patterns of Health and Disease among the Navajos.' In L. Lynch, ed., *The Cross-Cultural Approach to Health Behavior*, 83–110. Rutherford, N.J.: Farleigh Dickinson University Press.

Adamson, J.D., J.P. Moody, and A.F. Peart. 1949. 'Poliomyelitis in the Arctic.' *Canadian Medical Association Journal* 61:339–48.

Adelson, N. 2000. *Being Alive Well: Health and the Politics of Cree Well-being*. Toronto: University of Toronto Press.

AHF. *See* Aboriginal Healing Foundation.

Aldred, L. 2000. 'Plastic Shamans and Astroturf Sun Dances: New Age Commercialization of Native American Spirituality.' *American Indian Quarterly* 24(3):329–52.

310   References cited

Allison, M.J., ed. 1976. 'Paleopathology.' *Medical College of Virginia Quarterly* 12(2):39–86.

Allison, M.J., D. Mendoza, and A. Pezzia. 1973. 'Documentation of a Case of Tuberculosis in Pre-Columbian America.' *American Review of Respiratory Disease* 107:985–91.

Amnesty International. 2003. *Stolen Sisters: A Human Rights Response to Discrimination and Violence against Indigenous Women in Canada.* London: Amnesty International.

Anand, S.S., S. Yusuf, R. Jacobs, A.D. Davis, Q. Yi, H. Gerstein, P.A. Montague, and E. Lonn. 2001. 'Risk Factors, Atherosclerosis, and Cardiovascular Disease among Aboriginal People in Canada: The Study of Health Assessment and Risk Evaluation in Aboriginal Peoples (SHARE-AP).' *Lancet* 358:1147–53.

Anderson, J.E. 1969. 'The People of Fairty: An Osteological Analysis of an Iroquoian Ossuary.' *National Museum of Canada Bulletin* 193, *Contributions to Anthropology* 1961–1962 (Part I), Ottawa.

Anderson, R. 1991. 'The Efficacy of Ethnomedicine: Research Methods in Trouble.' *Medical Anthropology* 13:1–17.

Armelagos, G.J., K. Barnes, and J. Lin. 1996. 'Disease in Human Evolution: The Re-emergence of Infectious Disease in the Third Epidemiological Transition.' *AnthroNotes* 18(3):1–7.

Arnason, T., R. Hebda, and T. Johns. 1981. 'Use of Plants for Food and Medicine by Native Peoples of Eastern Canada.' *Canadian Journal of Botany* 59:2189–325.

Arriaza, B.T., W. Salo, A.C. Aufderheide, and T.A. Holcomb. 1995. 'Pre-Columbian Tuberculosis in Northern Chile: Molecular and Skeletal Evidence.' *American Journal of Physical Anthropology* 98:37–45.

Assembly of First Nations. 1979. *Brief Summary of Rights and Priorities in Indian Health.* Ottawa: National Commission of Inquiry on Indian Health, Assembly of First Nations.

– 1988. *Special Report: The National Indian Health Transfer Conference.* Ottawa: Assembly of First Nations.

Asuni, T. 1979. 'The Dilemma of Traditional Healing with Special Reference to Nigeria.' *Social Science and Medicine* 13(B):33–9.

Atcheson, D., D. Rodgers, C. Hellon, and P. Kehoe. 1969. *Survey of Mental Health Needs of the Northwest Territories.* Report to Medical Services Branch. Ottawa: Department of National Health and Welfare.

Auditor General of Canada. Various years. *Report of the Auditor General of Canada to the House of Commons.* Ottawa.

Ayotte, P., G. Carrier, and E. Dewailly. 1996. 'Health Risk Assessment for Inuit Newborns Exposed to Dioxin-Like Compounds through Breast Feeding.' *Chemosphere* 32:531–42.

Bailey, A. 1969. *The Conflict of European and Eastern Algonkian Cultures 1504–1700*. 2nd ed. Toronto: University of Toronto Press.

Balikci, A. 1963. 'Shamanistic Behavior among the Netsilik Eskimos.' *Southwestern Journal of Anthropology* 19:380–96.

Barkwell, P. 1981. 'The Medicine Chest Clause in Treaty No.6.' *Canadian Native Law Reporter* 4:1–23.

Barnes, G.E. 1979. 'Solvent Abuse: A Review.' *International Journal of Addictions* 14:1–26.

Barron, F. 1988. 'The Indian Pass System in the Canadian West, 1882–1935.' *Prairie Forum* 13(1):25–42.

Barron, F.L., and J. Garcea, eds. 1999. *Urban Indian Reserves: Forging New Relationships in Saskatchewan*. Saskatoon: Purich Publishing.

Bates, C., C. Van Dam, and D.F. Horrobin. 1985. 'Plasma Essential Fatty Acids in Pure and Mixed Race American Indians on and off a Diet Exceptionally Rich in Salmon.' *Prostaglandins and Leukotrienes in Medicine* 17:77–84.

Bates, J. 1982. 'Tuberculosis: Susceptibility and Resistance.' *American Review of Respiratory Disease* 125(3):20–4.

Bathurst, R.R. 2004. 'Archaeological Evidence of Intestinal Parasites from Coastal Shell Middens.' *Journal of Archaeological Science* 32(1):115–23.

– 2005. 'Human Settlement Implications of Parasites from Pacific Northwest Coast Archaeological Sites.' PhD diss., McMaster University, Hamilton.

Bathurst, R.R., and J.L. Barta. 2004. 'Molecular Evidence of Tuberculosis-Induced Hypertrophic Osteopathy in a 16th Century Iroquian Dog.' *Journal of Archaeological Science* 31:917–25.

Beardsley, G. 1941. 'Notes on Cree Medicines, Based on a Collection Made by I. Cowie in 1892.' *Michigan Academy of Science, Arts and Letters, Papers*, 83–496.

Beardy, E., and R. Coutts. 1996. *Voices from Hudson Bay: Cree Stories from York Factory*. Montreal: McGill-Queen's University Press.

Bearskin, S., and C. Dumont. 1991. 'The Cree Board of Health and Social Services of James Bay: The First TwelveYears – 1978–1990.' In B. Postl et al., eds, *Circumpolar Health 90: Proceedings of the 8th International Congress*, 123–5. Winnipeg: University of Manitoba Press.

Beattie, O., B. Apland, E.W. Blake, J.A. Cosgrove, S. Gaunt, S. Greer, A.P. Mackie, K.E. Mackie, D. Straathof, V. Thorp, and P.M. Troffe. 2000. 'The Kwäday Däy Ts'ínchí Discovery from a Glacier in British Columbia.' *Canadian Journal of Archaeology* 24:129–46.

Bell, R. 1886. 'The 'Medicine-Man' or Indian and Eskimo Notions of Medicine.' *Canada Medical and Surgical Journal*, 456–537.

Ben-Dor, S. 1966. *Makkovik: Eskimos and Settlers in a Labrador Community: A Con-*

trastive Study in Adaptation. St John's: Institute of Social and Economic Research, Memorial University of Newfoundland.

Bennion, L., and T.K. Li. 1976. 'Alcohol Metabolism in American Indians and Whites.' *New England Journal of Medicine* 294:9–13.

Berger, T. 1980. *Report of the Advisory Commission on Indian and Inuit Health Consultation*. Ottawa: Department of National Health and Welfare, Medical Services Branch.

Bernard, L., C. Lavallee, K. Gray-Donald, and H. Delisle. 1995. 'Overweight in Cree Schoolchildren and Adolescents Associated with Diet, Low Physical Activity, and High Television Watching.' *Journal of the American Dietetic Association* 95:800–2.

Bernardo, T.A., W. Salo, A.C. Aufderheide, and T.A. Holcomb. 1995. 'Pre-Columbian Tuberculosis in Northern Chile: Molecular and Skeletal Evidence.' *American Journal of Physical Anthropology* 98:37–45.

Bird, L., and M. Moore. 1991. 'The William Charles Health Centre of Montreal Lake Band: A Case Study of Transfer.' In B. Postl et al., eds, *Circumpolar Health 90: Proceedings of the 8th International Congress*, 20–5. Winnipeg: University of Manitoba Press.

Bjerregaard, P., E. Dewailly, T.K. Young, C. Blanchet, R.A. Hegele, S.E.O. Ebbesson, P.M. Risca, and G. Mulvad. 2003. 'Blood Pressure among the Inuit (Eskimo) Populations in the Arctic.' *Scandinavian Journal of Public Health* 31:92–9.

Bjerregaard, P., T.K. Young, and R.A. Hegele. 2003. 'Low Incidence of Cardiovascular Diseases among the Inuit – What Is the Evidence?' *Atherosclerosis* 166:351–7.

Black, F. 1966. 'Measles Endemicity in Insular Populations: Critical Community Size and Its Evolutionary Implications.' *Journal of Theoretical Biology* 11:207–11.

Black, L. 1969. 'Morbidity, Mortality and Medical Care in the Keewatin Area of the Central Arctic – 1967.' *Canadian Medical Association Journal* 101:35–41.

Black-Rogers, M. 1986. 'Varieties of "Starving": Semantics and Survival in the Subarctic Fur Trade, 1750–1850.' *Ethnohistory* 33:353–83.

Bobet, E. 1997. *Diabetes among First Nations People: Information from the 1991 Aboriginal Peoples Survey Carried Out by Statistics Canada*. Ottawa: Health Canada, Medical Services Branch.

Boeckx, R.L., B. Postl, and F.J. Coodin. 1977. 'Gasoline Sniffing and Tetraethyl Lead Poisoning in Children.' *Pediatrics* 60:140–5.

Boothroyd, L.J., L.J. Kirmayer, S. Spreng, M. Malus, and S. Hodgins. 2001. 'Completed Suicides among the Inuit of Northern Quebec, 1982–1996: A Case-Control Study.' *Canadian Medical Association Journal* 165:749–55.

Booz-Allen and Hamilton Canada Ltd. 1969. *Study of Health Services for Canadian Indians: Summary Report*. Ottawa: Department of National Health and Welfare.

Borah, W. 1976. 'The Historical Demography of Aboriginal and Colonial America: An Attempt at Perspective.' In W.H. Denevan, ed., *The Native Population of the Americas in 1492*, 13–34. Madison: University of Wisconsin Press.

Boston, P., S. Jordan, E. McNamara, K. Kozolanka, E. Bobbish-Rondeau, and H. Iserhoff. 1997. 'Using Participatory Action Research to Understand the Meanings Aboriginal Canadians Attribute to the Rising Incidence of Diabetes.' *Chronic Diseases in Canada* 18:5–12.

Boyd, R. 1992. 'Population Decline from Two Epidemics on the Northwest Coast.' In J.W. Verano and D.H. Ubelaker, eds, *Disease and Demography in the Americas*, 249–55. Washington, D.C.: Smithsonian Institution.

– 1999. *The Coming of the Spirit of Pestilence. Introduced Infectious Disease and Population Decline among Northwest Coast Indians, 1774–1874*. Vancouver: University of British Columbia Press.

Braun, M., D.C. Cook, and S. Pfeiffer. 1998. 'DNA from *Mycobacterium tuberculosis* Complex Identified in North American, Pre-Columbian Human Skeletal Remains.' *Journal of Archaeological Science* 25:271–7.

Brett, H.B. 1969. 'A Synopsis of Northern Medical History.' *Canadian Medical Association Journal* 100:521–5.

Briggs, J. 1970. *Never in Anger: Portrait of an Eskimo Family*. Cambridge, Mass.: Harvard University Press.

Brosch, R., S.V. Gordon, M. Marmiesse, P. Brodin, C. Buchrieser, K. Eiglmeier, T. Garnier, C. Gutierrez, G. Hewinson, K. Kremer, L.M. Parsons, A.S. Pym, S. Samper, D. van Soolingen, and S.T. Cole. 2002. 'A New Evolutionary Scenario for the *Mycobacterium tuberculosis* Complex.' *Proceedings of the National Academy of Sciences USA* 99(6):3684–9.

Brown, J. 1980. *Strangers in Blood: Fur Trade Families in Indian Country*. Vancouver: University of British Columbia Press.

Brown, J., and R. Brightman. 1988. *'The Orders of the Dreamed': George Nelson on Cree and Northern Ojibwa Religion and Myth, 1823*. Winnipeg: University of Manitoba Press.

Bruce, S.G., E. Kliewer, T.K. Young, T. Mayer, and A. Wajda. 2003. 'Diabetes among the Métis of Canada: Defining the Population, Estimating the Disease.' *Canadian Journal of Diabetes* 27:442–8.

Bruner, E. 1986. 'Ethnography as Narrative.' In V.W. Turner and E.M. Bruner, eds, *The Anthropology of Experience*, 139–55. Urbana: University of Illinois Press.

Bryce, P. 1907. 'Report of the Chief Medical Officer.' *Sessional Papers No. 27*, 7–8 Edward VII, A, 263–77.

– 1909. 'Report of the Superintendent of Health.' *Sessional Papers No. 27*, 7–8 Edward VII, A, 273–84.
– 1914. 'The History of the American Indians in Relation to Health.' *Ontario Historical Society* 12:128–41.
– 1922. *The Story of a National Crime: An Appeal for Justice to the Indians of Canada.* Ottawa: James Hope.
Buikstra, J. 1999. 'Paleoepidemiology of Tuberculosis in the Americas.' In G. Pálfi, O. Dutour, J. Deák, and I. Hutás, eds, *Tuberculosis Past and Present*, 479–94. Budapest: Golden Book Publisher Ltd, Tuberculosis Foundation.
Bull, W. 1934. *From Medicine Man to Medical Man: A Record of a Century and a Half of Progress in Health and Sanitation as Exemplified by Developments in Peel.* Toronto: G. McLeod.
Calam, B., M. Bass, and G. Deagle. 1992. 'Pap Smear Screening Rates: Coverage on the Southern Queen Charlotte Islands.' *Canadian Family Physician* 38:1103–9.
Canadian Diabetes Association (CDA). 2003. 'Clinical Practice Guidelines for the Prevention and Treatment of Diabetes in Canada.' *Canadian Journal of Diabetes* 27 (Supplement 2).
Canitz, B. 1989a. 'Northern Nurses: A Profession in Crisis.' *Musk-Ox* (37):175–83.
– 1989b. 'Nursing in the North: Challenge and Isolation.' In M. Crnkovich, ed., *'GOSSIP': A Spoken History of Women in the North*, 193–212. Ottawa: Canadian Arctic Resources Committee.
Cannon, A. 1995. 'The Ratfish and Marine Resource Deficiencies on the Northwest Coast.' *Canadian Journal of Archaeology* 19:49–60.
– 2001. 'Was Salmon Important in Northwest Coast Prehistory?' In S.C. Gerlach and M.S. Murray, eds, *People and Wildlife in Northern North America: Essays in Honor of R. Dale Guthrie*, 178–87. BAR International Series 944.
Cannon, C., H.P. Schwarcz, and M. Knyf. 1999. 'Marine-Based Subsistence Trends and the Stable Isotope Analysis of Dog Bones from Namu, British Columbia.' *Journal of Archaeological Science* 26:399–407.
Card, B., G. Hirabayashi, and C. French. 1963. *The Métis in Alberta Society.* Edmonton: University of Alberta and the Alberta Tuberculosis Association.
Carlson, C., G. Armelagos, and A. Magennis. 1992. 'Impact of Disease on the Precontact and Early Historic Populations of New England and the Maritimes.' In J.W. Verano and D.H. Ubelaker, eds, *Disease and Demography in the Americas*, 141–54. Washington, D.C.: Smithsonian Institution.
Carter, S.A. 1990. *Lost Harvests: Prairie Indian Reserve Farmers and Government Policy.* Montreal: McGill-Queen's University Press.
Caulfield, L.E., S.B. Harris, E.A. Whalen, and M.E. Sugamori. 1998. 'Maternal

Nutritional Status, Diabetes and Risk of Macrosomia among Native Canadian Women.' *Early Human Development* 50:293–303.

Chan, H.M, P.R. Berti, O. Receveur, and H.V. Kuhnlein. 1997. 'Evaluation of the Population Distribution of Dietary Contaminant Exposure in an Arctic Population Using Monte Carlo Statistics.' *Environmental Health Perspectives* 35:316–21.

Chandler, M.J., and C. Lalonde. 1998. 'Cultural Continuity as a Hedge against Suicide in Canada's First Nations.' *Transcultural Psychiatry* 35:191–219.

Churchill, W. 1990. 'Spiritual Hucksterism.' *Z Magazine* December: 94–8.

Clark, M., P. Riben, and E. Nowegesic. 2002. 'The Association of Housing Density, Isolation and Tuberculosis in Canadian First Nations Communities.' *International Journal of Epidemiology* 31:940–5.

Clarke, H. 1997. 'Research in Nursing and Cultural Diversity: Working with First Nations People.' *Canadian Journal of Nursing Research* 29(2):11–25.

Clements, F.E. 1932. 'Primitive Concepts of Disease.' *University of California Publications in American Archaeology and Ethnology* 32(2):185–252.

Coates, K.S. 1991. *Best Left as Indians: Native-White Relations in the Yukon Territory, 1840–1973*. Montreal: McGill-Queen's University Press.

Cohen, M.N. 1989. *Health and the Rise of Civilization*. New Haven: Yale University Press.

Cohen, M.N., and C. Crane-Kramer. 2003. 'The State and Future of Paleoepidemiology.' In C. Greenblatt and M. Spigelman, eds, *Emerging Pathogens: Archaeology, Ecology and Evolution of Infectious Disease*, 79–92. Oxford: Oxford University Press.

Cole, D., and Ira Chaikin. 1990. *An Iron Hand upon the People: The Law against the Potlatch on the Northwest Coast*. Vancouver: Douglas and McIntyre.

Commission on the Future of Health Care in Canada. 2002. *Building in Values: The Future of Health Care in Canada – Final Report*. Ottawa.

Connell, G., R Flett, and P. Stewart. 1991. 'Implementing Primary Health Care through Community Control: The Experience of Swampy Cree Tribal Council.' In B. Postl et al., eds, *Circumpolar Health 90: Proceedings of the 8th International Congress*, 44–6. Winnipeg: University of Manitoba Press.

Cook, S. 1973. 'The Significance of Disease in the Extinction of the New England Indians.' *Human Biology* 45:485–508.

Cook, S., and W. Borah. 1971. *Essays in Population History: Mexico and the Caribbean*. Berkeley: University of California Press.

Cooper, J. 1944. 'The Shaking Tent Rite among the Plains and Forest Algonquians.' *Primitive Man* 17(3):60–84.

Corrigan, C. 1946. 'Medical Practice among the Bush Indians of Northern Manitoba.'*Canadian Medical Association Journal* 54:220–3.

Craib, K.J.P., P.M. Spittal, E. Wood, N. Laliberte, R.S. Hogg, K. Li, K. Heath, M.W. Tyndall, M.V. O'Shaughnessy, and M.T. Schechter. 2003. 'Risk Factors for Elevated HIV Incidence among Aboriginal Injection Drug Users in Vancouver.' *Canadian Medical Association Journal* 168:19–24.

Crinnion, C., D.C. Merrett, and S. Pfeiffer. 2003. 'The Definition of the Moatfield People.' In R.F.Williamson and S. Pfeiffer, eds, *Bones of the Ancestors: The Archaeology and Osteobiography of the Moatfield Ossuary*, 223–40. Mercury Series. Archaeology Paper 163. Ottawa: Canadian Museum of Civilization.

Crosby, A.W. 1986. *Ecological Imperialism: The Biological Expansion of Europe, 900–1900*. Cambridge: Cambridge University Press.

Cruikshank, J. 1979. 'Athapaskan Women: Lives and Legends.' *Canadian Ethnology Service Paper* No. 57. Ottawa.

Culhane Speck, D. 1989. 'The Indian Health Transfer Policy: A Step in the Right Direction, or Revenge of the Hidden Agenda?' *Native Studies Review* 5(1):187–213.

Cuthand Goodwill, J. 1989. 'Indian and Inuit Nurses of Canada.' *Canadian Women's Studies* 10 (2, 3):117–23.

Cybulski, J.S. 1977. 'Cribra Orbitalia, a Possible Sign of Anemia in Early Historic Native Populations of the British Columbia Coast.' *American Journal of Physical Anthropology* 47(1):31–40.

– 1990. 'Human Biology.' In W. Suttles, ed., *Handbook of North American Indians. Vol 7. Northwest Coast*, 52–9. Washington, D.C.: Smithsonian Institution.

– 1994. 'Culture Change, Demographic History, and Health and Disease on the Northwest Coast.' In C.S. Larsen and G.R. Milner, eds, *In the Wake of Contact: Biological Responses to Conquest*, 75–85. New York: Wiley-Liss.

Dailey, R. 1968. 'The Role of Alcohol among North American Indian Tribes as Reported in the Jesuit Relations.' *Anthropologica*, NS 10(1):45–60.

Daniel, M., L.W. Green, S.A. Marion, D. Gamble, C.P. Herbert, and C. Hertzman. 1999. 'Effectiveness of Community-Directed Diabetes Prevention and Control in a Rural Aboriginal Population in British Columbia.' *Social Science and Medicine* 48:815–32.

Daniel, R. 1987. 'The Spirit and Terms of Treaty Eight.' In Richard Price, ed., *The Spirit of the Alberta Indian Treaties*, 47–100. Montreal: Institute for Research on Public Policy.

Daniel, T.M. 1981. 'An Immunochemist's View of the Epidemiology of Tuberculosis.' In J.E. Buikstra, ed., *Prehistoric Tuberculosis in the Americas*, 221–8. Evanston, Ill.: Northwestern University Archaeological Program.

Darnell, R. 1986. 'A Linguistic Classification of Canadian Native Peoples: Issues, Problems, and Theoretical Implications.' In R.B. Morrison and C.R. Wilson, eds, *Native Peoples: The Canadian Experience*, 22–44. Toronto: McClelland and Stewart.

Daveluy, C., C. Lavallee, M. Clarkson, and E. Robinson. 1994. *Santé Québec: A Health Profile of the Cree*. Montreal: Ministère de la Santé et des Services Sociaux.

Davey, K.W. 1974. 'Dental Therapists in the Canadian North.' *Journal of the Canadian Dental Association* 40:287–91.

Dean, H.J., T.K. Young, B. Flett, and P. Wood-Steiman. 1998. 'Screening for Type-2 Diabetes in Aboriginal Children in Northern Canada.' *Lancet* 352:1523–4.

Decker, J. 1988. 'Tracing Historical Diffusion Patterns: The Case of the 1780–8 Smallpox Epidemic among the Indians of Western Canada.' *Native Studies Review* 4(1–2):1–24.

– 1989. '"We Should Never Be Again the Same People": The Diffusion and Cumulative Impact of Acute Infectious Diseases Affecting the Natives on the Northern Plains of the Western Interior of Canada. 1774–1839.' PhD diss. York University, Toronto.

DeCoster, C., S. Peterson, K.C. Carriere, and P. Kasian. 1999. 'Assessing the Extent to Which Hospitals Are Used for Acute Care Purposes.' *Medical Care* 37 (Suppl. 6):JS151–66.

Delisle, H.F., and J.M. Ekoé. 1993. 'Prevalence of Non-Insulin-Dependent Diabetes Mellitus and Impaired Glucose Tolerance in Two Algonquin Communities in Quebec.' *Canadian Medical Association Journal* 48:41–7.

Denevan, W. 1976. *The Native Population of the Americas in 1492*. Madison: University of Wisconsin Press.

Denis, C. 1997. *We Are Not You: First Nations and Canadian Modernity*. Peterborough, Ont.: Broadview Press.

Densmore, F. 1929. *Chippewa Customs*. Bulletin 68, Bureau of American Ethnology. Washington, D.C.: Smithsonian Institution.

Department of Indian Affairs. 1882. *Sessional Papers*, No. 5, 195.

– 1908. 'Report of the Chief Medical Officer.' *Sessional Papers* No. 27.

– 1911. 'Report of the Department of Indian Affairs.' *Sessional Papers* No. 27.

Department of Indian Affairs and Northern Development (DIAND). 1989. *Fire Loss Report – 1989*. Ottawa: DIAND, Technical Services.

– 1990. *Impacts of the 1985 Amendments to the Indian Act (Bill C-J 1): Summary Report*. Ottawa: DIAND.

– 2000. *Comparison of Social Conditions, 1991 and 1996: Registered Indians, Registered Indians Living on Reserve and the Total Population of Canada*. Ottawa: DIAND.

– 2002. *Basic Departmental Data 2002*. Ottawa: DIAND.

Department of National Health and Welfare (DNHW). Various years. *Annual Report*. Ottawa: DNHW.

– 1974. *Report of the Interdepartmental Committee on the Nursing Group*. Ottawa: DNHW.

– 1975a. *Nutrition Canada: Eskimo Survey Report*. Ottawa: DNHW.

– 1975b. *Nutrition Canada: Indian Survey Report*. Ottawa: DNHW.

– 1983. *Report of the Task Force on Medical Officers* (Chair: K. Butler). Ottawa: DNHW.

– 1989–1992. *Health Transfer Newsletter*. Spring 1989; Fall 1989; Special Issue 1990; Winter 1992.

– 1991. *Health Status of Canadian Indians and Inuit – 1990*. Ottawa: DNHW, Medical Services Branch.

Deschamps, M., M. Band, and T.G. Hislop. 1992. 'Barriers to Cervical Cytology Screening in Native Women in British Columbia.' *Cancer Detection and Prevention* 16:337–9.

Dewailly, E., P. Ayotte, S. Bruneau, G. Lebel, P. Levallois, and J.P. Weber. 2001. 'Exposure of the Inuit population of Nunavik (Arctic Quebec) to Lead and Mercury.' *Archives of Environmental Health* 56:350–7.

Dewailly, E., C. Blanchet, S. Lemieux, L. Sauve, S. Gingras, P. Ayotte, and B.J. Holub. 2001. 'N-3 Fatty Acids and Cardiovascular Disease Risk Factors among the Inuit of Nunavik.' *American Journal of Clinical Nutrition* 74:464–73.

DIAND. *See* Department of Indian Affairs and Northern Development.

Dickason, O.P. 1992. *Canada's First Nations: A History of Founding Peoples from Earliest Times*. Toronto: McClelland and Stewart.

– 2002. *Canada's First Nations: A History of Founding Peoples from Earliest Times*. Don Mills: Oxford University Press.

Dickson, G. 1989. 'Iskwew: Empowering Victims of Wife Abuse.' *Native Studies Review* 5:115–35.

Dickson, J.H., M.P. Richards, R.J. Hebda, P.J. Mudie, O. Beattie, S. Ramsay, N.J. Turner, B.J. Leighton, J.M. Webster, N.R. Hobischak, G.S. Anderson, R.J. Troffe, and P.M. Wigen. 2004. 'Kwäday Dän Ts'ínchí, the First Ancient Body of a Man from North American Glacier: Reconstructing His Last Days by Intestinal and Biomolecular Analyses.' *The Holocene* 14(4):481–6.

DNHW. *See* Department of National Health and Welfare.

Dobbin, M. 1981. *The One-and-a-Half Men. The Story of Jim Brady and Malcolm Norris, Métis Patriots of the 20th Century*. Vancouver: New Star Books.

Dobyns, H. 1966. 'An Appraisal of Techniques for Estimating Aboriginal American Population with a New Hemispheric Estimate.' *Current Anthropology* 7:395–416.

– 1976. 'Scholarly Transformation: Widowing the "Virgin Land."' *Ethnohistory* 23:161–72.

– 1983. *Their Number Become Thin*. Knoxville: University of Tennessee Press.

– 1984. 'Native American Population Collapse and Recovery.' In W.R Swagerty, ed., *Scholars and the Indian Experience*, 17–35. Bloomington: Indiana University Press.

– 1989. 'More Methodological Perspectives on Historical Demography.' *Ethnohistory* 36(3):285–98.

– 1992. 'Native American Trade Centers as Contagious Disease Foci.' In J.W. Verano and D.H. Ubelaker, eds, *Disease and Demography in the Americas*, 215–22. Washington, D.C.: Smithsonian Institution Press.

Dorken, E., S. Grzybowski, and D.A. Enarson. 1984. 'Ten-Year Evaluation of a Trial of Chemoprophylaxis against Tuberculosis in Frobisher Bay, Canada.' *Tubercle* 65:93–9.

Doucette, S. 1989. 'The Changing Role of Nurses: The Perspective of Medical Services Branch.' *Canadian Journal of Public Health* 80:92–4.

Driver, H. 1969. *Indians of North America*. 2nd ed. Chicago: University of Chicago Press.

Duffy, R.Q. 1988. *The Road to Nunavut: The Progress of the Eastern Arctic Inuit since the Second World War*. Montreal: McGill-Queen's University Press.

Dunn, F.L. 1968. 'Epidemiological Factors: Health and Disease in Hunter-Gatherers.' In R.B. Lee and I. DeVore, eds, *Man the Hunter*, 221–8. Chicago: Aldine.

Dupras, T. 2003. 'The Moatfield Infant and Juvenile Skeletal Remains.' In R.F. Williamson and S. Pfeiffer, eds, *Bones of the Ancestors: The Archaeology and Osteobiography of the Moatfield Ossuary*, 295–308. Mercury Series. Archaeology Paper 163. Ottawa: Canadian Museum of Civilization.

Dyck, L.E. 1986. 'Are North American Indians Biochemically More Susceptible to the Effects of Alcohol?' *Native Studies Review* 2:85–9.

Dyck, N. 1986. 'An Opportunity Lost: The Initiative of the Reserve Agricultural Programme in the Prairie West.' In F.L. Barron and James B. Waldram, eds, *1885 and After: Native Society in Transition*, 121–37. Regina: Canadian Plains Research Centre.

Dyck, R.F. 2001. 'Mechanisms of Renal Disease in Indigenous Populations: Influences at Work in Canadian Indigenous Peoples.' *Nephrology* 6:3–7.

Dyck, R.F., and H. Cassidy. 1995. 'Preventing Non-Insulin-Dependent Diabetes among Aboriginal Peoples: Is Exercise the Answer?' *Chronic Diseases in Canada* 16:175–7.

Dyck, R.F., and L. Tan. 1994. 'Rates and Outcomes of Diabetic End-Stage Renal Disease among Registered Native People in Saskatchewan.' *Canadian Medical Association Journal* 150:203–8.

Edwards, G.T. 1980. 'Bella Coola Indian and European Medicines.' *The Beaver* (Winter): 5–11.

Egan, C. 1999. 'Inuit Women's Perceptions of Pollution.' PhD diss., University of Manitoba, Winnipeg.

Eisenberg, D., R. Kessler, C. Foster, F. Norlock, D. Calkins, and T. Delbanco. 1993. 'Unconventional Medicine in the United States.' New England Journal of Medicine 328:246–52.

Elias, P.D. 2002. *The Dakota of the Canadian Northwest: Lessons for Survival*. Regina: Canadian Plains Research Centre.

Ellestad-Sayed, J., F.H. Coodin, L.A. Dilling, and J.C. Haworth. 1979. 'Breast-feeding Protects against Infection in Indian Infants.' *Canadian Medical Association Journal* 120:295–8.

El-Najjar, M.Y. 1979. 'Human Treponematosis and Tuberculosis: Evidence from the New World.' *American Journal of Physical Anthropology* 51:599–618.

Eshleman, J.A., R.S. Malhi, and D.G. Smith. 2003. 'Mitochondrial DNA Studies of Native Americans: Conceptions and Misconceptions of the Population Prehistory of the Americas.' *Evolutionary Anthropology* 12:7–18.

Evers, S.E., E. McCracken, I. Antone, and G. Deagle. 1987. 'Prevalence of Diabetes in Indians and Caucasians Living in Southwestern Ontario.' *Canadian Journal of Public Health* 78:240–3.

Ewald, P.W. 2003. 'Evolution and Ancient Disease: The Roles of Genes, Germs, and Transmission Models.' In C. Greenblatt and M. Spigelman, eds, *Emerging Pathogens: Archaeology, Ecology and Evolution of Infectious Disease*, 117–24. Oxford: Oxford University Press.

Ewart, W. 1983. 'Causes of Mortality in a Subarctic Settlement (York Factory, Man.) 1714–1946.' *Canadian Medical Association Journal* 129:571–4.

Ewers, J. 1973. 'The Influence of Epidemics on the Indian Populations and Cultures of Texas.' *Plains Anthropologist* 18:104–15.

Favel-King, A. 1993. 'The Treaty Right to Health Care.' In Royal Commission on Aboriginal Peoples, *The Path to Healing*, 120–9. Ottawa: Royal Commission on Aboriginal Peoples.

Fecteau, R., J. Molnar, and G. Warwick. 1991. 'Iroquoian Village Ecology.' Paper presented at the 24th Annual Meeting of the Canadian Archaeology Association, St John's, Newfoundland.

Felton, J. 1959. 'Friend in Need.' *The Beaver* 290 (Summer):36–8.

Fenna, D., L. Mix, O. Schaefer, and J.A. Gilbert. 1971. 'Ethanol Metabolism in Various Racial Groups.' *Canadian Medical Association Journal* 105:472–5.

Ferguson, R. 1928. *Tuberculosis among the Indians of the Great Canadian Plains*. London: Adlard and Sons Limited.

– 1955. *Studies in Tuberculosis*. Toronto: University of Toronto Press.

Ferguson, R.G., and A.B. Sime. 1949. 'BCG Vaccination of Indian Infants in Saskatchewan.' *Tubercle* 30:5–11.

Fetherstonhaugh, R. 1940. *The Royal Canadian Mounted Police*. New York: Garden City Publishing Co.

First Nations Information Governance Committee. 2004. *First Nations and Inuit Regional Health Surveys*, 1997. Ottawa: National Aboriginal Health Organization.

Fisher, A.D. 1987. 'Alcoholism and Race: The Misapplication of Both Concepts to North American Indians.' *Canadian Review of Sociology and Anthropology* 24:81–98.

Fisher, R. 1977. *Contact and Conflict: Indian-European Relations in British Columbia, 1774–1890*. Vancouver: University of British Columbia Press.

Flannery, R. 1939. 'The Shaking-Tent Rite among the Montagnais of James Bay.' *Primitive Man* 17(1):11–16.

Fleming, A. nd. *An Arctic Hospital*. Toronto: The Arctic Mission.

Fleming, C.M. 1992. 'American Indians and Alaska Natives: Changing Societies Past and Present.' In M. Orlandi, ed., *Cultural Competence for Evaluators*, 147–71. Rockville, Md: U.S. Department of Health and Human Services.

Fleming, R., ed. 1940. *Minutes of Council Northern Department of Rupert Land, 1821–1831*. London: Hudson's Bay Record Society.

Ford, R. 1981. 'Ethnobotany in North America: An Historical Phytogeographic Perspective.' *Canadian Journal of Botany* 59:2178–88.

Fortuine, R. 1971. 'The Health of the Eskimos as Portrayed in the Earliest Written Accounts.' *Bulletin of the History of Medicine* 65(2):97–114.

– 1985. 'Lancets of Stone: Traditional Methods of Surgery among the Alaska Natives.' *Arctic Anthropology* 22(1):23–45.

– 1989. *Chills and Fever: Health and Disease in the Early History of Alaska*. Fairbanks: University of Alaska Press.

– 2005. *'Must We All Die?' Alaska's Enduring Struggle with Tuberculosis*. Fairbanks: University of Alaska Press.

Fossett, R. 2001. *In Order to Live Untroubled: Inuit of the Central Arctic, 1550–1940*. Winnipeg: University of Manitoba Press.

Foulkes, R.G. 1962a. 'Medics in the North: A History of the Contributions of the Royal Canadian Air Force to the Medical Care of Civilians in the Fort Nelson Area of British Columbia. Part 1.' *Medical Services Journal of Canada* 18 (7):523–50.

– 1962b. 'Medics in the North: A History of the Contributions of the Royal Canadian Air Force to the Medical Care of Civilians in the Fort Nelson Area of British Columbia. Part 3.' *Medical Services Journal of Canada* 18(9):675–86.

– 1962c. 'Medics in the North: A History of the Contributions of the Royal Canadian Air Force to the Medical Care of Civilians in the Fort Nelson Area of British Columbia. Part 4.' *Medical Services Journal of Canada* 18(10):736–52.

Four Directions International. 2002. *Mapping the Healing Journey: The Final Report of a National Research Project on Healing in Canadian Aboriginal Communities*. Lethbridge, Alta.: Four Worlds Institute for Human and Community Development.

Francis, D., and T. Morantz. 1983. *Partners in Furs: A History of the Fur Trade in Eastern James Bay, 1600–1870*. Montreal: McGill-Queen's University Press.

Franklin, J. 1969. *Narrative of a Journey to the Shore of the Polar Sea in the Years 1819, 20, 21, 22*. New York: Greenwood.

Friesen, B. 1985. 'Haddon's Strategy for Prevention: Application to Native House Fires.' In R. Fortuine, ed., *Circumpolar Health 84: Proceedings of the 6th International Symposium*, 105–9. Seattle: University of Washington Press.

Frost, W.H. 1939. 'The Age of Selection of Mortality from Tuberculosis in Successive Decades.' *American Journal of Hygiene* 30:91–6.

Fry, G. 1974. 'Ovum and Parasite Examination of Saltes Cave Human Paleofeces.' In P.J. Watson, ed., *Archeology of the Mammoth Cave Area*. New York: Academic Press.

Fuchs, M., and R. Bashshur. 1975. 'Use of Traditional Indian Medicine among Urban Native Americans.' *Medical Care* 13(11):915–27.

Fumoleau, R. 1973. *As Long as the Land Shall Last*. Toronto: McClelland and Stewart.

Gagnon, Y. 1989. 'Physicians' Attitudes toward Collaboration with Traditional Healers.' *Native Studies Review* 5(1):175–86.

Gallagher, R.P., and J.M. Elwood. 1979. 'Cancer Mortality among Chinese, Japanese, and Indians in British Columbia, 1964–73.' *National Cancer Institute Monographs* 53:89–94.

Garrison, V. 1977. 'Doctor, Espiritista or Psychiatrist?: Health-Seeking Behavior in a Puerto Rican Neighborhood of New York City.' *Medical Anthropology* 1(2):65–191.

Garro, L.C. 1987. 'Cultural Knowledge about Diabetes.' In T.K. Young, ed., *Diabetes in the Canadian Native Population: Biocultural Perspectives*, 97–109. Toronto: Canadian Diabetes Association.

– 1988a. 'Culture and High Blood Pressure: Understandings of a Chronic Illness in an Ojibwa Community.' *Arctic Medical Research* 47 (Suppl. 1):70–3.

– 1988b. 'Explaining High Blood Pressure: Variation in Knowledge about Illness.' *American Ethnologist* 15:98–119.

– 1988c. 'Resort to Folk Healers in a Manitoba Ojibwa Community.' *Arctic Medical Research* 47 (Suppl. 1):317–20

– 1990. 'Continuity and Change: The Interpretation of Illness in an Anishinaabe (Ojibway) Community.' *Culture, Medicine and Psychiatry* 14:417–54.

– 1991. 'Consultations with Anishinaabe (Ojibway) Healers in a Manitoba Community.' In B. Postl et al., eds, *Circumpolar Health 90: Proceedings of the 8th International Congress*, 213–16. Winnipeg: University of Manitoba Press.

– 1995. 'Individual or Societal Responsibility? Explanations of Diabetes in an Anishinaabe (Ojibway) Community.' *Social Science and Medicine* 40:37–46.

– 1996. 'Intracultural Variation in Causal Accounts of Diabetes: A Comparison of Three Canadian Anishinaabe (Ojibwa) Communities.' *Culture, Medicine and Psychiatry* 20:381–420.

Garro, L.C., and G.C. Lang. 1994. 'Explanations of Diabetes: Anishinaabe and Dakota Deliberate upon a New Illness.' In J.R. Joe and R.S. Young, eds, *Diabetes as a Disease of Civilization: The Impact of Culture Change on Indigenous Peoples*, 293–328. Berlin: Mouton de Gruyter.

Garro, L., J. Roulette, and R. Whitmore. 1986. 'Community Control of Health Care Delivery: The Sandy Bay Experience.' *Canadian Journal of Public Health* 77:281–4.

Garvin, J., ed. 1927. *Alexander Mackenzie: Voyages from Montreal*. Toronto: The Radisson Society of Canada.

Gaudette, L.A., R. Dufour, S. Freitag, and A.B. Miller. 1991. 'Cancer Patterns in the Inuit Population of Canada, 1970–1984.' In B.D. Postl et al., eds, *Circumpolar Health 90: Proceedings of the 8th International Congress on Circumpolar Health*, 443–6. Winnipeg: University of Manitoba Press.

Gaudette, L.A., S. Freitag, R. Dufour, and M. Baikie. 1996. 'Cancer in Circumpolar Inuit: Background Information for Cancer Patterns in Canadian Inuit.' *Acta Oncologica* 35:527–33.

Gaudette, L.A., R.-N. Gao, S. Freitag, and M. Wideman. 1993. 'Cancer Incidence by Ethnic Group in the Northwest Territories (NWT), 1969–1988.' *Health Reports* 5:23–32.

George, P., and B. Nahwegahbow. 1993. 'Anishinawbe Health.' In Royal Commission on Aboriginal Peoples, *The Path to Healing*, 241–3. Ottawa: Royal Commission on Aboriginal Peoples.

Gillis, D.C., J. Irvine, and L. Tan. 1991. 'Cancer Incidence and Survival of Saskatchewan Northerners and Registered Indians, 1967–1986.' In B.D. Postl et al., eds, *Circumpolar Health 90: Proceedings of the 8th International Congress*, 447–51. Winnipeg: University of Manitoba Press.

Gittelsohn, J., S.B. Harris, K. Burris, L. Kakagamic, L.T. Landman, and A. Sharma. 1996. 'Use of Ethnographic Methods for Applied Research on Diabetes among the Ojibwa-Cree in Northern Ontario.' *Health Education Quarterly* 23:365–82.

Gittelsohn, J., T.M.S. Wolever, S.B. Harris, R. Harris-Giraldo, A.J.G. Hanley, and B. Zinman. 1998. 'Specific Patterns of Food Consumption and Preparation Are Associated with Diabetes and Obesity in a Native Canadian Community.' *Journal of Nutrition* 128:541–7.

Glover, R., ed. 1958. *A Journey from Prince of Wales's Fort in Hudson's Bay to the Northern Ocean, 1769, 1770, 1771, 1772 by Samuel Hearne*. Toronto: Macmillan.

Godwin, M., M. Muirhead, J. Huynh, B. Helt, and J. Grimmer. 1999. 'Prevalence of Gestational Diabetes Mellitus among Swampy Cree Women in Moose Factory, James Bay.' *Canadian Medical Association Journal* 160:1299–302.

Goodman, J. 1981. *American Genesis*. New York: Summit Books.

Goodwill, J. Cuthand. *See* Cuthand Goodwill.

Goodwill, J., and N. Sluman. 1984. *John Tootoosis*. Winnipeg: Pemmican.

Graburn, N. 1969. *Eskimos without Igloos: Social and Economic Development in Sugluk*. Boston: Little, Brown.

Graham-Cumming, G. 1967. 'Health of the Original Canadians. 1867–1967.' *Medical Services Journal* 23(2):115–66.

Grant, J.W. 1984. *Moon of Wintertime: Missionaries and the Indians of Canada in Encounter since 1534*. Toronto: University of Toronto Press.

Green, C., J.F. Blanchard, T.K. Young, and J. Griffith. 2003. 'The Epidemiology of Diabetes in the Manitoba Registered First Nation Population.' *Diabetes Care* 26:1993–8.

Green, C., R.D. Hoppa, T.K. Young, and J.F. Blanchard. 2002. 'Geographic Analysis of Diabetes Prevalence in an Urban Area.' *Social Science and Medicine* 57:551–60.

Greenberg, J.H., C.G. Turner II, and S.L. Zegura. 1986. 'The Settlement of the Americas: A Comparison of the Linguistic, Dental, and Genetic Evidence.' *Current Anthropology* 27(5):477–98.

Gregory, D. 1989. 'Traditional Indian Healers in Northern Manitoba: An Emerging Relationship with the Health Care System.' *Native Studies Review* 5(1):163–74.

Grigg, E. 1958. 'The Arcana of Tuberculosis.' *American Review of Respiratory Disease* 78:151–72, 583–603.

Grinnell, G. 1972. *Blackfoot Lodge Tales: The Story of a Prairie People*. Williamstown, Mass.: Comer House. (Original publication 1892.)

Grygier, P.S. 1994. *A Long Way from Home: The Tuberculosis Epidemic among the Inuit*. Montreal: McGill-Queen's University Press.

Hackett, C. 1983. 'Problems in the Paleopathology of the Human Treponematosis.' In G.D. Hart, ed., *Diseases in Ancient Man*, 106–28. Toronto: Clarke Irwin.

Hackett, F.P. 1991. 'The 1819–20 Measles Epidemic: Its Origin, Diffusion and Mortality Effects upon the Indians of the Petit Nord.' MA thesis, University of Manitoba, Winnipeg.

– 2002. *A Very Remarkable Sickness: Epidemics in the Petit Nord, 1670 to 1846*. Winnipeg: University of Manitoba Press.

– 2004. 'Averting Disaster: The Hudson's Bay Company and Smallpox in Western Canada during the Late Eighteenth and Early Nineteenth Centuries.' *Bulletin of the History of Medicine* 78:575–609.

Hader, J. 1990. 'The Effect of Tuberculosis on the Indians of Saskatchewan, 1926–1965.' MA thesis, University of Saskatchewan, Saskatoon.

Hagey, R. 1984. 'The Phenomenon, the Explanations and the Responses: Metaphors Surrounding Diabetes in Urban Canadian Indians.' *Social Science and Medicine* 18:265–72.

Hallowell, A.I. 1942. *The Role of Conjuring in Saulteaux Society.* Philadelphia: University of Pennsylvania Press.

– 1963. 'Ojibwa World View and Disease.' In I. Galdston, ed., *Man's Image in Medicine and Anthropology*, 258–315. New York: International Universities Press.

Hamer, J., and J. Steinbring. 1980. 'Alcohol and the North American Indian: Examples from the Subarctic.' In J. Hamer and J. Steinbring, eds, *Alcohol and Native Peoples of the North*, 1–29. Washington, D.C.: University Press of America.

Hanley, A.J.G., S.B. Harris, J. Gittelsohn, T.M.S. Wolever, B. Saksvig, and B. Zinman. 2000. 'Overweight among Children and Adolescents in a Native Canadian Community: Prevalence and Associated Factors.' *American Journal of Clinical Nutrition* 71:693–700.

Harmon, D. 1911. *A Journal of Voyages and Travels in the Interior of North America.* Toronto: Courier Press.

Harper, R. [director], and J. Krepakevich [producer]. 1992. *Coppermine.* Ottawa: National Film Board of Canada.

Harris, H. 1997. 'Late Pleistocene Environments from Northern Northwest Coast Oral History.' Paper presented at the 50th Northwest Anthropological Conference, Ellensburg, Wa.

Harris, S.B., L.E. Caulfield, M.S. Sugamori, E.A. Whalen, and B. Henning. 2005. 'The Epidemiology of Diabetes in Pregnant Native Canadians: A Risk Profile.' *Diabetes Care* 20:1422–5.

Harris, S.B., J. Gittelsohn, A.J.G. Hanley, A. Barnie, T.M.S. Wolever, J. Gao, A. Logan, and B. Zinman. 2005. 'The Prevalence of NIDDM and Associated Risk Factors in Native Canadians.' *Diabetes Care* 20:185–97.

Hartney, P.C. 1981. 'Tuberculous Lesions in a Prehistoric Population Sample from Southern Ontario.' In J.E. Buikstra, ed., *Prehistoric Tuberculosis in the Americas*, 141–60. Evanston, Ill.: Northwestern University Archaeological Program.

Heagerty, J.J. 1928. *Four Centuries of Medical History in Canada.* Toronto: Macmillan.

Heal, G., R.K. Elwood, and J.M. FitzGerald. 1998. 'Acceptance and Safety of Directly Observed versus Self-Administered Isoniazid Preventive Therapy in

Aboriginal Peoples in British Columbia.' *International Journal of Tuberculosis and Lung Diseases* 2:979–83.

Health Canada. 1994. *Native Foods and Nutrition: An Illustrated Reference Manual.* Rev. ed. Ottawa: Health Canada, Medical Services Branch, Cat. No. H34–59/1994E.

– 1996. *Trends in First Nations Mortality, 1979–1993.* Ottawa: Health Canada, Medical Services Branch.

– 1999. *Ten Years of Health Transfer – First Nation and Inuit Control.* Ottawa: Health Canada, First Nations and Inuit Health Branch.

– 2001. *Unintentional and Intentional Injury Profile for Aboriginal People in Canada, 1990–1999.* Ottawa: Health Canada, First Nations and Inuit Health Branch, Cat. No. H35-4/8-1999.

– 2002. *Annual Report.* Ottawa: Health Canada, First Nations and Inuit Health Branch.

– 2003a. *Interim FNIHB Medical Transportation Policy Framework.* Ottawa: Health Canada, First Nations and Inuit Health Branch.

– 2003b. *Non-Insured Health Benefits Program: Annual Report 2002/2003.* Ottawa: Health Canada, First Nations and Inuit Health Branch.

– 2003c. *A Statistical Profile on the Health of First Nations in Canada.* Ottawa: Health Canada, First Nations and Inuit Health Branch.

– 2003d. *2003–2004 Estimates: Part III – Report on Plans and Priorities.* Ottawa: Health Canada.

– 2003e. 'Working Together to Close the Gaps.' *Health Policy Research.* Bulletin 5(1). Ottawa: Health Canada, Applied Research and Analysis Directorate.

– 2004. 'Transfer of Health Programs to First Nations and Inuit Communities.' In *Handbook 1. An Introduction to Three Approaches.* Ottawa: Health Canada, First Nations and Inuit Health Branch.

Hegele, R.A., H. Cao, S.B. Harris, A.J.G. Hanley, and B. Zinman. 1999. 'The Hepatic Nuclear Factor-1–Alpha G319S Variant Is Associated with Early Onset Type-2 Diabetes in Canadian Oji-Cree.' *Journal of Clinical Endocrinology and Metabolism* 84:1077–82.

Hegele, R.A., P.W. Connelly, A.J.G. Hanley, F. Sun, S.B. Harris, and B. Zinman. 1997. 'Common Genomic Variants Associated with Variation in Plasma Lipoproteins in Young Aboriginal Canadians.' *Arteriosclerosis, Thrombosis and Vascular Biology* 17:1060–6.

Hegele, R.A., F. Sun, S.B. Harris, C. Anderson, A.J.G. Hanley, and B. Zinman. 1999. 'Genome-Wide Scanning for Type-2 Diabetes Susceptibility in Canadian Oji-Cree, Using 190 Microsatellite Markers.' *Journal of Human Genetics* 44:10–14.

Hegele, R.A., T.K. Young, and P.W. Connelly. 1997. 'Are Canadian Inuit at

Increased Genetic Risk for Coronary Heart Disease?' *Journal of Molecular Medicine* 74:364–70.

Hellson, J. 1974. 'Ethnobotany of the Blackfoot Indians.' *Canadian Ethnology Service Paper* No. 19. Ottawa: National Museum of Canada.

Helm, J. 1980. 'Female Infanticide, European Diseases and Population Levels among Mackenzie Dene.' *American Ethnologist* 7:259–85.

Henderson, J. 1987. 'Factors Determining the State of Preservation of Human Remains.' In A. Boddington, A.N. Garland, and R.C. Janaway, eds, *Death, Decay and Reconstruction: Approaches to Archaeology and Forensic Sciences*, 43–54. Manchester: Manchester University Press.

Henige, D. 1990. 'Their Numbers Become Thick: Native American Historical Demography as Expiation.' In J.A. Clifton, ed., *The Invented Indian: Cultural Fictions and Government Policies*, 169–91. London: Transaction Publications.

Henry, A. 1976. *Travels and Adventures in Canada and the Indian Territories between the Years 1760 and 1776*. New York: Garland. (Original publication 1809.)

Herring, D.A. 1992. 'Toward a Reconsideration of Disease and Contact in the Americas.' *Prairie Forum* 17(2):153–65.

– 1993. '"There Were Young People and Old People and Babies Dying Every Week": The 1918–1919 Influenza Pandemic at Norway House.' *Ethnohistory* 41(1):73–105.

– 1994. 'The 1918 Influenza Epidemic in the Central Canadian Subarctic.' In A. Herring and L. Chan, eds, *Strength in Diversity: A Reader in Physical Anthropology*, 365–84. Toronto: Canadian Scholars' Press.

Herring, D.A., S. Abonyi, and R.D. Hoppa. 2003. 'Malnutrition among Northern Peoples of Canada in the 1940s: An Ecological and Economic Disaster.' In D.A. Herring and A. C. Swedlund, eds, *Human Biologists in the Archives*, 289–310. Cambridge: Cambridge University Press.

Herring, D.A., and R.D. Hoppa. 1997. 'Changing Patterns of Mortality Seasonality among the Western James Bay Cree.' *International Journal of Circumpolar Health* 56:121–33.

– 1999. 'Endemic Tuberculosis among Nineteenth Century Cree in the Central Canadian Subarctic.' *Perspectives in Human Biology* 4:189–99.

Herring, D.A., and S. Sattenspiel. 2003. 'Death in Winter: Spanish Flu in the Canadian Subarctic.' In H. Phillips and D. Killingray, eds, *The Spanish Influenza Pandemic of 1918–19: New Perspectives*, 156–72. London: Routledge.

Hiebert, S., E. Angees, T.K. Young, and J.D. O'Neil. 2001. 'The Evaluation of Transferred Health Care Services in Wunnimun Lake, Wapekeka and Kingfisher Lake First Nations: A Nursing Perspective.' *International Journal of Circumpolar Health* 60:473–8.

Hildes, J.A., and O. Schaefer. 1984. 'The Changing Picture of Neoplastic Disease in the Western and Central Canadian Arctic (1950–1980).' *Canadian Medical Association Journal* 130:25–33.

Hill, D.M. 2003. *Traditional Medicine in Contemporary Contexts: Protecting and Respecting Indigenous Knowledge and Medicine.* Ottawa: National Aboriginal Health Organization.

Hislop, T.G., H. Clarke, M. Deschamps, and R. Joseph. 1996. 'Cervical Cytology Screening: How Can We Improve Rates among First Nations Women in Urban British Columbia?' *Canadian Family Physician* 42:1701–8.

Hislop, T.G., M. Deschamps, P.R. Band, J.M. Smith, and H.F. Clarke. 1992. 'Participation in the British Columbia Cervical Cytology Screening Program by Native Indian Women.' *Canadian Journal of Public Health* 83:344–5.

Hislop, T.G., W.J. Threlfall, R.P. Gallagher, and P.R. Band. 1987. 'Accidental and Intentional Violent Deaths among British Columbia Native Indians.' *Canadian Journal of Public Health* 78:271–4.

Hoffecker, J.F., W.R. Powers, and T. Goebel. 1993. 'The Colonization of Beringia and the Peopling of the New World.' *Science* 259:46–53.

Holcomb, R.C. 1940. 'Syphilis of the Skull among Aleuts, and the Asian and North American Eskimo about Bering and Arctic Seas.' *U.S. Naval Medical Bulletin* 38:177–92.

Honigmann, J.J. 1948. *Foodways in a Muskeg Community.* Ottawa: Department of Northern Affairs and Natural Resources, Northern Coordination and Research Centre.

Hood, E., S.A. Malcolmson, L.T. Young, and S. Abbey. 1993. 'Psychiatric Consultation in the Eastern Canadian Arctic. I. Development and Evolution of the Baffin Psychiatric Consultation Service.' *Canadian Journal of Psychiatry* 38:23–7.

Hoppa, R.D. 1998. 'Mortality in a Northern Ontario Fur-Trade Community: Moose Factory – 1964.' *Canadian Studies in Population* 25:175–98.

Hopwood, V., ed. 1971. *David Thompson: Travels in Western North America, 1784–1812.* Toronto: Macmillan.

Horn, O.K., G. Paradis, L. Potvin, A.C. Macaulay, and S. Desrosiers. 2001. 'Correlates and Predictors of Adiposity among Mohawk Children.' *Preventive Medicine* 33:274–81.

Houston, S., A. Fanning, C.L. Soskolne, and N. Fraser. 1990. 'The Effectiveness of Bacille Calmette-Guerin (BCG) Vaccination against Tuberculosis.' *American Journal of Epidemiology* 131:340–8.

Howard, J. 1977. *The Plains-Ojibwa or Bungi: Hunters and Warriors of the Northern Prairies with Special Reference to the Turtle Mountain Band.* Lincoln, Nebr.: J. and L. Reprint Co. Reprints in Anthropology, vol. 7.

Hrdlicka, A. 1908. 'Contribution to the Study of Tuberculosis in the Indian.'

Transactions of the Sixth International Congress on Tuberculosis, Washington.
Vol. 3, Section 5, 480–93. Philadelphia: William F. Fell Co.

Hughes, C.C. 1996. 'Ethnopsychiatry.' In C.F. Sargent and T.M. Johnson, eds, *Medical Anthropology: Contemporary Theory and Method*, 131–50. Westport, Conn.: Praeger.

Hultkrantz, A. 1992. *Shamanic Healing and Ritual Drama: Health and Medicine in Native North American Religious Traditions*. New York: Crossroad.

Hurlich, M. 1983. 'Historical and Recent Demography of the Algonkians of Northern Ontario.' In A.T. Steegmann Jr, ed., *Boreal Forest Adaptations: The Northern Algonkians*, 143–200. New York: Plenum.

Hutchens, Alma. 1973. *Indian Herbalogy of North America*. Windsor: Merco.

Indian Association of Alberta. 1970. *Citizens Plus*. Edmonton: Indian Association of Alberta.

Innis, S.M., and H.V. Kuhnlein. 1987. 'The Fatty Acid Composition of Northern Canadian Marine and Terrestrial Mammals.' *Acta Medica Scandinavica* 222:105–9.

Jackes, M. 1983. 'Osteological Evidence of Smallpox: A Possible Case from Seventeenth Century Ontario.' *American Journal of Physical Anthropology* 60:75–81.

– 1986. 'The Mortality of Ontario Archaeological Populations.' *Canadian Journal of Anthropology* 5(2):33–47.

– 1988. *The Osteology of the Grimsby Site*. Edmonton: Department of Anthropology, University of Alberta.

Jacklin, K., and W. Warry. 2004. 'The Indian Health Transfer Policy: Toward Cost Containment or Self-Determination?' In M. Singer and A. Castro, eds, *Unhealthy Health Policy: A Critical Anthropological Examination*, 215–34. Walnut Creek, Calif.: Altamira Press.

Jenkins, D. 1977. 'Tuberculosis: The Native Indian Viewpoint on Its Prevention, Diagnosis, and Treatment.' *Preventive Medicine* 6:545–55.

Jenness, D. 1938. *The Sarcee Indians of Alberta*. Ottawa: National Museum of Canada. Bulletin 90.

– 1972. *Eskimo Administration: II. Canada*. Arctic Institute of North America Technical Paper No. 14. (Original publication 1964.)

Jetté, M. 1994. *Santé Québec: A Health Profile of the Inuit*. Montreal: Ministère de la Santé et des Services Sociaux.

Jilek, W.G. 1978. 'Native Renaissance: The Survival and Revival of Indigenous Therapeutic Ceremonials among North American Indians.' *Transcultural Psychiatric Research Reviews* 15:117–47.

– 1982a. 'Altered States of Consciousness in North American Indian Ceremonials.' *Ethos* 10:326–43.

- 1982b. *Indian Healing: Shamanic Ceremonialism in the Pacific Northwest Today.* Surrey, B.C.: Hancock House.

Jilek, W.G., and L. Jilek-Aall. 1982. 'Shamanic Symbolism in Salish Indian Rituals.' In I. Rossi, ed., *The Logic of Culture*, 127–36. South Hadley, Mass.: J.F. Bergen Publishers.

- 1991. 'Traditional Medicine and Mental Health Care.' In B. Postl et al., eds, *Circumpolar Health 90: Proceedings of the 8th International Congress*, 303–8. Winnipeg: University of Manitoba Press.

Jilek, W.G., and C. Roy. 1976. 'Homicide Committed by Canadian Indians and Non-Indians.' *International Journal of Offender Therapy Comparative Criminology* 20:201–16.

Jilek-Aall, L. 1976. 'The Western Psychiatrist and His Non-Western Clientele.' *Canadian Psychiatric Association Journal* 19:357–61.

- 1981. 'Acculturation, Alcoholism and Indian-Style Alcoholics Anonymous.' *Journal of Studies in Alcoholism* (Suppl. 9):143–58.

Johansson, S. 1982. 'The Demographic History of the Native Peoples of North America: A Selected Bibliography.' *Yearbook of Physical Anthropology* 25:133–52.

Johnson, J., and F. Johnson. 1993. 'Community Development, Sobriety and After-Care at Alkali Lake Band.' In Royal Commission on Aboriginal Peoples, *The Path to Healing*, 227–30. Ottawa: Royal Commission on Aboriginal Peoples.

Joraleman, D. 1982. 'New World Depopulation and the Case of Disease.' *Journal of Anthropological Research* 38(1):108–27.

Kaplan, B., and D. Johnson. 1964. 'The Social Meaning of Navaho Psychopathology and Psychotherapy.' In A. Kiev, ed., *Magic, Faith, and Healing: Studies in Primitive Psychiatry Today*, 203–29. New York: The Free Press.

Katzenberg, M.A. 1989. 'Stable Isotope Analysis of Archaeological Faunal Remains from Southern Ontario.' *Journal of Archaeological Science* 16(3):319–30.

- 1992. 'Changing Diet and Health in Pre- and Proto-Historic Ontario.' *MASCA Research Papers in Science and Archaeology* 9:23–31.

- 2000. 'Stable Isotope Analysis: A Tool for Studying Past Diet, Demography, and Life History.' In M.A. Katzenberg and S.R. Saunders, eds, *Biological Anthropology of the Human Skeleton*, 305–28. New York: Wiley-Liss.

Katzenberg, M.A., S.R. Saunders, and W.R. Fitzgerald. 1993. 'Age Differences in Stable Carbon and Nitrogen Isotope Ratios in a Population of Prehistoric Maize Horticulturalists.' *American Journal of Physical Anthropology* 90(3):267–81.

Katzenberg, M.A., and J.P. Schwarcz. 1986. 'Paleonutrition in Southern Ontario: Evidence from Strontium and Stable Isotopes.' *Canadian Journal of Anthropology* 5(2):15–21.

Kaufert, J., and W. Koolage. 1985. 'Culture Brokerage and Advocacy in Urban Hospitals: The Impact of Native Language Interpreters.' *Santé Culture Health* 3(2):3–8.

Keenleyside, A. 1990. 'Euro-American Whaling in the Canadian Arctic: Its Effects on Eskimo Health.' *Arctic Anthropology* 27(1):1–19.

– 1993. 'Skeletal Evidence of Health and Disease in Pre-Contact and Contact Period Alaskan Eskimos and Aleuts.' Paper presented at the 62nd Annual Meeting of the American Association of Physical Anthropologists, Toronto.

– 1994. 'Skeletal Evidence of Health and Disease in Pre- and Postcontact Alaskan Eskimos and Aleuts.' PhD diss., McMaster University, Hamilton.

– 2003. 'Changing Patterns of Health and Disease among the Aleuts.' *Arctic Anthropology* 40(1):48–69.

Kehoe, A. 1990. 'Primal Gaia: Primitivists and Plastic Medicine Men.' In J. Clifton, ed., *The Invented Indian: Cultural Fictions and Government Policies*, 193–209. New York: Transaction Publishers.

Kelm, M.E. 1998. *Colonizing Bodies: Aboriginal Health and Healing in British Columbia 1900–50*. Vancouver: University of British Columbia Press.

– 2005. 'Diagnosing the Discursive Indian: Medicine, Gender and the "Dying Race."' *Ethnohistory* 52(2):371–406.

Kennedy, D. 1984. 'The Quest for a Cure: A Case Study in the Use of Health Care Alternatives.' *Culture* 4(2):21–31.

Kidd, G. 1946. 'Trepanation among the Early Indians of British Columbia.' *Canadian Medical Association Journal* 55:513–15.

King, S.E., and S.J. Ulijaszek. 1999. 'Invisible Insults during Growth and Development: Contemporary Theories and Past Populations.' In R.D. Hoppa and C.M. FitzGerald, eds, *Human Growth in the Past: Studies from Bones and Teeth*, 161–82. Cambridge: Cambridge University Press.

Kirk, R., and E. Szathmary, eds. 1985. *Out of Asia: Peopling of the Americas and the Pacific*. Canberra: The Journal of Pacific History Inc.

Kirmayer, L.J., C. Fletcher, E. Corin, and L.J. Boothroyd. 1997. *Inuit Concepts of Mental Health and Illness: An Ethnographic Study*. Report No. 4. Montreal: Culture and Mental Health Research Unit, Institute of Family Psychiatry, Sir Mortimer B. Davis–Jewish General Hospital, and Department of Psychiatry, McGill University.

Kirmayer, L.J., M. Malus, and L.J. Boothroyd. 1996. 'Suicide Attempts among Inuit Youth: A Community Survey of Prevalence and Risk Factors.' *Acta Psychiatrica Scandinavica* 94:8–17.

Kleinman, A. 1980. *Patients and Healers in the Context of Culture*. Berkeley: University of California Press.

Knight, R. 1996. *Indians at Work: An Informal History of Native Labour in British Columbia 1848–1930*. Vancouver: New Star Books.

Konomi, N.E., K. Lebwohl, I. Mowbray, I. Tattersall, and D. Zhang. 2002. 'Detection of Mycobacterial DNA in Andean Mummies.' *Journal of Clinical Microbiology* 40(12):4738–40.

Kralt, J. 1990. 'Ethnic Origins in the Canadian Census, 1871–1986.' In S.S. Halli, F. Trovato, and L. Driedger, eds, *Ethnic Demography: Canadian Immigrant, Racial and Cultural Variations*, 13–29. Ottawa: Carleton University Press.

Krech, S., III. 1983a. 'Disease, Starvation, and Northern Athapaskan Social Organization.' *American Ethnologist* 5:710–32.

– 1983b. 'The Influence of Disease and the Fur Trade on Arctic Drainage Lowlands Dene, 1800–1850.' *Journal of Anthropological Research* 39(1):123–46.

Kriska, A.M., A.J.G. Hanley, S.B. Harris, and B. Zinman. 2001. 'Physical Activity, Physical Fitness, and Insulin and Glucose Concentrations in an Isolated Native Canadian Population Experiencing Rapid Lifestyle Change.' *Diabetes Care* 24:1787–92.

Kroeber, A.L. 1925. *Handbook of the Indians of California*. Bureau of American Ethnology Bulletin 78. Washington, D.C.

Kroeber, A.L. 1934. 'Native American Population.' *American Anthropologist* 36:1–25.

Kuhnlein, H.V., and O. Receveur. 1996. 'Dietary Change and Traditional Food Systems of Indigenous Peoples.' *Annual Review of Nutrition* 16:417–42.

Kuhnlein, H.V., and N.J. Turner. 1991. *Traditional Plant Foods of Canadian Indigenous Peoples: Nutrition, Botany and Use*. Philadelphia: Gordon and Breach.

Lamoureux, M., ed. 1991. *Domestic Violence in Aboriginal Communities: Reference Manual*. Quebec: Ministère de la Santé et des Services Sociaux.

LaPointe, K. 1986. 'Bureaucratic Bungling Separated Inuit.' *Saskatoon Star-Phoenix*, 23 September 1986, B:4.

Larocque, R. 1991. 'The Detection of Epidemics on Human Skeletal Remains: An Example from Huronia.' Paper presented at the 1991 Canadian Association for Physical Anthropology meeting, Hamilton.

Larsen, C.S., and G.R. Milner, eds. 1994. *In the Wake of Contact: Biological Responses to Conquest*. New York: Wiley-Liss.

Laughlin, W., A. Harper, and D. Thompson. 1979. 'New Approaches to the Pre- and Post-Contact History of Arctic Peoples.' *American Journal of Physical Anthropology* 51:579–88.

LaViolette, F. 1973. *The Struggle for Survival: Indian Cultures and the Protestant Ethic in British Columbia*. Toronto: University of Toronto Press.

Leiber, C.S. 1972. 'Metabolism of Ethanol and Alcoholism: Racial and Acquired Factors.' *Annals of Internal Medicine* 76:326–7.

Leighton, A. 1985. *Wild Plant Use by the Woods Cree of East-Central Saskatchewan.* Ethnology Service Paper No. 101. Ottawa: National Museum of Canada.

Lemchuk-Favel, L., and R. Jock. 2004. 'Aboriginal Health Systems in Canada: Nine Case Studies.' *Journal of Aboriginal Health* 1(1):28–51.

Levine, S., M. Eastwood, and Q. Rae-Grant. 1974. 'Psychiatry Service to Northern Indians: A University Project.' *Canadian Psychiatric Association Journal* 9:343–9.

Levy, J.E., and S. Kunitz. 1974. *Indian Drinking: Navajo Practices and Anglo-American Theories.* New York: Wiley and Sons.

Levy, J.E., R. Neutra, and D. Parker. 1987. *Hand Trembling, Frenzy Witchcraft, and Moth Madness: A Study of Navajo Seizure Disorders.* Tucson: University of Arizona Press.

Lewis, R.G. 1980. 'Cultural Perspectives on Treatment Modalities with Native Americans.' In M. Bloom, ed., *Life Span Development: Bases for Preventive and Interventive Healing*, 458–64. New York: MacMillan.

Long, J., and C. Merbs. 1981. 'Coccidioidomycosis: A Primate Model.' In J.E. Buikstra, ed., *Prehistoric Tuberculosis in the Americas*, 69–83. Evanston, Ill.: Northwestern University Archaeological Program.

Longclaws, L., G.E. Barnes, L. Grieve, and R. Dumoff. 1980. 'Alcohol and Drug Use among the Brokenhead Ojibwa.' *Journal of Studies in Alcohol* 41:21–36.

Lopatin, I. 1960. 'Origin of the Native American Steam Bath.' *American Anthropologist* 62:977–93.

Lucier, C., J. VanStone, and D. Keats. 1971. 'Medical Practice and Human Anatomical Knowledge among the Noatak Eskimos.' *Ethnology* 10(3):251–64.

Lux, M.K. 1992. 'Prairie Indians and the 1918 Influenza Epidemic.' *Native Studies Review* 8(1):23–33.

– 2001. *Medicine That Walks: Disease, Medicine, and Canadian Plains Native People, 1880–1940.* Toronto: University of Toronto Press.

Lynch, G.I. 1991. 'Movement toward Professional Excellence – Medical Services Branch Indian Health.' In B. Postl et al., eds, *Circumpolar Health 90: Proceedings of the 8th International Congress*, 173–6. Winnipeg: University of Manitoba Press.

Macaulay, A.C., S.B. Harris, L. Levesque, M. Cargo, E. Ford, J. Salsberg, A. McComber, R. Fiddler, and R. Kirby. 2003. 'Primary Prevention of Type 2 Diabetes: Experiences of Two Aboriginal Communities in Canada.' *Canadian Journal of Diabetes* 27:464–75.

Macaulay, A.C., L.T. Montour, and N. Adelson. 1988. 'Prevalence of Diabetic and Atherosclerotic Complications among Mohawk Indians of Kahnawake, PQ.' *Canadian Medical Association Journal* 139:221–4.

Macaulay, A.C., G. Paradis, and L. Powin. 1997. 'The Kahnawake Schools Diabetes Prevention Project: Intervention, Evaluation and Baseline Results of a Diabetes Primary Prevention Program with a Native Community in Canada.' *Preventive Medicine* 26:779–90.

Mackenzie, A. 1971. *Voyages from Montreal on the River St Laurence through the Continent of North America to the Frozen and Pacific Oceans in the Years 1789–1793.* Edmonton: Hurtig.

MacMillan, H.L., C.A. Walsh, E. Jamieson, M.Y. Wong, E.J. Faries, J. McCue, A.B. MacMillan, D.D. Offord, and the Technical Advisory Committee of the Chiefs of Ontario. 2003. 'The Health of Ontario First Nations People: Results from the Ontario First Nations Regional Health Survey.' *Canadian Journal of Public Health* 94:168–72.

Malchy, B., M.W. Enns, T.K. Young, and B.J. Cox. 1997. 'Suicide among Manitoba's Aboriginal People, 1988 to 1994.' *Canadian Medical Association Journal* 156:1133–8.

Mandelbaum, D.G. 1935. Unpublished Field Notebooks. Saskatchewan Archives Board, Regina.

– 1979. *The Plains Cree: An Ethnographic, Historical, and Comparative Study.* Regina: Canadian Plains Research Centre.

Mandryk, C.A.S., H. Josenhans, D.W. Fedje, and R.W. Mathewes. 2001. 'Late Quaternary Paleoenvironments of Northwestern North America: Implications for Inland versus Coastal Migration Routes.' *Quaternary Science Reviews* 20:301–4.

Manson, S., J. Beals, T. O'Nell, J. Piasecki, D. Bechtold, E. Keane, and M. Jones. 1996. 'Wounded Spirits, Ailing Hearts: PTSD and Related Disorders among American Indians.' In A.J. Marsella, M.J. Friedman, E.T. Gerrity, and R.M. Scurfield, eds, *Ethnocultural Aspects of Posttraumatic Stress Disorder: Issues, Research, and Clinical Applications,* 225–83. Washington, D.C.: American Psychological Association.

Mao, Y., B.W. Moloughney, R. Semenciw, and H. Morrison. 1992. 'Indian Reserve and Registered Indian Mortality in Canada.' *Canadian Journal of Public Health* 83:350–3.

Mao, Y., H. Morrison, R. Semenciw, and D. Wigle. 1986. 'Mortality on Canadian Indian Reserves 1976–1983.' *Canadian Journal of Public Health* 77:263–8.

Marchand, J.F. 1943. 'Tribal Epidemics in the Yukon.' *Journal of the American Medical Association* 123:1019–20.

Marrett, L.D., and M. Chaudhry. 2003. 'Cancer Incidence and Mortality in Ontario First Nations, 1968–1991 (Canada).' *Cancer Causes and Control* 14:259–68.

Marshall, I. 1977. 'An Unpublished Map Made by John Cartwright between 1768–1773 Showing Beothuk Indian Settlements and Artifacts and Allowing a New Population Estimate.' *Ethnohistory* 24(3):223–49.

– 1981. 'Disease as a Factor in the Demise of the Beothuk Indians.' *Culture* 1(1):71–7.

Martens, P., R. Bond, L. Jebamani, C. Burchill, N. Roos, and S. Derksen, et al. 2002. *The Health and Health Care Use of Registered First Nations People Living in Manitoba: A Population-Based Study.* Winnipeg, Manitoba Centre for Health Policy, University of Manitoba.

Martens, P., and T.K. Young. 1997. 'Determinants of Breastfeeding in Four Canadian Ojibwa Communities: A Decision-Making Model.' *American Journal of Human Biology* 9:579–93.

Martens, T., B. Daily, and M. Hodgson. 1988. *Characteristics and Dynamics of Incest and Child Sexual Abuse, with a Native Perspective.* Edmonton: Nechi Institute.

Maundrell, C. 1942. 'Indian Health: 1867–1940.' MA thesis, Queen's University, Kingston.

May, P.A. 1984. 'Explanations of Native American Drinking: A Literature Review.' In R. Hornby and R. Dana, eds, *Mni Wakan and the Sioux: Respite, Release and Recreation,* 13–27. Brandon: Justin Publishing.

Mayhall, J.T. 1992. 'Techniques for the Study of Dental Morphology.' In S.R. Saunders and M.A Katzenberg, eds, *Skeletal Biology of Past Peoples: Research Methods,* 59–78. New York: Wiley-Liss.

McCaa, R. 2002. 'Paleodemography of the Americas from Ancient Times to Colonialism and Beyond.' In R.H. Steckel and J.C. Rose, eds, *The Backbone of History: Health and Nutrition in the Western Hemisphere,* 94–126. Cambridge: Cambridge University Press.

McCarthy, F. 1912. 'The Influence of Race in the Prevalence of Tuberculosis.' *Boston Medical and Surgical Journal* 166:207–13.

McGhee, R. 1992. 'Before Columbus: Early European Visitors to the Shores of the "New World."' *The Beaver* 72(3):6–23.

McGrath, J. 1988. 'Social Networks of Disease Spread in the Lower Illinois Valley: A Simulation Approach.' *American Journal of Physical Anthropology* 77:483–96.

– 1991. 'Biological Impact of Social Disruption Resulting from Epidemic Disease.' *American Journal of Physical Anthropology* 84:407–20.

McHardy, M., and E. O'Sullivan. 2004. *First Nations Community Well-Being in Canada: The Community Well-Being Index (CWB), 2001.* Ottawa: Department of Indian Affairs and Northern Development, Strategic Research and Analysis Directorate, QS-7067–000–EE-A1.

McKennan, R. 1965. *The Chandalar Kutchin.* Technical Paper No. 17. Calgary: Arctic Institute of North America.

McKeown, T. 1988. *The Origins of Human Disease.* Oxford: Blackwell.

McLean, J. 1889. *The Indians of Canada: Their Manners and Customs*. Toronto: William Briggs.

McMillan, A.D. 1995. *Native Peoples and Cultures in Canada*. 2nd ed. Vancouver: Douglas and McIntyre.

McMillan, A.D., and E. Yellowhorn. 2004. *First Peoples in Canada*. Vancouver: Douglas and McIntyre.

McNeill, W.H. 1976. *Plagues and Peoples*. New York: Penguin.

Meijer-Drees, L. 2002. *The Indian Association of Alberta: A History of Political Action*. Vancouver: University of British Columbia Press.

Meiklejohn, C. 2002. *Human Remains, Drifting River/Lwiski, Manitoba (EhMc-18)*. Winnipeg. Report to the Manitoba Historic Resources Branch.

Meiklejohn, C., and D.C. Merrett. 2002. *Human Remains, Pakatawakan Bay 2, Pakatawakan Lake, Manitoba (HgLr-3)*. Winnipeg. Report to the Manitoba Historic Resources Branch.

– 2004. *Human Remains, Valley River Burial 1, Valley River, Manitoba (EiMg-3)*. Winnipeg. Report to the Manitoba Historic Resources Branch.

Meister, C. 1976. 'Demographic Consequences of Euro-American Contact on Selected American Indian Populations and Their Relationship to the Demographic Transition.' *Ethnohistory* 23(2):161–72.

Merbs, C.F. 1963. 'Patterns of Pathology in Eskimos and Aleuts.' *American Journal of Physical Anthropology* 19(1):103 (abstract).

– 1992. 'A New World of Infectious Disease.' *Yearbook of Physical Anthropology* 35:3–42.

Merbs, C.F., and W. Wilson. 1960. 'Anomalies and Pathologies of the Sadlermiut Eskimo Vertebral Column.' *National Museum of Canada Bulletin, Contributions to Anthropology, Part 1*, 154–80.

Merbs, C.F., W. Wilson, and W.S. Laughlin. 1961. 'The Vertebral Column of the Sadlermiut Eskimos.' *American Journal of Physical Anthropology* 19(1):103 (abstract).

Merrett, D.C. 2003. 'Maxillary Sinusitis among the Moatfield People.' In R.F. Williamson and S. Pfeiffer, eds, *Bones of the Ancestors: The Archaeology and Osteobiography of the Moatfield Ossuary*, 241–62. Mercury Series, Archaeology Paper 163. Ottawa: Canadian Museum of Civilization.

Merrett, D.C., T. Garlie, C. Meiklejohn, L. Larcombe, B.M. Rothschild, and B. Waddell. 2003. 'Treponemal Infection among an Early Manitoba Boreal Forest Population (ca. 2000 BP): Evidence from Whaley Cairn (EbKx-10).' Paper presented at the Paleopathology Association, Annual Meeting, Tempe, Arizona.

Merriwether, D.A., F. Rothhammer, and R.E. Ferrell. 1995. 'Distribution of the Four Founding Lineage Haplotypes in Native Americans Suggests a Single

Wave of Migration for the New World.' *American Journal of Physical Anthropology* 98:411–30.

Mignone, J. 2003. *Measuring Social Capital: A Guide for First Nations Communities.* Winnipeg, Centre for Aboriginal Health Research, University of Manitoba.

Millar, W. 1992. 'Place of Birth and Ethnic Status: Factors Associated with Smoking Prevalence among Canadians.' *Health Reports* 1:7–24.

Millar, W. 1997. 'Use of Alternative Health Care Practitioners by Canadians.' *Canadian Journal of Public Health* 88(3):154–8.

Miller, J.R. 1989. *Skyscrapers Hide the Heavens: A History of Indian-White Relations in Canada.* Toronto: University of Toronto Press.

– 1996. *Shingwauk's Vision: A History of Native Residential Schools.* Toronto: University of Toronto Press.

Miller, V. 1976. 'Aboriginal Micmac Population: A Review of the Evidence.' *Ethnohistory* 23(2):117–27.

– 1982. 'The Decline of Nova Scotia Micmac Population, AD 1600–1850.' *Culture* 2(3):107–20.

Mitchell, P. 2003. 'The Archaeological Study of Epidemic and Infectious Disease.' *World Archaeology* 35(2):171–9.

Moerman, D.E. 1983. 'Physiology and Symbols: The Anthropological Implications of the Placebo Effect.' In L. Romanucci-Ross, D. Moerman, and L. Tancredi, eds, *The Anthropology of Medicine: From Culture to Method*, 156–67. New York: Praeger.

– 1986. *Medicinal Plants of North America.* Technical Reports, No. 19. Ann Arbor: University of Michigan Museum of Anthropology.

– 1995. *Native American Ethnobotany.* Portland, Ore.: Timber Press.

– 2002. *Meaning, Medicine and the 'Placebo Effect.'* Cambridge: Cambridge University Press.

Moffat, T., and A. Herring. 1999. 'The Historical Roots of High Rates of Infant Death in Aboriginal Communities in Canada in the Early Twentieth Century: The Case of Fisher River, Manitoba.' *Social Science and Medicine* 48:1821–32.

Moffatt, M. 1987. 'Land Settlements and Health Care: The Case of the James Bay Cree.' *Canadian Journal of Public Health* 78:223–7.

Molto, J.E. 1999. 'A Treponematosis "Endemic" to the Precontact Population of the Cape Region of Baja California Sur.' In O. Dutour, G. Pálfi, J. Bérato, and J.-P. Brun, eds, *L'origine de la syphilis en Europe. Avant ou après 1493?*, 176–84. Paris: Editions Errance.

Molto, J.E., and F.J. Melbye. 1984. 'Treponemal Disease from Two Seventeenth Century Iroquois Sites in Southern Ontario.' Paper presented at the 1984 Paleopathology Association meeting, Philadelphia.

Montour, L.T., A.C. Macaulay, and N. Adelson. 1989. 'Diabetes Mellitus in

Mohawks of Kahnawake, PQ: A Clinical and Epidemiologic Description.' *Canadian Medical Association Journal* 141:549–52.

Mooney, J. 1928. 'The Aboriginal Population of America North of Mexico.' In J.R Swanton, ed., *Smithsonian Miscellaneous Collections* 80(7). Washington, D.C.: Smithsonian Institution.

Moore, M., H. Forbes, and L. Henderson. 1990. 'The Provision of Primary Health Services under Band Control: The Montreal Lake Case.' *Native Studies Review* 6(1):153–64.

Moore, P.E. 1946. 'Indian Health Services.' *Canadian Journal of Public Health* 37:140–2.

– 1956. 'Medical Care of Canada's Indians and Eskimos.' *Canadian Journal of Public Health* 47(6):227–36.

– 1974. 'The Modern Medicine Man.' In M. Van Steensel, ed., *People of Light and Dark*, 132–6. Ottawa: Department of Indian Affairs and Northern Development.

Moore, P.E., H.D. Kruse, F.F. Tisdall, and R.S. Corrigan. 1946. 'Medical Survey of Nutrition among the Northern Manitoba Indian.' *Canadian Medical Association Journal* 54:223–33.

Morice, A. 1900–1. 'Dene Surgery.' *Transactions of the Canadian Institute* 7:15–27.

Morris, A. 1880. *The Treaties of Canada with the Indians*. Repr. 1979. Toronto: Coles.

Morrison, R.B., and C.B.Wilson. 2004. *Native Peoples: The Canadian Experience*. Toronto: Oxford University Press.

Morrison, W. 1985. *Showing the Flag: The Mounted Police and Canadian Sovereignty in the North, 1894–1925*. Vancouver: University of British Columbia Press.

Morse, S.S. 1993. 'Examining the Origins of Emerging Viruses.' In S.J. Morse, ed., *Emerging Viruses*, 10–28. Oxford: Oxford University Press.

Muckle, G., P. Ayotte, E. Dewailly, S.W. Jacobson, and J.L. Jacobson. 2001. 'Prenatal Exposure of the Northern Quebec Inuit Infants to Environmental Contaminants.' *Environmental Health Perspectives* 109:1291–9.

Mulcahy, G., and Y. Lunham-Armstrong. 1998. 'A First Nations Approach to Healing.' In S. Madu and P. Baguma, eds, *Quest for Psychotherapy in Modern Africa*, 240–56. Sovenga, South Africa: UNIN Press.

Murray, R. 1990. *Future Directions for Health Care in Saskatchewan. Report of the Saskatchewan Commission on Directions in Health Care*. Regina: Government of Saskatchewan.

Myers, T., M.C. Liviana, R. Cockerill, W.M. Victor, and S.L. Bullock. 1993. *Ontario First Nations AIDS and Health Lifestyle Survey*. Toronto: University of Toronto, Department of Health Administration.

Nabigon, H., and A.-M. Mawhiney. 1996. 'Aboriginal Theory: A Cree Medicine

Wheel Guide for Healing First Nations.' In F. Turner, ed., *Social Work Treatment: Interlocking Theoretical Approaches*, 4th ed., 18–38. New York: Free Press.

National Aboriginal Health Organization (NAHO). 2004a. *First Nations and Inuit Regional Health Surveys, 1997: A Synthesis of the National and Regional Reports*. Ottawa: NAHO.

– 2004b. *Preliminary Findings of the First Nations Regional Longitudinal Health Survey (RHS) 2002–03: Adult Survey*. Ottawa: NAHO.

– 2004c. *What First Nations Think about Their Health and Health Care: The National Aboriginal Health Organization's Public Opinion Poll on First Nations Health and Health Care in Canada*. Ottawa: NAHO.

Neel, J.V., A.B. Weder, and S. Julius. 1998. 'Type II Diabetes, Essential Hypertension, and Obesity as a "Syndrome of Impaired Genetic Homeostasis": The "Thrifty Genotype" Hypothesis Enters the 21st Century.' *Perspectives in Biology and Medicine* 42:44–74.

Newbold, K.B. 1997. 'Aboriginal Physician Use in Canada: Location, Orientation and Identity.' *Health Economics* 6:197–207.

Newman, M.T. 1976. 'Aboriginal New World Epidemiology and Medical Care, and the Impact of Old World Disease Imports.' *American Journal of Physical Anthropology* 45:667–72.

Norris, M.J. 1990. 'The Demography of Aboriginal People in Canada.' In S.S. Halli, F. Trovato, and L. Driedger, eds, *Ethnic Demography: Canadian Immigrant, Racial and Cultural Variations*, 33–59. Ottawa: Carleton University Press.

Northwest Territories. 2004. *Summary Report:2002 NWT School Tobacco Survey*. Yellowknife: Government of the Northwest Territories.

Noymer, A., and M. Garenne. 2003. 'Long-Term Effects of the 1918 "Spanish" Influenza Epidemic on Sex Differentials of Mortality in the USA: Exploratory Findings from Historical Data.' In H. Phillips and D. Killingray, eds, *The Spanish Influenza Pandemic of 1918–19: New Perspectives*, 202–17. London: Routledge.

Nunavut Department of Health and Social Services. 2004. *Nunavut Report on Comparable Health Indicators*. Iqaluit: Department of Health and Social Services.

Ogborn, M.R., L. Hamiwka, E. Orrbine, D.S. Newburg, A. Sharma, P.N. McLaine, P. Orr, and P. Rowe. 1998. 'Renal Function in Inuit Survivors of Epidemic Hemolytic-Uremic Syndrome.' *Pediatric Nephrology* 12:485–8.

Omran, A.R. 1971. 'The Epidemiological Transition: A Theory of the Epidemiology of Population Change.' *Millbank Memorial Fund Quarterly* 49:509–38.

O'Neil, J.D. 1985. 'Community Control over Health Problems: Alcohol Prohibition in a Canadian Inuit Village.' In R. Fortuine, ed., *Circumpolar Health 84: Proceedings of the 6th International Symposium*, 340–3. Seattle: University of Washington Press.

– 1986. 'The Politics of Health in the Fourth World: A Northern Canadian Example.' *Human Organization* 45:119–28.

– 1988. 'Referrals to Traditional Healers: The Role of Medical Interpreters.' In D. Young, ed., *Health Care Issues in the Canadian North*, 29–38. Edmonton: Boreal Institute for Northern Studies.

– 1990. 'The Impact of Devolution on Health Services in the Baffin Region, NWT: A Case Study.' In G. Dacks, ed., *Devolution and Constitutional Development in the Canadian North*, 157–93. Ottawa: Carleton University Press.

– 1993. 'Aboriginal Health Policy for the Next Century: A Discussion Paper for the Royal Commission on Aboriginal Peoples.' In Royal Commission on Aboriginal Peoples, *The Path to Healing: Report of the National Round Table on Aboriginal Health and Social Issues*. Ottawa: Royal Commission on Aboriginal Peoples.

Ontario Ministry of Health. 1994. *New Directions: Aboriginal Health Policy for Ontario*. Toronto: Ontario Ministry of Health.

Oosten, J.G. 1986. 'Male and Female in Inuit Shamanism.' *Etudes Inuit Studies* 10(1–2):115–31.

Ortner, D.J. 1992. 'Skeletal Paleopathology: Probabilities, Possibilities, and Impossibilities.' In J.W. Verano and D.H. Ubelaker, eds, *Disease and Demography in the Americas*, 5–13. Washington, D.C.: Smithsonian Institution Press.

Osgood, C. 1931. *The Ethnography of the Great Bear Lake Indians*. Bulletin No. 70. Ottawa: National Museum of Canada.

– 1936. *Contributions to the Ethnography of the Kutchin*. New Haven: Yale University Press.

Pálfi, G., O. Dutour, J. Deák, and I. Hutás, eds. 1999. *Tuberculosis Past and Present*. Budapest: Golden Book Publisher Ltd, Tuberculosis Foundation.

Palkovich, A. 1981. 'Demography and Disease Patterns in a Protohistoric Plains Group: A Study of the Mobridge Site (39 WW 1).' *Plains Anthropologist* 26 (Memoir 17):71–84.

Pastore, R. 1987. 'Fishermen, Furriers, and Beothuks: The Economy of Extinction.' *Man in the Northeast* 33:47–62.

– 1989. 'The Collapse of the Beothuk World.' *Acadiensis* 19(1):52–71.

Patterson, D.K. 1984. *A Diachronic Study of Dental Palaeopathology and Attritional Status of Prehistoric Ontario Pre-Iroquois and Iroquois Populations*. Mercury Series, Archaeological Survey of Canada Paper 122. Ottawa: National Museum of Man.

Peart, A.F., and F.P.Nagler. 1954. 'Measles in the Canadian Arctic, 1952.' *Canadian Journal of Public Health* 45:146–57.

Pelz, M., H. Merskey, C. Brant, P.G.R. Patterson, and G.F.D. Heseltine. 1981.

'Clinical Data from a Psychiatric Service to a Group of Native People.' *Canadian Journal of Psychiatry* 26:345–8.

Penner, Keith (Chair). 1983. *Indian Self-Government in Canada: Report of the Special Committee on Indian Self-Government*. Ottawa: House of Commons.

Peterson, J., and J.S.H. Brown, eds. 1985. *The New People: Being and Becoming Métis in North America*. Winnipeg: University of Manitoba Press.

Pettipas, K. 1994. *Severing the Ties That Bind: Government Repression of Indigenous Religious Ceremonies on the Prairies*. Winnipeg: University of Manitoba Press.

Pfeiffer, S. 1984. 'Paleopathology in an Iroquoian Ossuary, with Special Reference to Tuberculosis.' *American Journal of Physical Anthropology* 65:181–9.

– 1986. 'Morbidity and Mortality in the Uxbridge Ossuary.' *Canadian Journal of Anthropology* 5(2):23–31.

– 1991. 'Is Paleopathology a Relevant Predictor of Contemporary Health Patterns?' In D.J. Ortner and A.C. Aufderheide, eds, *Human Paleopathology: Current Syntheses and Future Options*, 12–17. Washington, D.C.: Smithsonian Institution Press.

– 2003. 'The Health of the Moatfield People as Reflected in Palaeopathological Features.' In R.F. Williamson and S. Pfeiffer, eds, *Bones of the Ancestors: The Archaeology and Osteobiography of the Moatfield Ossuary*, 189–204. Mercury Series, Archaeology Paper 163. Ottawa: Canadian Museum of Civilization.

Pfeiffer, S., and S.I. Fairgrieve. 1994. 'Evidence from Ossuaries: The Effect of Contact on the Health of Iroquoians.' In C.S. Larsen and G.R. Milner, eds, *In the Wake of Contact: Biological Responses to Conquest*, 47–61. New York: Wiley-Liss.

Pfeiffer, S., and P. King. 1983. 'Cortical Bone Formation and Diet among Protohistoric Iroquoians.' *American Journal of Physical Anthropology* 60:23–8.

Pfeiffer, S., and R.F. Williamson. 2003. 'Summary and Conclusions. What We Learned from Studying Our Ancestors.' In R.F. Williamson and S. Pfeiffer, eds, *Bones of the Ancestors: The Archaeology and Osteobiography of the Moatfield Ossuary*, 333–48. Mercury Series. Archaeology Paper 163. Ottawa: Canadian Museum of Civilization.

Piché, V., and M.V. George. 1973. 'Estimates of Vital Rates for the Canadian Indians, 1960–1970.' *Demography* 10(3):367–82.

Pocklington, T. 1991. *The Government and Politics of the Alberta Métis Settlements*. Regina: Canadian Plains Research Centre.

Potvin, L., S. Desrosiers, M. Trifonopoulos, N. Leduc, M. Rivard, A.C. Macaulay, and G. Paradis. 1999. 'Anthropometric Characteristics of Mohawk Children Aged 6–11 Years: A Population Perspective.' *Journal of the American Dietetic Association* 99:955–61.

Prat, J.G.I., and S.M.F. de Souza. 2003. 'Prehistoric Tuberculosis in America:

Adding Comments to a Literature Review.' *Mem Inst Oswaldo Cruz, Rio de Janerio* 98 (Suppl. 1):151–9.

Press, I. 1969. 'Urban Illness: Physicians, Curers and Dual Use in Bogota.' *Journal of Health and Social Behavior* 10:209–18.

Preston, R. 1975. 'Cree Narrative: Expressing the Personal Meanings of Events.' Canadian Ethnology Service Paper No. 30. Ottawa: National Museums of Canada.

– 1986. 'Twentieth-Century Transformations of the West Coast Cree.' In W. Cowan, ed., *Proceedings of the Seventeenth Annual Algonquian Conference*, 238–51. Ottawa: Carleton University.

Price, J.A. 1975. 'An Applied Analysis of North American Indian Drinking Patterns.' *Human Organization* 34:17–26.

Price, W.A. 1934. 'Why Dental Caries with Modern Civilizations? VIII. Field Studies on Modernized Indians in Twenty Communities of the Canadian and Alaskan Pacific Coast.' *Dental Digest* 40:81–4.

Proulx, J., and S. Perrault. 2000. *No Place for Violence: Canadian Aboriginal Alternatives*. Halifax: Fernwood.

Public Health Agency of Canada. 2004a. *HIV/AIDS among Aboriginal Peoples in Canada: A Continuing Concern*. Ottawa: Public Health Agency of Canada.

– 2004b. *Tuberculosis in Canada 2002*. Ottawa: Public Health Agency of Canada.

Ramenofsky, A.F. 1987. *Vectors of Death: The Archaeology of European Contact*. Albuquerque: University of New Mexico Press.

Ramenofsky, A.F., A.K. Wilbur, and A.C. Stone. 2003. 'Native American Disease History: Past, Present and Future Directions.' *World Archaeology* 35(2):241–57.

Ray, A.J. 1974. *Indians in the Fur Trade: Their Role as Hunters, Trappers and Middlemen in the Lands Southwest of Hudson Bay, 1660–1870*. Toronto: University of Toronto Press.

– 1975. 'Smallpox: The Epidemic of 1837–38.' *The Beaver* 306(2):8–13.

– 1976. 'Diffusion of Diseases in the Western Interior of Canada, 1830–1950.' *Geographical Review* 66(2):139–57.

– 1984. 'William Todd: Doctor and Trader for the Hudson's Bay Company, 1816–51.' *Prairie Forum* 9(1):13–26.

– 1990. *The Canadian Fur Trade in the Industrial Age*. Toronto: University of Toronto Press.

– 1996. *I Have Been Here since the World Began: An Illustrated History of Canada's Native People*. Toronto: Lester Publishing Limited and Key Porter Books.

Ray, A., J. Miller, and F. Tough. 2000. *Bounty and Benevolence: A History of Saskatchewan Treaties*. Montreal: McGill-Queen's University Press.

RCAP. *See* Royal Commission on Aboriginal Peoples.

Read, J., and F.L. Strick. 1969. 'Medical Education and the Native Canadian: An

Example of Mutual Symbiosis.' *Canadian Medical Association Journal* 100:515–20.

Reading, J. 1996. *Eating Smoke: A Review of Non-Traditional Uses of Tobacco among Aboriginal People*. Ottawa: Health Canada.

Receiver General for Canada. Various years. *Public Accounts of Canada*. Ottawa.

Reed, T.E. 1985. 'Ethnic Differences in Alcohol Use, Abuse, and Sensitivity: A Review with Genetic Interpretation.' *Social Biology* 32:195–209.

Reed, T.E., H. Kalant, R.J. Gibbins, B.M. Kapur, and J.G. Rankin. 1976. 'Alcohol and Acetaldehyde Metabolism in Caucasians, Chinese and Amerinds.' *Canadian Medical Association Journal* 115:851–5.

Reff, D. 1991. *Disease, Depopulation and Culture Change in Northwestern New Spain, 1518–1764*. Salt Lake City: University of Utah Press.

Remington, G., and B.F. Hoffman. 1984. 'Gas Sniffing as a Form of Substance Abuse.' *Canadian Journal of Psychiatry* 29:31–5.

Rheinhard, K. 1992. 'Parasitology as an Interpretive Tool in Archaeology.' *American Antiquity* 57:231–45.

Rheinhard, K., J. Ambler, and M. McGuffie. 1985. 'Diet and Parasitism in Dust Devil Cave.' *American Antiquity* 50:819–24.

Rich, E., ed. 1938. *Journal of Occurrences in the Athabasca Department by George Simpson, 1820 and 1821, and Report*. London: Hudson's Bay Record Society.

– 1949. *James Isham's Observations on Hudson's Bay, 1743 and Notes and Observations on a Book Entitled 'A Voyage to Hudson's Bay in the Dobbs Galley, 1749.'* London: Hudson's Bay Record Society.

– 1951–2. Cumberland and Hudson House Journals, 1775–1782. London: Hudson's Bay Record Society.

Rideout, M., and R. Menzies. 1994. 'Factors Affecting Compliance with Preventive Treatment for Tuberculosis at Mistassini Lake, Quebec, Canada.' *Clinical and Investigative Medicine* 17:31–6.

Riley, T.J. 1993. 'Ascarids, American Indians, and the Modern World: Parasites and the Prehistoric Record of a Pharmacological Tradition.' *Perspectives in Biology and Medicine* 36:369–75.

Ritenbaugh, C., and C. Goodby. 1989. 'Beyond the Thrifty Gene: Metabolic Implications of Prehistoric Migration into the New World.' *Medical Anthropology* 11:227–36.

Ritzenthaler, R. 1963. 'Primitive Therapeutic Practices among the Wisconsin Chippewa.' In I. Galdston, ed., *Man's Image in Medicine and Anthropology*, 316–34. New York: International Universities Press.

Robb, J.C. 1988. 'Legal Impediments to Traditional Indian Medicine.' In D. Young, ed., *Health Care Issues in the Canadian North*, 134–9. Edmonton: Boreal Institute for Northern Studies.

Robinson, E.J. 1988. 'The Health of the James Bay Cree.' *Canadian Family Physician* 34:1606–13.

Robinson, E., Y. Gebre, J. Pickering, B. Petawabano, B. Superville, and C. Lavallee. 1995. 'Effect of Bush Living on Aboriginal Canadians of the Eastern James Bay Region with Non-Insulin-Dependent Diabetes Mellitus.' *Chronic Diseases in Canada* 16:144–8.

Robitaille, N., and R. Choiniere. 1985. *An Overview of Demographic and Socioeconomic Conditions of the Inuit in Canada*. Ottawa: Department of Indian Affairs and Northern Development, Research Branch, Corporate Policy.

Rode, A., and R.J. Shephard. 1992. *Fitness and Health of an Inuit Community: Years of Cultural Change*. Ottawa: Department of Indian Affairs and Northern Development, Circumpolar and Scientific Affairs Directorate, Publ. No. 92–05.

Rodriguez, S., E. Robinson, and K. Gray-Donald. 1999. 'Prevalence of Gestational Diabetes among James Bay Cree Women in Northern Quebec.' *Canadian Medical Association Journal* 160:1293–7.

Romaniuk, A., and V. Piché. 1972. 'Natality Estimates for the Canadian Indians by Stable Population Models, 1900–1969.' *Canadian Journal of Sociology and Anthropology* 9:1–20.

Rosenberg, T., O. Kendall, J.F. Blanchard, S. Martel, C. Wakelin, and M. Fast. 1997. 'Shigellosis on Indian Reserves in Manitoba, Canada: Its Relationship to Crowded Housing, Lack of Running Water, and Inadequate Sewage Disposal.' *American Journal of Public Health* 87:1547–51.

Ross, C.A., and B. Davis. 1986. 'Suicide and Parasuicide in a Northern Canadian Native Community.' *Canadian Journal of Psychiatry* 31:331–4.

Ross, W.G. 1977. 'Whaling and the Decline of Native Populations.' *Arctic Anthropology* 14(2):138–59.

– 1984. *An Arctic Whaling Diary: The Journal of Captain George Comer in Hudson Bay, 1903–1905*. Toronto: University of Toronto Press.

Roth, E. 1981. 'Sedentism and Changing Fertility Patterns in a Northern Athapascan Isolate.' *Journal of Human Evolution* 10:413–25.

Rothschild, B.M. 1992. 'Advances in Detecting Disease in Earlier Human Populations.' In S.R. Saunders and M.A. Katzenberg, eds, *Skeletal Biology of Past Peoples: Research Methods*, 131–52. New York: Wiley-Liss.

Rothschild, B.M., L.D. Martin, G. Lev, H. Bercovier, G.K. Bar-Gal, C. Greenblatt, H. Donoghue, M. Spigelman, and D. Brittain. 2001. '*Mycobacterium tuberculosis* Complex DNA from an Extinct Bison Dated 17,000 Years before the Present.' *Clinical Infectious Disease* 33:305–11.

Rowe, P.C., E. Orrbine, M. Ogborn, G.A. Wells, W. Winther, H. Lior, D. Manuel, and P.N. McLaine. 1998. 'Epidemic *Escherichia coli* 0157: H7 Gastroenteritis and Hemolytic-Uremic Syndrome in a Canadian Inuit Community: Intestinal Illness in Family Members as a Risk Factor.' *Journal of Pediatrics* 124:21–6.

Royal Commission on Aboriginal Peoples (RCAP). 1993. *The Path to Healing: Report of the National Round Table on Aboriginal Health and Social Issues.* Ottawa: Royal Commission on Aboriginal Peoples.

– 1995. *Choosing Life: Special Report on Suicide among Aboriginal People.* Ottawa: Royal Commission on Aboriginal Peoples.

– 1996. *Final Report.* Vol. 3. Ottawa: Royal Commission on Aboriginal Peoples.

Salisbury, R.F. 1986. *A Homeland for the Cree: Regional Development in James Bay, 1971–1981.* Montreal: McGill-Queen's University Press.

Salo, W.L., A.C. Aufderheide, J. Buikstra, and T.A. Holcomb. 1994. 'Identification of *Mycobacterium tuberculosis* DNA in a Pre-Columbian Peruvian Mummy.' *Proceedings of the National Academy of Sciences USA* 91:2091–4.

Salter, E.M. 1984. 'Skeletal Biology of Cumberland Sound, Baffin Island, N.W.T.' PhD diss., University of Toronto.

Sattenspiel, S. 2003. 'Infectious Diseases in the Historical Archives: A Modeling Approach.' In D.A. Herring and A.C. Swedlund, eds, *Human Biologists in the Archives*, 234–65. Cambridge: Cambridge University Press.

Saunders, S.R. 1988. *The MacPherson Site: Human Burials, a Preliminary Descriptive Report.* Hamilton: Department of Anthropology, McMaster University.

Saunders, S.R., and F.J. Melbye. 1990. 'Subadult Mortality and Skeletal Indicators of Health in Late Woodland Ontario Iroquois.' *Canadian Journal of Archaeology* 14:1–14.

Saunders, S.R., P.G. Ramsden, and D.A. Herring. 1992. 'Transformation and Disease: Precontact Ontario Iroquoians.' In J. Verano and D. Ubelaker, eds, *Disease and Demography in the America*, 117–26. Washington, D.C.: Smithsonian Institution Press.

Schaefer, O. 1959. 'Medical Observations and Problems in the Canadian Arctic.' *Canadian Medical Association Journal* 81:248–53.

– 1977. 'Are Eskimos More or Less Obese Than Other Canadians? A Comparison of Skinfold Thickness and Ponderal Index in Canadian Eskimos.' *American Journal of Clinical Nutrition* 30:1623–8.

Schaefer, O., J.A. Hildes, L.M. Medd, and D.G. Cameron. 1975. 'The Changing Pattern of Neoplastic Disease in Canadian Eskimos.' *Canadian Medical Association Journal* 112:1399–404.

Schaeffer, C.E. 1969. *Blackfoot Shaking Tent.* Occasional Paper No. 5. Calgary: Glenbow Museum.

Schindler, D.L. 1985. 'Anthropology in the Arctic: A Critique of Racial Typology and Normative Theory.' *Current Anthropology* 26:475–500.

Scholtissek, C. 1994. 'Source for Influenza Pandemics.' *European Journal of Epidemiology* 4(10):455–8.

Schurr, T.G., and S.T. Sherry. 2004. 'Mitochondrial DNA and Y Chromosome Diversity and the Peopling of the Americas: Evolutionary and Demographic Evidence.' *American Journal of Human Biology* 16:420–39.

Schwarcz, H.P., P.J. Melbye, M.A. Katzenberg, and M. Knyf. 1985. 'Stable Isotopes in Human Skeletons of Southern Ontario: Reconstructing Paleodiet.' *Journal of Archaeological Science* 12:187–206.

Schwartz, L. 1969. 'The Hierarchy of Resort in Curative Practices: The Admiralty Islands, Melanesia.' *Journal of Health and Social Behavior* 10:201–9.

Scott, K.A., and A.M. Myers. 1988. 'Impact of Fitness Training on Native Adolescents' Self-Evaluations and Substance Use.' *Canadian Journal of Public Health* 79:424–9.

Scott-McKay-Bain Health Panel. 1989a. *Companion Documents*. Toronto.

– 1989b. *From Here to There, Steps Along the Way: Achieving Health for All in the Sioux Lookout Zone*. Toronto.

Seaby, S. 1983. *Native Healer Program, Lake of the Woods Hospital, Kenora. Evaluation Report* (unpublished).

Shadomy, H. 1981. 'The Differential Diagnosis of Various Fungal Pathogens and Tuberculosis in the Prehistoric Indians.' In J.E. Buikstra, ed., *Prehistoric Tuberculosis in the Americas*, 25–34. Evanston, Ill.: Northwestern University Archaeological Program.

Shah, B.R., J.E. Hux, and B. Zinman. 2000. 'Increasing Rates of Ischemic Heart Disease in the Native Population of Ontario, Canada.' *Archives of Internal Medicine* 160:1862–6.

Shaw, W. 1923. 'Medical Experiences among the Kwquithlih Indians along Discovery Passage.' *Canadian Medical Association Journal* 13:657–9.

Sherley-Spiers, S.K. 1989. 'Dakota Perceptions of Clinical Encounters with Western Health Care Providers.' *Native Studies Review* 5(1):41–51.

Silver, S.M., and J.P. Wilson. 1988. 'Native American Healing and Purification for War Stress.' In J.P. Wilson, Z. Harel, and B. Kahana, eds, *Human Adaptation to Extreme Stress: From the Holocaust to Vietnam*, 337–55. New York: Plenum Press.

Singer, M., and S. Clair. 2003. 'Syndemics and Public Health: Reconceptualizing Disease in Bio-Social Context.' *Medical Anthropology Quarterly* 17(4):423–41.

Skinner, M., and A.H. Goodman. 1992. 'Anthropological Uses of Developmental Defects of Enamel.' In S.R. Saunders and M.A. Katzenberg, eds, *Skeletal Biology of Past Peoples: Research Methods*, 153–74. New York: Wiley-Liss.

Sluman, N., and J. Goodwill. 1982. *John Tootoosis: Biography of a Cree Leader*. Ottawa: Golden Dog Press.

Smith, D. 1973. *Inkonze: Magico-Religious Beliefs of Contact-Traditional Chipewyan Trading at Fort Resolution, NWT, Canada.* Ethnology Division Paper No. 6. Ottawa: National Museum of Canada.

Smith, D.G. 1993. 'The Emergence of "Eskimo Status": An Examination of the "Eskimo Disk List System" and Its Social Consequences, 1925–1970.' In J.B. Waldram and Noel Dyck, eds, *Anthropology, Public Policy and Native Peoples in Canada*, 41–74. Montreal: McGill-Queen's University Press.

Snow, D. 1992. 'Diseases and Population Decline in the Northeast.' In J.W. Verano and D.H. Ubelaker, eds, *Disease and Demography in the Americas*, 177–86. Washington, D.C.: Smithsonian Institution Press.

Snow, D., and K. Lanphear. 1987. 'European Contact and Indian Depopulation in the Northeast: The Timing of the First Epidemics.' *Ethnohistory* 35:15–35.

Southern, B. 1990. 'An Assessment of Bone Quality and Age-Related Patterns of Bone Loss among Iroquoian Populations.' Paper presented at the Canadian Archaeological Association Meeting, Whitehorse, Yukon.

Southesk, Earl of. 1875. *Saskatchewan and the Rocky Mountains. A Diary and Narrative of Travel, Sport, and Adventure during a Journey through the Hudson's Bay Company's Territories, in 1859–1860.* Toronto: James Campbell and Son.

Speck, D. Culhane. *See* Culhane Speck.

Starna, W.A., G.R. Hammell, and W.L. Butts. 1984. 'Northern Iroquoian Horticulture and Insect Infestation: A Cause for Village Removal.' *Ethnohistory* 31(3):197–207.

Statistics Canada. 1993a. *Age and Sex:1991 Aboriginal Data.* Ottawa: Statistics Canada, Cat. No. 94–327.

– 1993b. *Language, Tradition, Health, Lifestyle and Social Issues: 1991 Aboriginal Peoples Survey.* Ottawa: Statistics Canada, Cat. No. 89–533.

– 1993c. *Schooling, Work and Related Activities, Income, Expenses and Mobility:1991 Aboriginal Peoples Survey.* Ottawa: Statistics Canada, Cat. No. 89–534.

– 2001. *Aboriginal Peoples in Canada.* Canadian Centre for Justice Statistics Profile Series. Ottawa: Statistics Canada.

– 2003. *Aboriginal Peoples of Canada: A Demographic Profile.* 2001 Census: Analysis Series. Ottawa, Statistics Canada.

– 2004. *Comparable Health Indicators – Canada, Provinces, and Territories.* Ottawa: Statistics Canada, Cat. No. 82, 401–XIE.

Stead, W.W. 1997. 'The Origin and Erratic Global Spread of Tuberculosis: How the Past Explains the Present and Is the Key to the Future.' *Clinics in Chest Medicine* 18(1):65–77.

Steckel, R.H., and J.C. Rose. 2002a. 'Conclusions.' In R.H. Steckel and J.C. Rose, eds, *The Backbone of History: Health and Nutrition in the Western Hemisphere*, 583–9. Cambridge: Cambridge University Press.

– 2002b. 'Introduction.' In R.H. Steckel and J.C. Rose, eds, *The Backbone of History: Health and Nutrition in the Western Hemisphere*, 3–10. Cambridge: Cambridge University Press.

– 2002c. 'Patterns of Health in the Western Hemisphere.' In R.H. Steckel and J.C. Rose, eds, *The Backbone of History: Health and Nutrition in the Western Hemisphere*, 563–79. Cambridge: Cambridge University Press.

Steckel, R.H., and J.C. Rose, eds. 2002d. *The Backbone of History: Health and Nutrition in the Western Hemisphere*. Cambridge: Cambridge University Press.

Steckel, R.H., P.W. Sciulli, and J.C. Rose. 2002. 'A Health Index from Skeletal Remains.' In R.H. Steckel and J.C. Rose, eds, *The Backbone of History: Health and Nutrition in the Western Hemisphere*, 61–93. Cambridge: Cambridge University Press.

Steinbock, R. 1976. *Paleopathological Diagnosis and Interpretation*. Springfield, Ill.: Charles C. Thomas.

Stephens, M. 1991. 'The Special Premedical Studies Program – Review of Ten Years of Experience.' In B. Postl et al., eds, *Circumpolar Health 90: Proceedings of the 8th International Congress*, 134–7. Winnipeg: University of Manitoba Press.

Stephens, M.C., P. Mirwaldt, and S. Matusik. 1998. 'Premedical Program Effective in Increasing Admissions to Health Professional Schools.' *International Journal of Circumpolar Health* 57 (Suppl. 1):87–90.

Stewart, D.A. 1936. 'The Red Man and the White Plague.' *Canadian Medical Association Journal* 35:674–6.

Stewart, T.D. 1932. 'The Vertebral Column of the Eskimos.' *American Journal of Physical Anthropology* 17:123–36.

– 1973. *The People of America*. New York: Charles Scribner's Sons.

– 1979. 'Patterning of Skeletal Pathologies and Epidemiology.' In William S. Laughlin and Albert B. Harper, eds, *The First Americans: Origins, Affinities, and Adaptations*, 257–74. New York: Gustav Fischer.

Stock, J., and Willmore, K. 2003. 'Body Size, Bone Mass and Biomechanical Analyses of the Adult Post-Cranial Remains.' In R.F. Williamson and S. Pfeiffer, eds, *Bones of the Ancestors: The Archaeological and Osteobiography of the Moatfield Ossuary*, 309–32. Mercury Series. Archaeology Paper 163. Ottawa: Canadian Museum of Civilization.

Stone, E.L. 1926. 'Health and Disease at the Norway House Indian Agency.' Repr. in *Native Studies Review* 5(1):237–56 (1989).

– 1935. 'Canadian Indian Medical Services.' *Canadian Medical Association Journal* 33:82–5.

Storey, R. 1992. *Life and Death in the Ancient City of Teotihuacan: A Modern Paleodemographic Synthesis*. Tuscaloosa: University of Alabama Press.

Stuart-Macadam, P. 1992. 'Porotic Hyperostosis: A New Perspective.' *American Journal of Physical Anthropology* 87:39–47.

Suttles, W. 1968. 'Coping with Abundance: Subsistence on the Northwest Coast.' In R.B. Lee and I. DeVore, eds, *Man the Hunter*, 56–68. Chicago: Aldine.

Swartz, L. 1988. 'Healing Properties of the Sweatlodge Ceremony.' In D.E. Young, ed., *Health Care Issues in the Canadian North*, 102–7. Edmonton: Boreal Institute for Northern Studies.

Szathmary, E.J. 1985. 'Peopling of North America: Clues from Genetic Studies.' In R. Kirk and E. Szathmary, eds, *Out of Asia: Peopling of the Americas and the Pacific*, 79–104. Canberra: The Journal of Pacific History.

– 1990. 'Diabetes in Amerindian Populations: The Dogrib Studies.' In G. Armelagos and A.C. Swedlund, eds, *Health and Disease of Populations in Transition*, 75–103. New York: Bergin and Garvey.

– 1993. 'Genetics of Aboriginal North Americans.' *Evolutionary Anthropology* 1:202–20.

– 1994. 'Non-Insulin Dependent Diabetes Mellitus among Aboriginal North Americans.' *Annual Review of Anthropology* 23:457–82.

Szathmary, E.J., and N. Holt. 1983. 'Hyperglycemia in Dogrib Indians of the N.W.T, Canada: Association with Age and a Centripetal Distribution of Body Fat.' *Human Biology* 55:493–515.

Szathmary, E.J., and N.S. Ossenberg. 1978. 'Are the Biological Differences between North American Indians and Eskimos Truly Profound?' *Current Anthropology* 19:673–701.

Thistle, P.C. 1986. *Indian-European Trade Relations in the Lower Saskatchewan River Region to 1840*. Winnipeg: University of Manitoba Press.

Thornton, R. 1987. *American Indian Holocaust and Survival: A Population History since 1492*. Norman: University of Oklahoma Press.

Thornton, R., T. Miller, and J. Warren. 1991. 'American Indian Population Recovery Following Smallpox Epidemics.' *American Anthropologist* 93(1):28–45.

Thorpe, E.L.M. 1989. *The Social Histories of Smallpox and Tuberculosis in Canada*. University of Manitoba Anthropology Papers, No. 30. Winnipeg: University of Manitoba.

Thouez, J.-P., P. Foggin, and A. Rannou. 1990. 'Correlates of Health-Care Use: Inuit and Cree of Northern Quebec.' *Social Science and Medicine* 30(1):25–34.

Tillson, T. 2002. 'Acknowledging Native Healing Tradition: Medicine Wheel Offers Sacred Approach to Treating Addiction.' *Journal of Addiction and Mental Health* 5(2):13.

Timpson, J. 1984. 'Indian Mental Health: Changes in the Delivery of Care in Northwestern Ontario.' *Canadian Journal of Psychiatry* 29:234–41.

Tisdall, F.F., and E.C. Robertson. 1948. 'Voyage of the Medicine Men.' *The Beaver* 28:42–6.

Titley, E. 1986. *A Narrow Vision: Duncan Campbell Scott and the Administration of Indian Affairs in Canada*. Vancouver: University of British Columbia Press.

Titley, K.C. 1973. 'Sioux Lookout Dental Care Project: A Progress Report.' *Journal of the Canadian Dental Association* 39:793–6.

Titley, K.C., and D.H. Bedard. 1986. 'An Evaluation of a Dental Care Program for Indian Children in the Community of Sandy Lake: Sioux Lookout Zone, 1973–1983.' *Journal of the Canadian Dental Association* 52:923–8.

Tjepkema, M. 2002. 'The Health of the Off-Reserve Aboriginal Population.' *Health Reports* 13 (Suppl.):73–88.

Tonelli, M., B. Hemmelgarn, B. Manns, G. Pylypchuk, C. Bohm, K. Yeates, S. Gourishankar, and J.S. Gill. 2004. 'Death and Renal Transplantation among Aboriginal People Undergoing Dialysis.' *Canadian Medical Association Journal* 171:577–82.

Torbert, K.W. 1990. 'Dental Therapists in Canada.' *Canadian Journal of Community Dentistry* (February):10–11.

Travers, K.D. 1995. 'Using Qualitative Research to Understand the Sociocultural Origins of Diabetes among Cape Breton Mi'kmaq.' *Chronic Diseases in Canada* 16:140–3.

Trigger, B.G. 1985. *Natives and Newcomers: Canada's 'Heroic Age' Reconsidered*. Montreal: McGill-Queen's University Press.

Triggs-Raine, B.L., R.D. Kirkpatrick, S.L. Kelly, L.D. Norwuay, P.A. Cattini, K. Yamagata, A.J.G. Hanley, B. Zinman, S.B. Harris, P.H. Barrett, and R.A. Hegele. 2002. 'HNF-1α G319S, a Transactivation-Deficient Mutant, Is Associated with Altered Dynamics of Diabetes Onset in an Oji-Cree Community.' *Proceedings of the National Academy of Sciences USA* 99:4614–9.

Trimble, J., S. Manson, N. Dinges, and B. Medicine. 1984. 'American Indian Concepts of Mental Health: Reflections and Directions.' In P. Pederson, N. Sartorius, and A. Marsella, eds, *Mental Health Services: The Cross-Cultural Context*, 199–220. Beverly Hills: Sage.

Tuck, J.A. 1976. *Newfoundland and Labrador Prehistory*. Ottawa: National Museum of Man.

Tuck, J.A., and R.T. Pastore. 1985. 'A Nice Place to Visit, but ... Prehistoric Human Extinctions on the Island of Newfoundland.' *Canadian Journal of Archaeology* 9(1):69–80.

Turner, D.G., II. 1985. 'The Dental Search for Native American Origins.' In R. Kirk and E. Szathmary, eds, *Out of Asia: Peopling of the Americas and the Pacific*, 31–78. Canberra: The Journal of Pacific History.

Ubelaker, D.H. 1976. 'Prehistoric New World Population Size: Historical Review and Current Appraisal of North American Estimates.' *American Journal of Physical Anthropology* 45:661–5.

– 1988. 'North American Indian Population Size, AD 1500 to 1985.' *American Journal of Physical Anthropology* 77:289–94.

– 1992. 'North American Indian Population Size: Changing Perspectives.' In J.W. Verano and D.H. Ubelaker, eds, *Disease and Demography in the Americas*, 169–76. Washington, D.C.: Smithsonian Institution Press.

Upton, L. 1977. 'The Extermination of the Beothuks of Newfoundland.' *Canadian Historical Review* 58(2):133–53.

van der Merwe, N.J., S. Pfeiffer, and R.F. Williamson. 2003. 'The Diet of the Moatfield People.' In R.F. Williamson and S. Pfeiffer, eds, *Bones of the Ancestors: The Archaeology and Osteobiography of the Moatfield Ossuary*, 205–22. Mercury Series. Archaeology Paper 163. Ottawa: Canadian Museum of Civilization.

Van Kirk, S. 1980. *'Many Tender Ties': Women in Fur-Trade Society, 1670–1870*. Winnipeg: Watson and Dwyer.

Van Oostdam, J., A. Gilman, E. Dewailly, P. Usher, B. Wheatley, H.V. Kuhnlein, S. Neve, J. Walker, B. Tracy, M. Feeley, V. Jerome, and B. Kwavnick. 1999. 'Human Health Implications of Environmental Contaminants in Arctic Canada: A Review.' *Science of the Total Environment* 230:1–82.

van Rooyen, C. 1968. 'Serologic Surveys of Arctic Populations and Some Virus Diseases of Interest.' *Archives of Environmental Health* 17:547–54.

Vanast, W.J. 1991a. 'The Death of Jennie Kanajuq: Tuberculosis, Religious Competition and Cultural Conflict in Coppermine, 1929–31.' *Etudes Inuit Studies* 15(1):75–104.

– 1991b. '"Hastening the Day of Extinction": Canada, Quebec, and the Medical Care of Ungava's Inuit, 1867–1967.' *Etudes Inuit Studies* 15(2):55–84.

Vecsey, C. 1983. *Traditional Ojibwa Religion and Its Historical Changes*. Philadelphia: American Philosophical Society.

Verano, J.W., and D.H. Ubelaker, eds. 1992. *Disease and Demography in the Americas*. Washington, D.C.: Smithsonian Institution Press.

Vivian, R.P., C. McMillan, and P.E. Moore. 1948. 'The Nutrition and Health of the James Bay Indian.' *Canadian Medical Association Journal* 59:505–18.

Vizenor, G. 1990. *Crossbloods: Bone Courts, Bingo, and Other Reports*. Minneapolis: University of Minnesota Press.

Vogel, V. 1970. *American Indian Medicine*. Norman: University of Oklahoma Press.

Von Hunnius, T. 2004. 'Applying Skeletal, Histological and Molecular Techniques to Syphilitic Skeletal Remains from the Past.' PhD diss., McMaster University, Hamilton.

Waldram, J.B. 1990a. 'Access to Traditional Medicine in a Western Canadian City.' *Medical Anthropology* 12:325–48.

– 1990b. 'The Persistence of Traditional Medicine in Urban Areas: The Case of Canada's Indians.' *American Indian and Alaska Native Mental Health Research* 4(1):9–29.

– 1990c. 'Physician Utilization and Urban Native People in Saskatoon, Canada.' *Social Science and Medicine* 30(5):579–89.

– 1993. 'Aboriginal Spirituality: Symbolic Healing in Canadian Prisons.' *Culture, Medicine and Psychiatry* 17:345–62.

– 1997. *The Way of the Pipe: Aboriginal Spirituality and Symbolic Healing in Canadian Prisons.* Peterborough, Ont.: Broadview Press.

– 2000. 'The Efficacy of Traditional Medicine: Current Theoretical and Methodological Issues.' *Medical Anthropology Quarterly* 14(4):306–625.

– 2004. *Revenge of the Windigo: The Construction of the Mind and Mental Health of North American Aboriginal Peoples.* Toronto: University of Toronto Press.

Waldram, J.B., J. Whiting, B. Habbick, and N. Kordner. 2000. 'Cultural Understandings and the Use of Traditional Medicine among Urban Aboriginal People with Diabetes in Saskatoon, Canada.' *Canadian Journal of Diabetes Care* 24(2):31–8.

Wall, D. 1926. *Report of Medical Service to Indians Located along the Line of the Canadian National Railways from Cochrane, Ont., to La Tuque, Quebec, June to October.* Repr. in *Native Studies Review* 5(1):257–75 (1989).

Warry, W. 1998. *Unfinished Dreams: Community Healing and the Reality of Aboriginal Self-Government.* Toronto: University of Toronto Press.

Warwick, G. 1984. *Reconstructing Ontario Iroquoian Village Organization.* Mercury Series, Archaeological Survey of Canada Papers 124. Ottawa: National Museum of Man.

Way, J.E., III. 1978. 'An Osteological Analysis of a Late Thule / Early Historic Labrador Eskimo Population.' PhD diss., University of Toronto.

Weaver, S.M. 1972. *Medicine and Politics among the Grand River Iroquois: A Study of the Non-Conservatives.* Ottawa: National Museums of Canada.

– 1981. *Making Canadian Indian Policy: The Hidden Agenda, 1968–1970.* Toronto: University of Toronto Press.

– 1986. 'Indian Policy in the New Conservative Government, Part I: The Nielson Task Force of 1985.' *Native Studies Review* 2(1):1–43.

Weiser, J. 1999. 'Adapting Traditional Healing Practices.' *AIDS-Action* 46:7.

Welsch, R. 1983. 'Traditional Medicine and Western Medical Options among the Ningerum of Papua-New Guinea.' In L. Romanucci-Ross, D. Moerman, and L. Tancredi, eds, *The Anthropology of Medicine: From Culture to Method*, 32–53. New York: Praeger.

Wenman, W.M., M.R. Jofres, L.V. Tataryn, and the Edmonton Perinatal Infection Group. 2004. 'A Prospective Cohort Study of Pregnancy Risk Factors and Birth Outcomes in Aboriginal Women.' *Canadian Medical Association Journal* 171:585–9.

Wheatley, B., and G. Paradis. 1996. 'Balancing Human Exposure, Risk and Reality: Questions Raised by the Canadian Aboriginal Methylmercury Program.' *Neurotoxicology* 17:241–9.

Wherrett, G.J. 1965. *Tuberculosis in Canada*. Ottawa: Queen's Printer.

White, J.P., P.S. Maxim, and P.C. Whitehead. 2000. *Social Capital, Social Cohesion and Population Outcomes in Canada's First Nations Communities*. Report No. 00–7. London, Ont.: Population Studies Centre, University of Western Ontario.

Whitmore, T. 1992. *Disease and Death in Early Colonial Mexico: Simulating Amerindian Depopulation*. Boulder, Colo.: Westview Press.

Widmer, L., and A.J. Perzigian. 1981. 'Skeletal Lesions in Prehistoric Populations from North America.' In J.E. Buikstra, ed., *Prehistoric Tuberculosis in the Americas*, 99–113. Evanston, Ill.: Northwestern University Archaeological Program.

Wiebe, J. 1970. 'Health Service Delivery Problems in Northern Canada.' *Canadian Journal of Public Health* 61:481–7.

Wigmore, M., and D. McCue. 1991. 'No Information on a Forgotten People: How Healthy Are Native People in Canada When They Live Off Reserve?' In B.D. Postl et al., eds, *Circumpolar Health 90: Proceedings of the 8th International Congress*, 90–3. Winnipeg: University of Manitoba Press.

Williams, G., ed. 1969. *Andrew Graham's Observations on Hudson's Bay 1767–91*. London: Hudson's Bay Historical Society.

Williamson, K.J. 2000. 'Celestial and Social Families of the Inuit.' In R. Laliberte, B. Settee, J. Waldram, R. Innes, B. Macdougall, L. McBain, and F.L. Barron, eds, *Expressions in Canadian Native Studies*, 125–44. Saskatoon: University of Saskatchewan Extension Press.

Williamson, R.F., and S. Pfeiffer. 2003. *Bones of the Ancestors: The Archaeological and Osteobiography of the Moatfield Ossuary*. Mercury Series. Archaeology Paper 163. Ottawa: Canadian Museum of Civilizations.

Willows, N.D., E. Dewailly, and K. Gray-Donald. 2000. 'Anemia and Iron Status in Inuit Infants in Northern Quebec.' *Canadian Journal of Public Health* 91:407–10.

Willows, N.D., J. Morel, and K. Gray-Donald. 2000. 'Prevalence of Anemia among James Bay Cree Infants of Northern Quebec.' *Canadian Medical Association Journal* 162:323–6.

Wilson, K., and M.W. Rosenberg. 2002. 'Exploring the Determinants of Health for First Nations Peoples in Canada: Can Existing Frameworks Accommodate Traditional Activities?' *Social Science and Medicine* 55:2017–31.

Wilson, R., L.H. Krefting, P. Sutcliffe, and L. Van Bussel. 1992. 'Incidence and Prevalence of End-Stage Renal Disease among Ontario's James Bay Cree.' *Canadian Journal of Public Health* 83:143–6.

Wolever, T.M.S., S. Hamad, J. Gittelsohn, J. Gao, A.J.G. Hanley, and S.B. Harris. 1997. 'Low Dietary Fiber and High Protein Intakes Associated with Newly Diagnosed Diabetes in a Remote Aboriginal Community.' *American Journal of Clinical Nutrition* 66:1470–4.

Wolff, P.H. 1973. 'Vasomotor Sensitivity to Alcohol in Diverse Mongoloid Populations.' *American Journal of Human Genetics* 25:193–9.

Wood, J.W., G.R. Milner, H.C. Harpending, and K.M. Weiss. 1992. 'The Osteological Paradox: Problems of Inferring Prehistoric Health from Skeletal Samples.' *Current Anthropology* 33(4):343–70.

Woods, C. 1977. 'Alternative Curing in a Changing Medical Situation.' *Medical Anthropology* 1(3):25–54.

World Health Organization. 1978. *Primary Health Care: Report of the International Conference on Primary Health Care, Alma-Ata, USSR, 6–12 September 1978.* Geneva: World Health Organization.

– 2000. *World Health Report 2000.* Geneva: World Health Organization.

– 2001. *Legal Status of Traditional Medicine and Complementary/Alternative Medicine: A Worldwide Review.* Geneva: World Health Organization.

Yang, D.Y., A. Cannon, and S.R. Saunders. 2004. 'DNA Species Identification of Archaeological Salmon Bone from the Pacific Northwest Coast of North America.' *Journal of Archaeological Science* 31:619–31.

York, G. 1989. *The Dispossessed: Life and Death in Native Canada.* London: Vintage U.K.

Young, D.E., G. Ingram, and L. Swartz. 1989. *Cry of the Eagle: Encounters with a Cree Healer.* Toronto: University of Toronto Press.

Young, D.E., L. Swartz, G. Ingram, and J. Morse. 1988. 'The Psoriasis Research Project: An Overview.' In D.E. Young, ed., *Health Care Issues in the Canadian North*, 76–88. Edmonton: Boreal Institute for Northern Studies.

Young, D.E., and L.L. Smith. 1992. *The Involvement of Canadian Native Communities in Their Health Care Program: A Review of the Literature since the 1970s.* Edmonton: University of Alberta, Canadian Circumpolar Institute.

Young, T.K. 1979. 'Changing Patterns of Health and Sickness among the Cree-Ojibwa of Northwestern Ontario.' *Medical Anthropology* 3:191–223.

– 1981. 'Primary Health Care for Isolated Indians in Northwestern Ontario.' *Public Health Reports* 96:391–7.

– 1984. 'Indian Health Services in Canada: A Sociohistorical Perspective.' *Social Science and Medicine* 18(3):257–64.

- 1988a. 'Are Subarctic Indians Undergoing the Epidemiologic Transition?' *Social Science and Medicine* 26:659–71.
- 1988b. *Health Care and Cultural Change: The Indian Experience in the Central Subarctic.* Toronto: University of Toronto Press.
- 1991. 'Prevalence and Correlates of Hypertension in a Subarctic Indian Population.' *Preventive Medicine* 20:474–85.
- 1994. *The Health of Native Americans: Toward a Biocultural Epidemiology.* New York: Oxford University Press.
- 1996a. 'Obesity, Central Fat Patterning, and Their Metabolic Correlates among the Inuit of the Central Canadian Arctic.' *Human Biology* 68:245–63.
- 1996b. 'Sociocultural and Behavioural Determinants of Obesity among Inuit in the Central Canadian Arctic.' *Social Science and Medicine* 43:165–7.
- 2003. 'Review of Research on Aboriginal Populations in Canada: Relevance to Their Health Needs.' *British Medical Journal* 327:419–22.
- 2005. *Population Health: Concepts and Methods.* 2nd ed. New York: Oxford University Press.
Young, T.K., and N.W. Choi. 1985. 'Cancer Risks among Residents of Manitoba Indian Reserves, 1970–79.' *Canadian Medical Association Journal* 132:1269–72.
Young, T.K., H.J. Dean, B. Flett, and P. Wood-Steiman. 2000. 'Childhood Obesity in a Population at High Risk for Type 2 Diabetes.' *Journal of Pediatrics* 136:365–9.
Young, T.K., and J.W. Frank. 1983. 'Cancer Surveillance in a Remote Indian Population in Northwestern Ontario.' *American Journal of Public Health* 73:515–20.
Young, T.K., J.M. Gerrard, and J.D. O'Neil. 1999. 'Plasma Phospholipid Fatty Acids in the Central Canadian Arctic: Biocultural Explanations for Ethnic Differences.' *Journal of Physical Anthropology* 109:9–18.
Young, T.K., and E.S. Hershfield. 1986. 'A Case-Control Study to Evaluate the Effectiveness of Mass BCG Vaccination among Canadian Indians.' *American Journal of Public Health* 76:783–6.
Young, T.K., J.M. Kaufert, J.K. McKenzie, et al. 1989. 'Excessive Burden of End-Stage Renal Disease among Canadian Indians: A National Survey.' *American Journal of Public Health* 79:756–8.
Young, T.K., E. Kliewer, J.F. Blanchard, and T. Mayer. 2000. 'Monitoring Disease Burden and Preventive Behaviour with Data Linkage: Cervical Cancer among Aboriginal People in Manitoba, Canada.' *American Journal of Public Health* 90:1466–8.
Young, T.K., P. Martens, S.P. Taback, E.A.C. Sellers, H.J. Dean, M. Cheang, and B. Flett. 2002. 'Type 2 Diabetes Mellitus in Children: Prenatal and Early Infancy Risk Factors among Native Canadians.' *Archives of Pediatrics and Adolescent Medicine* 156:651–5.

Young, T.K., L.L. McIntyre, J. Dooley, and J. Rodriguez. 1985. 'Epidemiologic Features of Diabetes Mellitus among Indians in Northwestern Ontario and Northeastern Manitoba.' *Canadian Medical Association Journal* 132:793–7.

Young, T.K., M.E. Moffatt, and J.D. O'Neil. 1993. 'Cardiovascular Diseases in a Canadian Arctic Population.' *American Journal of Public Health* 83:881–7.

Young, T.K., Y.P. Nikitin, E.V. Shubnikov, et al. 1995. 'Plasma Lipids in Two Indigenous Arctic Populations with Low Risk for Cardiovascular Diseases.' *American Journal of Human Biology* 5(7):223–6.

Young, T.K., J. Reading, B. Elias, and J.D. O'Neil. 2000. 'Type-2 Diabetes in Canada's First Nations: Status of an Epidemic in Progress.' *Canadian Medical Association Journal* 163:561–6.

Young, T.K., C.D. Schraer, E.V. Shubnikoff, E.J. Szathmary, and Y.P. Nikitin. 1992. 'Prevalence of Diagnosed Diabetes in Circumpolar Indigenous Populations.' *International Journal of Epidemiology* 21:730–6.

Young, T.K., and G. Sevenhuysen. 1989. 'Obesity in Northern Canadian Indians: Patterns, Determinants, and Consequences.' *American Journal of Clinical Nutrition* 49:786–93.

Young, T.K., E.J. Szathmary, S. Evers, and B. Wheatley. 1990. 'Geographical Distribution of Diabetes among the Native Population of Canada: A National Survey.' *Social Science and Medicine* 31:129–39.

Zegura, S. 1985. 'The Initial Peopling of the Americas: An Overview.' In R. Kirk and E. Szathmary, eds, *Out of Asia: Peopling of the Americas and the Pacific*, 1–18. Canberra: The Journal of Pacific History.

Zimmerly, D. 1975. *Cain's Land Revisited: Culture Change in Central Labrador, 1775–1972*. St John's: Memorial University of Newfoundland, Institute of Social and Economic Research.

Zimmerman, M.R., and A.C Aufderheide. 1984. 'The Frozen Family of Utqiagvik: The Autopsy Findings.' *Arctic Anthropology* 21(1):53–64.

Zimmerman, M.R., and G.S. Smith. 1975. 'A Probable Case of Accidental Inhumation of 1600 Years Ago.' *Bulletin of the New York Academy of Medicine* 51 (2nd ser.):828–37.

Zimmerman, M.R., E. Trinkaus, and M. LeMay, et al. 1981. 'The Paleopathology of an Aleutian Mummy.' *Archives of Pathology and Laboratory Medicine* 105(12):638–41.

Zimmerman, M.R., M.R. Yeatman, H. Sprinz, and W. Titterington, et al. 1971. 'Examination of an Aleutian Mummy.' *Bulletin of the New York Academy of Medicine* 47(1):80–103.

Zink, A.R., W. Grabner, and A.G. Nerlich. 2005. 'Molecular Identification of Human Tuberculosis in Recent and Historic Bone Tissue Samples: The Role of

Molecular Techniques for the Study of Historical Tuberculosis.' *American Journal of Physical Anthropology* 126:32–47.

Zink, A.R., C. Sola, U. Reischl, W. Grabner, N. Rastogi, H. Wolf, and A.G. Nerlich. 2003. 'Characterization for *Mycobacterium tuberculosis* Complex DNAs from Egyptian Mummies by Spoligotyping.' *Journal of Clinical Microbiology* 41(1):359–67.

Zubek, E. 1994. 'Traditional Native Healing: Alternative or Adjunct to Modern Medicine?' *Canadian Family Physician* 40:1923–31.

Index